4

EDITION

Ethical Decision Making in Nursing and Health Care

The Symphonological Approach

James H. Husted ■ Gladys L. Husted

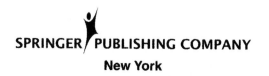

SPRINGER PUBLISHING COMPANY

New York

James H. Husted is an independent scholar. He is a member of the American Philosophical Association and the North American Spinoza Society. He has been a member of the high IQ societies, Mensa and Intertel. He was the philosophy expert for Dial-An-M for Mensa, as well as the philosophy editor of *Integra,* the journal of Intertel. He guest lectures on bioethics at Duquesne University in the BSN, MSN, and PhD programs. He writes and presents workshops in the area of bioethics.

Gladys L. Husted, RN, MSN, PhD, CNE, is a professor emeritus of nursing at Duquesne University, Pittsburgh, Pennsylvania. She received a master's in nursing education from the University of Pittsburgh, where she also completed her PhD in curriculum and supervision. She was awarded the title of School of Nursing Distinguished Professor in 1998. She has retired from full-time employment at Duquesne University but continues to teach part-time in the MSN and PhD programs. Her main area of expertise is in bioethics, where she writes, presents workshops, consults, and does research. Her other areas of expertise are in curriculum design, instructional strategies, and theory development. Dr. Husted's Web site can be accessed at www.nursing.duq.edu/faculty/husted/index.html.

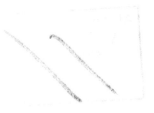

Springer Publishing Company, LLC
11 West 42nd Street
New York, NY 10036
www.springerpub.com

Acquisitions Editor: Allan Graubard
Production Editor: Tenea Johnson
Cover design: Joanne E. Honigman
Composition: Aptara Inc.

10/5 4 3

Library of Congress Cataloging-in-Publication Data

Husted, James H.
    Ethical decision making in nursing and health care : the symphonological approach / by James H. Husted, Gladys L. Husted. — 4th ed.
       p. ; cm.
    Gladys L. Husted's name appears first on the previous edition.
    Includes bibliographical references and index.
    ISBN 978-0-8261-1512-6 (pbk.)
    1. Nursing ethics.   2. Nursing — Decision making.   I. Husted, Gladys L.   II. Title.
[DNLM: 1. Ethics, Nursing — Case Reports.   2. Ethics, Nursing — Nurses' Instruction.
3. Decision Making — Case Reports.   4. Decision Making — Nurses' Instruction.
5. Models, Theoretical — Case Reports.   6. Models, Theoretical — Nurses' Instruction.
WY 85 H972e 2008]
RT85.H87   2008
174'.2 — dc22   2007029676

Printed in the United States of America by Offset Paperback Manufacturers, Inc.

Contents

Section I: The Basics of Bioethical Decision Making

Section II: Beyond the Basics—An Extended Perspective

Section III: Case Study Analyses

List of Case Study Dilemmas

List of Figures

List of Tables

Preface

Practice-Based Bioethics

Symphonia is a Greek word meaning "agreement." *Symphonology* is the study of agreements and the elements necessary to forming agreements. For our purposes in the health care arena, symphonology is the study of agreements between health care professionals and patients. It is a study of the ethical implications of the health care professional/patient agreement.

As a practice-based ethic appropriate to practicing professionals, symphonology includes standards of behavior—those preconditions necessary to agreement and professional interaction, requiring contextual understanding and application for optimal interactions in the health care setting.

Much has been written about optimum care for the patient. Although patient care is indispensable, in fact, central to professional bioethics, in this book we also concentrate on the welfare of the health care professional. A very high degree of personal development and emotional fulfillment for the professional is possible through bioethics, another aspect central to the patient's well-being.[1] And we recognize that these two aspects of the health care system can be made to "walk together" through a symphonological ethic.

Although ethical problems faced by nurses are the primary focus here, there are cases throughout the book that speak to other health care professions—pharmacists, physical therapists, physicians, social workers, dieticians, and so on. As such, the theory we present is applicable to any health care profession. The only adjustment required is the role considered—the education and experience of each professional involved. The theory is also applicable to any patient population, regardless of age, disease, competency, and cultural background.

Overview

Ethics originally was meant to be a search for, or a science of, the good life. The first major ethicist of the Western world, Socrates (464–399 BC), described ethics as an examination of life—as a way of making life worth living.

From this point on, ethics assumes three aspects.

First, as mentioned, there was Socrates whose project was twofold: (1) to discover appropriate definitions of ethical terms, and thus to allow people, when thinking about ethics, to know what they were thinking about (so far this project has been largely unsuccessful) and (2) to understand ethics as contextualized. That is to say, we should recognize that actions that are right in one circumstance may be wrong in another. For example, stealing the gun of a person in need of defending himself against an assassin is an evil action. But stealing the gun of an assassin is a good and praiseworthy action. Thus, a blanket condemnation of theft is a mistake. The context determines its ethical quality.

Second, there was Plato (427–347 BC), who shifted the theme of ethics from the good life—a life worth living— to "The Good." Ultimately, this shift displaced concern for the good life, nearly driving it out of ethics. This was a tragedy: Concern for life is central to the health care setting—the realm of bioethics. Concern for the good life is central to human existence—the realm of ethics—and of achievement and flourishing.

Plato set himself the task of discovering how we came to know the meaning of words and the nature of the things they signify. He resolved this problem by reference to a "World of Forms." In this world the souls of humans dwell prior to their birth. Here there is a perfect example of everything to be found on earth. Men and women have an eternity to learn the names and natures of all these things.

However, the ordeal of birth causes them to forget what they had learned in the "World of Forms." What is experienced as learning in our early life simply consists in recollection of what we originally learned in the "World of Forms." The most important of the Forms is the "form of the Good." No one can gain a clear idea of the nature of this "Form." As a result, man's ethical existence is simply a struggle to gain an understanding of the nature of the "Good."

Third, there was Aristotle (483–322 BC), who brought ethics out of Plato's prenatal, extraterrestrial world into the world of living women and men. The concerns of human life become the subject matter of ethics once again.

Aristotle's theory of ethics as a science of successful living and Socrates' emphasis on context has not yet played a dominant role in ethics or even bioethics. But hopefully they will.

As an example of Aristotle's perspective, we can do no better than refer to his doctrine of the "Golden Mean" which we will discuss at greater length. According to Aristotle, a virtue is a middle ground between two extremes which are vices. The "Golden Mean" consists of three possible attitudes. One attitude is a deficit. It is less than what is called for in the situation; for example, a nurse shows indifference to her patient when he needs her attention. The second attitude is an excess; for example, when a nurse is overbearing and controlling in relation to her patient when he needs a sense of being able to control his situation. The virtue that is a mean between these two vices is nurturing. A nurse is not indifferent but attentive. A nurse is attentive but not domineering. A nurse who is attentive is nurturing. A nurse who is nurturing is a virtuous nurse.

The interest of Socrates and Aristotle in defining, understanding, and living by the meaning of ethical terms has largely been forgotten. Plato's quixotic and tragic theory of ethics as a search for an unknown and unknowable "Good" has become the almost exclusive concern of ethics.

A practice-based ethic, the topic of this book, will be kindly disposed to Aristotle's view and Socrates' contextualism.

A Small Digression

As you go through the book time and time again your attention will be called to the importance of the implicit. What is left unsaid but implied in what is explicitly spoken is sometimes more informative than what is spoken. The nature of a circumstance at any given moment may be revealing of why the circumstance is as it is and not otherwise. This may be the most important thing the circumstance reveals—that which it reveals implicitly. Here are two questions. The answers will come much later in the book; at which time you will know far more about bioethics than you do at present.

Question: "What is the first agreement that anyone ever forms?"

The second question is: "Are there bad, harmful, destructive agreements?" The answer is yes, there are. The deeper and much more important question is: "What is the worst agreement a person can make?"

The Return to Life and Flourishing

In this book, we return to a concern for life. Like the ethicists of the past, we include in "life" a concern for flourishing—the achievement of happiness. We approach life as men and women experience it, as a journey accompanied by tears and smiles, by conflict and harmony. We begin amid life in all its complexity, discussing what we bring to life's journey—human virtues,[2] their relation to the health care setting, their development, and what they make possible. Along the way, we offer brief parables and vignettes to illustrate, from different perspectives, points that are to come.

We discuss individual rights, the necessary foundation for an ethic of human life and the most confused question in ethics. Essential questions prevail: "What is an ethical agent?" and "What is possible to an ethical agent?"

As individuals, a majority of the achievements possible to us come through cooperation with others. And this cooperation occurs through agreement (thus, the name *Symphonology*). Nowhere is this better illustrated than in the professional agreement between nurse and patient. For each—nurse and patient—nowhere are the values to be achieved greater than through this agreement.

From this vantage, we then analyze the decline of ethics from an individual pursuit into an exclusively social context: where societal standards dictate whether something is right or wrong. Then we analyze the absurd idea that the emotions of the individual provide the only possible guide to the resolutions of complex ethical dilemmas. Here, ethics has reached a dead end.

This is not a reason for you to ignore questions of right and wrong; quite the contrary. It is an overarching reason to understand your ethical beliefs. If you do not understand why you consider one action right and another action wrong, your disadvantage is obvious. You will not be able to interact on an equal footing with your colleagues, whose rationalizations can seem quite plausible. You will not be able to objectively and effectively defend the actions you take. You will have no objective means of moral self-defense.

We have included numerous dilemmas in this book as a way of providing you, the reader, practice in ethical decision making. We offer resolutions to most of these dilemmas, realizing that "being there" may change the information sought and, therefore, alter the resolution found. For the purpose of *practicing* ethical decision making, we suggest that you deal with the context as it is presented.

In this book, we cover a plethora of bioethical dilemmas from bedwetting to euthanasia. We demonstrate the relevance of bioethical standards to these (and by extension to all) bioethical dilemmas. We examine how to define and understand bioethical standards in different contexts in order to use them effectively in ethical decision making.

This approach will bring you to the center of the bioethical environment. The ethical decision-making process presented throughout the book will enable you, upon entering a nursing career, to quickly find yourself at home in your profession.

Because all the key concepts listed in the chapters are terms that require precise definitions, we have provided a glossary for your use.

Notes

1. The pronoun "she" is used to designate the health care professional. This convention is for the reader's ease of understanding and to keep understanding in context. The singular is preferred to the plural or indeterminate because professionals are individuals, and a practice-based ethic is, and ought to be, an individualistic ethic. On the other hand, we almost invariably use the pronoun "he" to designate the patient, again for the same reason.
2. There are certain subjects we will return to numerous times. This is especially true of "virtue," "individual rights," and bioethical standards. The reason for this is that these facts serve different functions in different aspects of the nurse/patient interaction—or because the later discussions will be easier to understand after the material that has been presented.

Digital Supplement

New to this edition is a digital supplement for educators who adopt this book for classroom use. This online teacher's manual, which can be obtained from Springer Publishing Company, LLC, provides a wealth of information for instructors to plan their teaching activities and to enhance active learning for students. It will assist faculty in preparing for class, and in decreasing preparation time.

The online teacher's manual includes:

- **Chapter Summaries:** To assist faculty in quickly identifying chapter themes and purposes.
- **Major Focus Areas:** To help in identifying key elements in each chapter and to pinpoint content essential to classroom instruction.
- **Classroom Activities:** To enhance active engagement of the learner through classroom activities (2–4 activities are included per chapter that can be used in a traditional or online class format). Directions are included for conducting these activities.
- **PowerPoint Slidesets:** To enable faculty to link to important elements in each chapter through power point presentations and to assist faculty in class preparation.
- **Test-bank:** To enhance the evaluative process through providing test questions for each chapter. The test-bank questions at the end of each chapter use the two types of questions that now appear on the NCLEX exam—"single answer" and "select all that apply."

How faculty use this information, especially the activities, depends on classroom variables: level of students, time available, and what fits best with class discussions.

Acknowledgments

We wish to acknowledge our gratitude to the following people:

Our students, who served as a crucible for refining the dominant ideas in this book.

Melanie (Lizzie) and Allena (Nicci), who remind us of the seriousness of play and the appropriateness of play to seriousness.

Sharen and David Custer for their enthusiasm and friendship.

Kirsten and Gary Kalwaytis for sharing adventures.

Tabitha and Rich Riggio for always being there.

Our Wine Group for all the oenological experiences.

Jim Costello for his encouragement.

Allan Graubard for his editorial assistance.

And finally to Charlie-Charlie, to whom this book is dedicated.

The Basics of Bioethical Decision Making

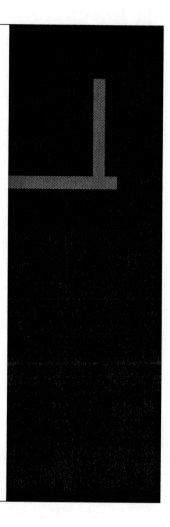

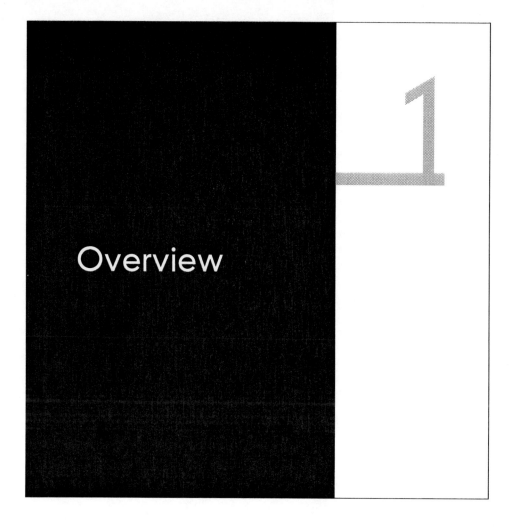

Overview

The Paradox of the Hammer

A paradox is a description of a state of affairs that:

- apparently cannot exist, but which, in fact, can exist, or
- apparently can exist, but, which in fact, cannot.

Paradoxes and dilemmas are very similar, but paradoxes are generally more difficult. Looking at paradoxes will make dilemmas much easier. This paradox is our first step. It is easy but it illustrates an important principle.

The famous ethicist, Benedict Spinoza, proposes two facts, apparently contradictory to each other.

- In order to make a hammer, it is necessary for a person to be able to work iron.
- In order for a person to be able to work iron, he needs a hammer.

Therefore, it seems that no one can work iron, and there can be no such thing as a hammer. For a person must have a hammer in order to make a hammer. But a person must be able to make a hammer in order to have a hammer. Therefore, it seems that it is impossible either to make or to have a hammer.

The Purpose of Ethics

Ethics, like every science, arose from the necessity of analyzing and coming to understand some part of our world. It is that part of our world that involves making decisions and taking actions in the face of adversity or opportunity.

Ethics deals with alternatives. For an interpersonal ethic, an ethic of interacting, the central alternative is between that which is beneficial and that which is harmful. In a strictly ethical context, that which makes life more perfect is beneficial. That which makes life less perfect is harmful.

> Ethics deals with alternatives. For an interpersonal ethic, an ethic of interacting, the central alternative is between that which is beneficial and that which is harmful. In a strictly ethical context, that which makes life more perfect is beneficial. That which makes life less perfect is harmful.

Ethics is a study of how decisions and actions move a human life from a state of lesser perfection (well-being and flourishing) to a state of greater perfection, or how decisions prevent a human life from moving from a state of greater perfection to a state of lesser perfection.

In the context of an individual's life, and discounting the possible influences of unpredictable fortune, a failed life is one that, at the end, one looks back on with regret for the way one has lived it. A successful life is a life that one experiences as having been lived well. A rational ethical system is a science of living well.

Resolution of the Paradox

It seems that it is impossible either to make or to have a hammer.

Yet, people do have hammers. People are able to work iron and to make hammers. "Hammersmiths" began with whatever assets they had ready at hand, no doubt stones. They perfected these assets, more and more, until they had a primitive type of hammer. With this they were able to work iron—primitively.

The better they became at working iron, the better hammer they were able to produce. The better hammer they could produce, the better they became at working iron.

So, without a hammer, they were able to work iron and produce a hammer.

The Process of Understanding

The process of achieving an understanding of oneself, is very similar to the process of making a hammer. In her earliest years, a person learns what a person is by observing persons, that is, by observing the nature of mature, independent people. By learning what a person is, she discovers her own nature; she comes to know what she is—a person. As with Spinoza's hammer, learning is a seesaw process—back and forth—from other people back to herself, from herself on to other people. In learning what other people are, she comes to understand what she is in ways that she could not without her understanding of other people. In learning what she is, she comes to understand other people in ways that she could not without self-understanding.

She knows others as persons before she knows herself. All of these persons are unique and difficult to understand. In order to understand them, she can compare their similarities and differences to herself, taking herself as a standard or yardstick by which she can measure their various characteristics. Then she can measure her own characteristics by taking what she has learned at any given stage of development, of the natures of others, that is, of persons as a standard or yardstick by which she can measure her own characteristics.

Persons

It is inescapably necessary for every person to make and act on the basis of decisions and agreements. It is powerfully advantageous for nurses to understand the nature and function of decisions and agreements in human interactions. It is desirable for every person to understand the nature and the lives of the persons who make decisions and agreements. For a nurse who would pursue her profession with great skill she needs some knowledge of:

- Her patient's desires—the things he reacts to, and how he reacts to them.
- His reasoning—the ways in which he seeks, or fails to seek, understanding.
- His life—the way he sees himself in the present moment, his expectations of the future, and how he acts in relation to these expectations. (Memories of the past must be handled discreetly. These may have a negative effect on his self-image, his expectations, and his actions).
- His purposes—the changes he is actually attempting to bring about in his life.
- His agency (his ability to initiate action, sustain action, and achieve his goals)—the successes and failures of his actions reveal this.

In order to gain understanding of oneself, one must observe others and discover the meanings that things have for others and how they came to have these meanings. To learn about oneself, one must begin by observing those in a more developed state. Then, through observing others, one can discover what characteristics people have in common. After this, the only task is to discover how these characteristics are expressed in each individual person and in oneself. This discovery will reveal the formative power of these characteristics in the person by whom they are expressed in action.

After a period of development, by observing others, a person gains a better understanding of herself by noting her similarities to, and differences from, these other persons.

Then she looks into herself and gains a better understanding of others by observing how they are similar to, and different from, her. This process continues and expands until the observer has gained a multifaceted competence.

Then she looks into herself and gains a better understanding of others by observing how they are similar to, and different from, her.

A health care professional sharpens her understanding of her patient's characteristics by observing herself. She observes:

■ Her desire for the awareness of who she is and the desire to sustain and develop herself.
■ Her power to act for herself in order to realize her own purposes and to lead a successful life.
■ Her need for a true and objective understanding of her world.
■ Her need to control her time and effort.
■ Her desire to attain good and to avoid harm.
■ Her desire to devote herself to what she values.

Through these observations, she gains a better understanding of herself. Then she observes others and discovers:

■ The pleasure others take in being who and what they are.
■ Their desire for freedom and the pleasure they take in acting on their freedom.
■ The actions they are motivated to take to gain a true and objective understanding of their world.
■ The pleasure they take in controlling their time and effort.
■ The actions they take in order to achieve benefit and to avoid harm.
■ The actions they take in order to devote themselves to what they value.

Through this process, she gains a better understanding of others. She becomes able to act confidently and to justify her actions. The process continues and expands until she reaches her fullest ethical understanding—the widest understanding she is able to gain of herself and of others. The more knowledge she gains of herself, the greater her understanding of others. The more knowledge she gains of others, the greater her understanding of herself.

The Discovery of Practical Reason

Every field of study has a purpose. Human beings desired to navigate the seas; someone created astronomy. Curious about living things, someone created biology. Someone created mathematics for the purpose of computation. Someone created medicine from a need to alleviate suffering and to heal. Every science and every art arises from imagination and reason. These are inspired by curiosity and need.

Every science and every art arises from imagination and reason. These are inspired by curiosity and need.

In order for a new science to be discovered, certain conditions are necessary:

1. The science must yield very abstract and general knowledge. There can be no science of crab apple trees. The discovery of how the speed of hair growth can be predicted will not constitute a science. These subjects are too narrow. Science is concerned with very broad areas of human interest.
2. There must be a purpose for the discovery. If it does not fill a need, it cannot be a science. There is no scientific way to harness flying horses. There is no possibility of anyone needing to harness a flying horse.
3. It must be possible to make the discovery. There must be something out in the world to be discovered. There can be no science of time travel. So far, at least, no one has made progress toward time travel.
4. The discoverer must love the pursuit of knowledge and have a tireless curiosity concerning the subject matter.

The demands of successful living are the natural principles of ethics. For instance, an individual requires the virtue of courage—a willingness to meet the demands that a human life encounters—in order to live successfully. This makes courage one of the natural principles of ethics.

In a derivative way, ethics also involves a study of the interactions between ethical agents. This study is made in terms of right and wrong. It deals with the practical conditions of interaction. These are the conditions under which one agent has, or has not, the right to expect to benefit from the action of another.

The Desert Island as an Ethical Laboratory

Would one need to be concerned with ethics if one was marooned alone on a desert island?

One's survival is an ethical concern. If one does not survive, one will have no concerns. Survival is the fundamental ethical concern.

One's survival on the desert island might well depend on the development of certain virtues (the strength of one's character; habits established on rational desires) and the overcoming of certain vices (the weakness of one's character; habits established on irrational desires).

One will need strength of character—fortitude. Along with this, one will need the virtue of an orientation onto reality—objectivity, or the awareness necessary to establish her understanding of her situation. She will need to develop the art and the habit of clear thinking. These virtues will have to be permeated with the virtue of purposiveness—industry.

There must be integrity (self-interest) added to the virtues of the agent's actions, and fidelity (self-interest) to her life. Fidelity to these values and fidelity to life are central ethical concepts. They are constituted of:

- Fidelity—objectivity (This is what is here), watchfulness (Is this all that is here?), imagination (What else could be brought into being here?).
- Purpose—determination (I must complete this task), wisdom (I must discover what I can do), prudence (I will not attempt the purposeless or the impossible), integrity (I will not betray what I value, what I know is true, or what I am).

▓ Pride—the pleasure one takes in one's virtues; needed to nurture the other virtues.

If one would need these virtues, then one would need ethics, for these virtues are ethics.

It is not necessary to have two or more people involved to rely on the science of ethics. In fact, if an individual marooned on a desert island did not need ethical awareness, no one ever, under any circumstances, would have any need for ethics. What is needed by a person in a downtown crowd, is needed more so by a person marooned and alone. We must all make decisions to make life better, to avoid allowing life to deteriorate, to survive, and to attempt, always, to achieve happiness.

Ethics has to do with benefit (the benefit of a person is that which assists her efficient functioning as the kind of being she is) and harm (in relation to an ethical agent the harmful is that which weakens her efficient functioning as the kind of being she is—a goal directed agent). One alone, marooned on a desert island, where survival is a constant concern, will have to be concerned with benefit and harm. That which sustains survival is the highest good. That which ends survival is the most basic evil. One alone on a desert island has to be concerned with ethics. Anyone, anywhere who has to be concerned with survival and flourishing (living a successful and rewarding life) needs to be concerned with ethics.

Ethics is a system of standards to motivate, determine, and justify actions taken in the pursuit of vital (essentially related to the preservation or enhancement of life) and fundamental (essential to the nature and causal powers of a thing; revealing a thing as the kind of thing it is) goals. An agent's pursuit of his vital and fundamental goals is a definite concern and perhaps his only concern on this island.

Symphonology, which is a system of ethics based on the terms and presuppositions of agreement, is concerned with ethical decisions and agreements.

> Symphonology, which is a system of ethics based on the terms and presuppositions of agreement, is concerned with ethical decisions and agreements.

On the desert island, one would have no one with whom to make an agreement. Therefore, it seems, one would have no need of ethics! But, one would be herself on the desert island. She would need to make agreements with herself. These agreements, however, are decisions, and on a desert island one will find many occasions to make decisions concerning vital and fundamental values—ethical decisions. One needs ethics before joining others and after parting from them. One needs ethics when walking across a street.

Being marooned would be a test of character. It would force one to develop efficiency at ethical decision making.

The Health Care Setting as an Ethical Laboratory

Human action is behavior that expresses the nature of a human being. It is behavior directed by reason. In ethics this is known as *agency*. The human possessing agency is known as an *agent*. In nursing, the human who has lost agency is known as a *patient*.

A patient comes into the health care setting because he has lost his power of agency—his power to take actions. A nurse is there to supply his agency—to do for him the things that need to be done, and that, because of his disability or lack of knowledge, he cannot do.

When an ethic is fully developed it can outline what is appropriate to human motivations and value-oriented action and how these relate to the human condition. It can examine the processes of decision making and the ways in which agents reach, or fail to reach, their goals. It can concern itself with the nature of the goals that agents pursue and pursue together. It can discover the ways these goals might best be pursued. Ethics examines the right and wrong of the decisions and choices agents make regarding their actions and interactions.

Ethics can and ought to have a practical purpose. This purpose is to guide practical affairs (action). And action has a purpose; its purpose being the flourishing of the acting agent. For bioethics the purpose is increasing or recapturing the patient's ability to flourish and, in some cases, to survive.

> When an ethic is fully developed it can outline what is appropriate to human motivations and value-oriented action and how these relate to the human condition.

Bioethics

Bioethics places particular emphasis on situations where one person is extremely vulnerable, where the goals to be pursued are crucial, and where the dilemmas to be resolved are extraordinarily complex. (Husted & Husted, in press)

"Bioethics should not tell [patients] what to do, but it should provide them with tools and skills in reasoning and ways to improve their own decisions" (Perring, 2005, p. 63). This includes nurses helping them in this process.

Bioethics is ethics as it relates to the health care professions. It came into existence as an independent discipline around 1970: "the vocabulary of the moral—of right and wrong—has been added to the vocabulary of scientific medicine—of fact and content" (Cassell, 1984, p. 35).

The fundamental background of an appropriate bioethics, which forms its essential nature, is:

- The nature and needs of humans as living, thinking beings.
- The purpose and function of a health care system in a human society.
- An increased awareness of the essential ethical dignity of individual human beings.

> Bioethics is ethics as it relates to the health care professions. It came into existence as an independent discipline around 1970: "the vocabulary of the moral—of right and wrong—has been added to the vocabulary of scientific medicine—of fact and content" (Cassell, 1984, p. 35).

All this forms the appropriate nature of the biomedical context. The needs and conditions of people who enter this context do not invite the nonobjective, the purposeless, or the arbitrary. The interpersonal relationships of health care professionals and patients give added dimension to this context. The values, which the biomedical sciences offer those who can profit from them, are complex and vitally important. At the same time, the threat to a patient's values is very real. The relationship between the health care professional and patient is extraordinarily intimate.

For this reason, the emphasis for bioethics should not be on what a nurse's actions are, but on her character. As Tunna and Conner (1993) have said of nurses:

> A degree of misdirection exists in contemporary nursing ethics. The focus is almost exclusively on what nurses ought to do with little emphasis on how the nurses, themselves, should be. Consequently, practitioners may believe that character is not an issue and that doing the right thing (according to rules predetermined by others) is what matters. (pp. 25–26)

Patients entrust nurses with their health, well-being, and life. Nurses, practicing nursing, make an implicit promise that the patient is justified in believing that the nurse will be worthy of this trust. Character can, and rule following cannot, justify a patient's confidence.

Practice-Based Versus More of the Same

Every health care professional should ask herself whether a professional ethic exists to increase her pride in, and enthusiasm for, the practice of her profession and to serve her patient's life, health, and well-being; or, whether bioethics can be nothing more than more of the same—a repetition of the generalized and irregular ethical ideas the nurse was offered as an alternative to guilt feelings and disapproval.

That which is the goal of practice ought to be the goal of ethics. Ethics, as well as practice, can heal disabilities and nurture the resources needed for successful living.

> That which is the goal of practice ought to be the goal of ethics.

Like the interaction between players on a professional sports team, the ideal interaction between a nurse and a patient is an uninterrupted series of intelligible (where nurse and patient are both aware of what is going on), causal (where nurse and patient are in control of events and nothing necessary waits on chance), sequences (their interactions are not disconnected and episodic).

Bioethics, like all of ethics, can be a defense against others, so that they will not lead the ethical agent in to wrongdoing. Or, a means by which the agent can defend herself against herself doing what is wrong. Or, it can be a positive means, as a way to increase success in the health care arena. It ought to be easy to see that the last perspective is more rewarding, more productive, and more mature. This is the perspective taken by a practice-based ethic. Bioethical decision making is a skill, and, like every skill, practice improves performance. And when performance is improved, the well-being of patients is improved.

A practice-based ethical decision maker is very much like a skilled pool player. An unskilled pool player merely attempts to put a ball into a pocket. An unskilled decision maker decides on what seems best at the time and acts on it. A skilled pool player sets up shots and tries to put a ball into a pocket while leaving the cue ball in such a position that it will be easy to make the next shot. A skilled decision maker makes decisions purposefully. A skilled nurse makes decisions based on the needs and purposes of her patient and on what is necessary to accomplish them. A skilled decision maker does not exert intense mental effort in order to make arrhythmic ethical decisions, but masters the process of bioethical decision making as a skill. She will not assume that the intuitive "knowledge" and the instinctual behavior that she has been conditioned to by her childhood training is adequate to the interaction with patients in the health care setting.

Four False Starts

The four most prominent ethical systems today are:

- Deontology: A duty ethic. The standard by which an ethical action is measured is by whether it is a response to a duty; without any regard for the consequences of action. This is often coupled with intuition and a "moral sense" as the sources of one's awareness of one's duty.

 A "moral sense" is supposedly an analog with our five senses. It is a fantastic creation that supposedly shows us immediately what is right and what is wrong. All of us, including embezzlers, serial killers, child abusers, torturers, kidnappers, and other out-of-sync members of society, have this moral sense. Can you imagine what they might do if we did not have it?

- Utilitarianism: An ethics of utility, utility being defined as "the greatest good for the greatest number." The standard by which an ethical action is measured is whether, in the circumstances, it brought about the greatest good for the largest possible number of beneficiaries. This precludes concern for one's individual patient.
- Social relativism: The sentiments (opinions) of society determine what is right or wrong, beneficial or harmful, meaning hypocrisy is the guide to ethical actions. Nothing true, good, or beautiful is created by society. Much of what is true, good, or beautiful is destroyed by society. That which (various segments of) society preaches is absurd. That which they practice is often disgusting. (Relativists do not specify which shall be the standard.) It is difficult to identify their (or its) true sentiments without reference to their (or its) actions.
- Emotivism: Emotivists subscribe to ethical nonnaturalism—the theory that ethics has nothing to do with the world we live in. In other words, we cannot find right and wrong in reality. They also embrace ethical noncognitivism—ethical terms cannot be defined or understood. Ethical decision making is a matter of taste (or convenience). Therefore, the only possible source of ethical guidance is from our emotions.

In the health care system, something somewhat more sophisticated than this is desirable. Instead of an inhibitor of action (duty), an action taken on the world stage (utility), an action that will win a smile from the neighbors (social relativism), or a system that we learned from the higher primates (emotivism), what is called for is a way to restore action and interaction on the part of a patient. The nurse can assist in providing this but not through these systems.

The standards of symphonology are not chosen arbitrarily. They become objects of awareness through discovery. They signify internal and external realities that are essential to human development, fulfillment, and flourishing.

This brief overview of the contemporary systems (see chapter 11 for an extensive analysis) is offered to help motivate readers to entertain the idea that something different, more relevant, and beneficial is possible to guide nursing practice. Ethical analysis and interaction are inspired and guided by optimal nursing practice. They link up in attitude, approach, and relationship. They each begin in agreement. Agreement and competence are manifested in intelligible, causal sequences. The final goal of each is survival and flourishing—the conditions of successful living.

Obligation

The word profession comes from a Latin term meaning "to make a public declaration."

The difference between a nurse and a restaurant worker, a prima donna at the opera, an interior decorator, and a sales clerk is that the nurse is a professional and the others are not. The nurse has professed that she will be a nurse. She will take on the responsibilities and obligations of a professional.

This suggests a couple questions:

■ What are her obligations?
■ What is the source of her obligation?

To explore these questions, which are ethical or metaethical questions, another series of questions will be helpful.

"You have a duty to perform action A."

"Yes, but do I have an obligation to perform action A?"

Unless every past, present, and future ethicist who did not subscribe to a duty ethic, if all the ethicists today who ridicule an ethics of duty are completely disoriented, it does not follow that if one is told that she has a duty, that her question is meaningless; and from being told that she has a duty, there must be such things as "duties" and it must follow that she has an obligation.

Another question: "If action A would bring about the greatest good for the greatest number, do I have an obligation to perform action A?"

Many intelligibly speaking ethicists ridicule this idea. In order to attempt to bring about the greatest good for the greatest number, one might have to perform atrocious action B. It is not self evident that one would have an obligation to do this. Then, again, Thomas Edison produced utility, but he did not have an obligation to do this. This question is not meaningless.

"I have a powerful emotion urging me to take ethical action A. But do I have an obligation to take action A?"

This question is quite meaningful. It has never been shown that an urge produces an obligation.

"Society expects you to take action A."

"But do I have an obligation to take action A?" It is impossible to know what society wants. The majority of people in any society might very well want things that could not rationally be recognized as ethically justifiable. Naïve ethical decision makers accept the sentiments of society as ethical standards or give lip service to this. Many ethicists, speaking intelligibly, would disagree. The sentiments of society do not establish an obligation. This is a meaningful question.

This question of whether it is warmer in the city or in the summer is a meaningless question. The questions of whether one has an obligation to do one's duty or to bring about utility, or to be led by the desires of society or one's emotions are meaningful questions. Each one can have a valid idea behind it.

The advocates of each ethical system ridicules the others and calls attention to their numerous ethical and logical flaws. And, in this, each one is entirely right.

> The questions of whether one has an obligation to do one's duty or to bring about utility, or to be led by the desires of society or one's emotions are meaningful questions.

Then, should a profession involve obligation? Can a professional be a professional without obligation? Should a professional be aware of an obligation? And, if a professional's obligation is not to her subconscious or to society, to what is her obligation?

"You made an agreement to take action A."

"Yes, but do I have an obligation to take action A?" This question does not make any sense. To make an agreement is to take on an obligation. So the discussion breaks down to: "You took on an obligation", "Yes, but "have I taken on an obligation?" This obviously makes no sense.

Trust

> *Being intertwined with other human beings, our life is characterized by encountering one another with natural trust. To trust is to lay oneself open to the other person. . . . Human beings should protect another's life when it is entrusted to them [as a nurse would with a patient]. (Fegran, Helseth, & Slettebo, 2006, p. 58)*

If a nurse exclusively practiced one of the contemporary ethical systems, she would not deserve a patient's trust. She has not taken on any obligation. None of the contemporary ethical systems offer anything sufficient to justify that trust. The patient is a marginal factor in her ethical concerns. If this nurse enters into an informal discussion of the contemporary ethical system of her choice, this will not inspire trust. If the discussion is with a patient, it might inspire panic.

There are two perspectives on ethical action infusing the contemporary ethical systems. These are never expressed openly but they are the basis of these systems. The first is a tautological perspective, that is, you ought to do X because you ought to do X. The other perspective is the subjective, that is, I know it just because I know it. These threaten the intelligibility and the sequentiality of interaction. They completely undermine causality, that is, control. They make ethical action a matter of purposeless ritual. They involve two implicit claims. The first, a claim of infallibility and the second, derived from the first, a rejection of any recourse to reason and analysis. Each perspective is an implicit admission of the decision maker's incompetence.

A nurse's trustworthiness is revealed in her ability to deal with things rationally and responsibly as they arise. Just knowing that their nurse is a professional ordinarily will inspire a patient's feeling of confidence. This trust is a moral asset. It validates a nurse's pride in herself and her practice. When her pride is eroded away, all the ethical value her profession offers to her goes with it.

> A nurse's trustworthiness is revealed in her ability to deal with things rationally and responsibly as they arise.

A nurse makes a professional agreement to meet the obligations of the profession. A nurse should always be aware of the nature and the beneficiary of those obligations.

A profession cannot not involve obligation.

A nurse takes on an obligation through an agreement—expressed in her professing that she is a professional. This agreement is the source of her obligation.

> Her obligation is guaranteed by her character.

Her obligation is guaranteed by her character.

Study Guide

1. Discuss the meaning of the hammer to nursing practice.
2. Why is it important to understand yourself? What if you did not, what then?
3. There are two definitions proposed for ethics. What does each offer? What does it mean to practice?
4. Do you need ethics in a situation in which you are all alone? Why?
5. What does it mean to say that ethics is based on agreement? What if it were not?

References

Fegran, L., Helseth, S., & Slettebo, A. (2006). Nurses as moral practitioners encountering parents in neonatal intensive care units. *Nursing Ethics, 13*, 51–64.

Husted, G. L., & Husted, J. H. (2004). Ethics and the advanced practice nurse. In L. A. Joel (Ed.), *Advanced practice nursing* (pp. 639–661). Philadelphia: Davis.

Husted, G. L., & Husted, J. H. (in press). The ethical experience of caring for vulnerable populations: The symphonological approach. In M. de Chesnay (Ed.), *Caring for the vulnerable: Perspectives in nursing theory, practice, and research*. Boston: Jones and Bartlett.

Perring, C. (2005). Expanding the repertoire of bioethics: What next? *The American Journal of Bioethics, 5*, 63–65.

Tunna, K., & Conner, M. (1993). You are your ethics. *The Canadian Nurse, 89*, 25–26.

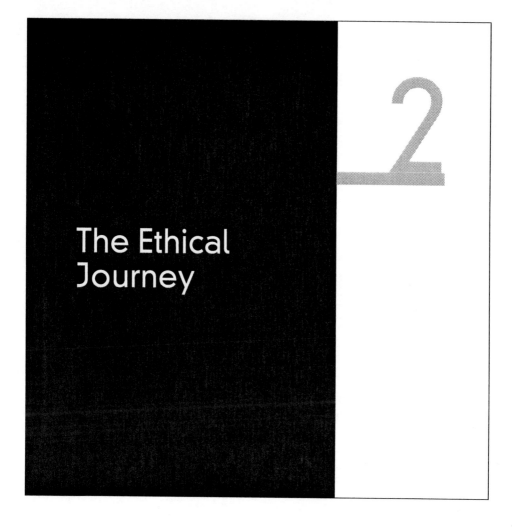

The Ethical Journey

In the nature of action or interaction, it is possible for intentions to be right and consequences to go wrong. Unknown conditions and unforeseeable events are never irrelevant to the consequences of action or interaction. It is also possible, although extremely unusual, for intentions to be wrong and consequences to be favorable. Evasion, deception, and coercion, by their natures, do not tend to serve human action and life.

For all of these reasons, ethics has traditionally been called "the practical science." The ability to engage in processes of ethical analysis is known as *practical reason*. "[Since] ethics is fundamentally a practical discipline [it is] concerned with what we should do and how we should live" (Churchill, 1989, p. 28).

Ethics has traditionally been called "the practice science." The ability to engage in processes of ethical analysis is known as *practical reason*.

Decision and Direction

An unflawed ethical decision is one that:

- One is going to act upon (it is more than theorizing).
- Will guide one's actions to a justifiable end.
- Actually affects one's life and one's character over a span of time.
- Will give one a reason to believe that one's actions will make life better (one's patient's life and one's own).
- Will enable one to change one's direction as one acts upon it.

This last point is especially important. There is a difference between being able to change the direction of actions when the direction proves to be mistaken and being tied into a course of action without having the awareness or the power to change it. This difference matters in whatever one does in one's life.

To be able to change one's direction is, of course, indispensable to clinical practice. It is also indispensable to a symphonological ethical system. One whose professional practice is such that, once the direction of action is set it is unchangeable, is to that extent incompetent. The same is no less true of one's ethical practice. A professional has a responsibility to interact with patients in order to assist them in avoiding avoidable failures and bringing about their sustained success in the health care system.

This points to an indispensable criterion for a professional ethic:

A nurse has a responsibility to interact with a patient as a person—as one thinking, desiring, feeling human being with another. A professional does credit to herself and her profession only when she remembers that she is a human being; her patient is a human being; and she acts as one human being with another.

> A professional does credit to herself and her profession only when she remembers that she is a human being; her patient is a human being; and she acts as one human being with another.

Human beings can make mistakes. A human being can make a decision and come to realize that she has made the wrong decision. When this happens, there are three things she can do:

1. She can make herself unconscious and refuse to let herself know that her decision is a bad one.
2. She can subtly change the definition of one or more terms describing what she is doing so that she can falsify it to herself or others.
3. She can change her direction.

Under contemporary ethical systems—nonpractice-based ethics—this latter alternative can only happen by accident, and it seldom happens.

Self-Determination

Art does not tolerate "anyhow", "in general", "approximately". "More or less" is the enemy of art. (Stanislavski, 1963, p. 108)

2.1

The journey.

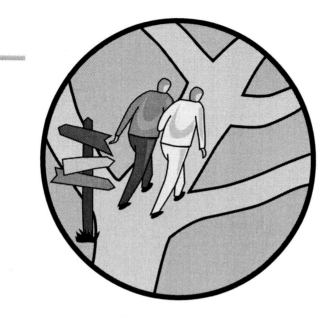

This quote often describes how a nurse sees her patient. A nurse knows, or comes to know, a great deal about patients, but knows about this patient only in terms of "more or less." Not, "Don is..." but "This type of patient is..." But a patient knows far more about his own life and values than his nurse does. This is why the patient is the final authority and why a nurse must strive to learn as much as possible about her patient.

A nurse may have a blueprint of generalized knowledge of persons, conditions, and generalities. This is invaluable. It will consist of knowledge, not of a specific patient, but of wide ranging abstractions.

Picture a person's arrival at forks in a road (Figure 2.1). There are, perhaps, five or six directions she can take. It was her generic knowledge that allowed her to get this far, but now to get to her destination she will need more specific knowledge, which she does not have. The nurse at the patient's crossroads is bewildered and probably unaware that she is bewildered. But, the patient has the necessary, narrower, and more specific knowledge. The patient is a person who knows, or who can come to know, which of the forks to take.

> A patient knows far more about his own life and values than his nurse does. This is why the patient is the final authority and why a nurse must strive to learn as much as possible about her patient.

When a nurse's professional action is effective, it is intelligible. It is obvious that she knows what she is doing. What she is doing is under her control and, therefore, under her patient's control. She is an efficient cause. Her actions are connected in a chain of sequences. These sequences are linked together by her concern for her patient's well-being and her sustained awareness. She is not comforted by acting on the basis of possibly irrelevant, generalized abstractions. When a system does not require sustained awareness, the system does not encourage any broader concern. It produces episodic interactions based on something outside of their relationship.

Justification

An ethical decision by which the nurse's patient loses the advantages of interacting within intelligible causal sequences is a flawed decision. The loss of intelligible causal sequences inspires the feeling of having lost control and being at the mercy of chance.

Human action and human life are enormously enhanced through objective and rational ethical interactions. This type of interaction will produce a series of sequential interactions that make understanding and continuing progress possible. A nonobjective and irrational ethical system will produce quite the opposite. Intelligibility will be only apparent. Causal efficacy will be hampered by unease and resentment. Interactions will arise spontaneously and then dwindle away into distrust. Ethical agents will not devote their causal abilities to bring things about on a productive and continuing basis.

An appropriate ethical decision is one that:

- Preserves the intelligibility that is found in the circumstance.
- Enables the nurse (and therefore the patient) to retain control of the events involved in a purposive process.
- Supports the continuation of causal chains that tend to enable the patient to realize his purpose.

By an appropriate ethical decision we mean nothing more than a decision that, when carried out into action, sustains intelligible causal sequences. It is a decision that is successful. The action it produces sustains progress.

By a justifiable ethical decision we mean nothing more than a decision that a nurse or patient can explain in terms of, or as related to, an agreed upon purpose. It is one that enables them to be capable of explaining the reasons for their decision and subsequent actions.

> In order to develop the ability to make justifiable practice-based bioethical decisions, a nurse must have a sound ethical orientation toward her role. This must be derived from the nature and purpose of her profession.

Within a practice-based bioethic, if a health care professional can develop the ability to objectively justify (explain) ethical decisions, she has, by that very fact, developed the ability to make appropriate decisions (decisions that will foreseeably work). And it seems impossible that she could develop an ability to make appropriate decisions consistently if she does not possess the ability to objectively justify her decisions.

In order to develop the ability to make justifiable practice-based bioethical decisions, a nurse must have a sound ethical orientation toward her role. This must be derived from the nature and purpose of her profession. Such an ethical orientation and the relation between her ethical system and her professional role make hers a practice-based ethical system. If she has this orientation, she can begin any ethical journey with calm assurance.

A justification is a description in terms of how an action can foreseeably achieve a purpose—the purpose formulated in a decision or agreement. To perform an operation, it is justifiable to use a scalpel. It would not be justifiable to use a retractor, or forceps, without a scalpel. These would not achieve the purpose. They would not make the operation possible. To fight a staph infection it is justifiable to use an antibiotic. It would not be justifiable to beat a drum, excise the affected part, or apply a tourniquet. This refers to technical justification, which is not our topic here. Our topic is ethical justification. An ethical justification is a description in terms of how an action assists the development or happiness of a human by preserving and/or enhancing his life, or how an action does not fail to respect his rights.

> An ethical justification is a description in terms of how an action assists the development or happiness of a human by preserving and/or enhancing his life, or how an action does not fail to respect his rights.

Purpose and Justification

It is necessary to justify ethical actions in terms of ethical purposes. It is also necessary to justify ethical purposes. If the actions necessary to accomplish a purpose are inappropriate given the context, then, of course, the purpose is not justifiable. If the actions, for instance, would violate someone's rights, they are, to say the least, inappropriate. An ethical purpose is not justified if the time and resources necessary to achieve it could be devoted to more vital and fundamental purposes—if it requires time and effort that could be devoted to pursuing greater values. A justifiable action, then, is an action that will foreseeably accomplish a justifiable purpose.

A perceptual and concrete-level example of the justifiable is: All things being equal, to catch a ride to a restaurant 10 miles from home, knowing you will have to walk 10 miles back may not be easy to justify rationally. In comparison, walking 1 mile to a restaurant and 1 mile back is easy to justify. The first action will bring one from a state of greater perfection (hungry but energetic) to a state of lesser perfection (well fed but exhausted). The second action will bring one from a state of lesser perfection (hungry but energetic) to a state of greater perfection (well fed, relaxed, and still energetic).

> It is necessary to justify ethical actions in terms of ethical purposes. It is also necessary to justify ethical purposes.

To act in a way that will foreseeably undermine one's own life or the life of one's patient is not justifiable. To act in a way that will foreseeably undermine the conditions that make agency possible is not justifiable. To act in a way that will foreseeably strengthen the agency and enhance the patient's life is justifiable.

> To act in a way that will foreseeably strengthen the agency and enhance the patient's life is justifiable.

If that which one's patient desires increases the ability to achieve that which is desirable, then this desire is justified. If it decreases this ability, then it is not. To act against one's knowledge and awareness when this action will affect the life of one's patient or one's own life cannot be justified. It is justifiable to act only when one knows what one is doing and that what one is doing makes sense.

Desire, Reason, and Justification

Without a motivating desire, nothing is important. Desire, itself, is important. Desire keeps us knowledgeable about ourselves. In a very strong sense, our desires sum up the evidence of who we are. We relate to things in the world through various forms of desire (or aversion—the desire to avoid). Without our relation to things in the world we would be aware of nothing. Desire, however, does not tell us about the conditions under which we desire something, whether we can achieve that which we desire, or the best foreseeable way to do this. Therefore, desire must always be subject to reason. Reason is an instrument our nature has given us to determine what is truly desirable and the best means of achieving it.

> Therefore, desire must always be subject to reason. Reason is an instrument our nature has given us to determine what is truly desirable and the best means of achieving it.

Reason, or unreason, writes our biography. Reason gives human life all of its meaning. The betrayal of reason brings life its tragedy. A decision must always be justified through the exercise of reason. It cannot be justified through desire alone. Desire alone will not produce intelligible decisions or actions. Desire responds to outside stimuli. It does not express the character of an agent. An agent is one whose actions are motivated and guided by reason. In itself, desire is not a virtue. Reason—and only reason—has the resources necessary to define desire, to defend itself, and to defend an agent's capacity to desire and to act.

> A purpose must always be achieved through the exercise of reason. It cannot be achieved through desire alone.

A purpose must always be achieved through the exercise of reason. It cannot be achieved through desire alone—unless one is a monkey who has spotted a banana. Even then, one must take care to avoid contact with a hungry tiger. And assume every tiger is hungry.

Role of Patient and Nurse

A patient is one who has lost or suffered a decrease in agency; one who is unable to take the actions his survival or flourishing requires. The fact that patients are persons who have suffered a decrease in their agency and are vulnerable is established by the fact that they are patients. As patients they remain vulnerable; more vulnerable than they were before they became patients. *Health care professionals possess an undesirable degree of power over patients.* They may be tempted to take actions that can be justified only through rationalization. They are sometimes motivated to take irrelevant, ritualistic actions. They often have little concern for the ethical meaning of their actions. They may see little need for ethical doubt or analysis. Their ethical concerns may be misguided. This increases the potential vulnerability of patients. The nurse (or any health care professional) is the agent of a patient, doing for the patient (given her education and experience) what he would do for himself if he were able. As the agent of a patient, a nurse must decrease in every way open to her, the vulnerability of the patient.

Mr. Dietrich is hospitalized. All his desires and intentions have been interrupted. As with every human being, the processes of thought, choice, decision, and action are natural to Mr. Dietrich. But now he cannot translate thought into action.

Mr. Dietrich's power of agency is nullified, and all his purposeful and goal-directed actions are frustrated. To seek values and to arrange these values into a more perfect life is natural to all humans. But Mr. Dietrich can only seek to rid himself of disvalues.

Mr. Dietrich expects beneficence from his nurse. He cannot know, and he probably would not believe, that his nurse would make an ethical decision involving him without knowing, objectively, why that decision was made. To do so would be a failure of beneficence. Mr. Dietrich, like every patient, assumes beneficence on the part of his nurse.

> Health care professionals possess an undesirable degree of power over patients.
>
> The nurse (or any health care professional) is the agent of a patient, doing for the patient (given her education and experience) what he would do for himself if he were able.

Mr. Dietrich is in the final stages of cancer. He probably will not live out the week. His physician has ordered physical therapy for him. Mr. Dietrich does not want to go to therapy. His nurse assumes that the physician has some reason for the therapy and decides that she will not question his decision. In this, she is not acting as the agent for Mr. Dietrich.

Can the nurse justify her decision? She has no reason to believe that it was an appropriate decision for the physician to make. In fact, it seems obvious that it is an inappropriate decision—irrelevant, at best, to Mr. Dietrich's circumstances. Physicians do sometimes make inappropriate decisions based on idea or facts irrelevant to a patient's values and circumstances.

Mr. Dietrich would have no reason to imagine that his nurse has no clear awareness of the relationship between the decision to make him endure the pain of therapy and the purposes that are appropriate to his context. There is no ethical justification for Mr. Dietrich's nurse to remain unaware. Yet, all too often, ethical decisions suffer this sort of defect. We all know this. But we do not like to think about it. All the same, a nurse has an ethical responsibility to think about it.

Generally, a nurse will learn from experience what is to be done. But no one can function well without an open and clear awareness of what she is doing and why she is doing it. In addition, the nurse's role as the agent of her patient is difficult. Her environment is filled with distractions. Even under conditions that make foreseeably appropriate ethical decisions impossible, a nurse can make ethical decisions that are justifiable. These are decisions made in crisis conditions on the basis of what the circumstances, her preexisting knowledge,

> Generally, a nurse will learn from experience what is to be done. But no one can function well without an open and clear awareness of what she is doing and why she is doing it.

and her present awareness allow. These are the best decisions that can be made, although they cannot be made with perfect assurance, serenity, or consistency. This is all that can ever be asked of a nurse: That she made a decision that was justified by her effective analysis of the circumstances, her preexisting knowledge, and her present awareness.

> Anxiety and dependency do not justify ethical decisions.

Justifiable ethical decision making is not impossible. It is not even difficult in most situations. But it is impossible on the basis of hunches and intuitions. It is also impossible on the basis of tradition or laws. These "imply a psychology of moral motivation in which anxiety and dependence are the primary [ethical] motivators" (van Hooft, 1990, p. 210). Anxiety and dependency do not justify ethical decisions.

The Departure

One day, many thousands of years ago, two cavemen passed each other on a forest pathway. One caveman struck the other with a club and knocked him down. There was nothing unusual about this. It had happened between cavemen many times before and it has happened between cavemen many times since. (It happens all the time.) But this day, something world-historic happened. The victim, holding his bloodied head, looked up and asked the fateful question, "Why did you do that?" This was history's first demand for an ethical justification.

Unfortunately for the children of cavemen, on that day the aggressor caveman did not bother to reply. At that time, cavemen did not spend much time analyzing ethical dilemmas. (Nor do they today.)

Thousands of years later, the same event occurred on an even more remarkable day, but with one noteworthy difference: The aggressor, a thoughtful chap as cavemen go, replied to his victim's query with the remark: "I harm you so that you will have no power to harm me. It is terribly unfortunate that you and I cannot leave each other alone, each of us free to do what he wants to do. Someday, we ought to give some thought to this."

> Rights is: The product of an implicit agreement among rational beings, made and held by virtue of their rationality, not to obtain actions nor the products or conditions of action from one another, except through voluntary consent objectively gained.

More time passed. During this passage of time, the human race began to form the idea of individual rights—the right to be left alone. It is an idea with a very rocky history and one that is far from completely formed. But it is a reality. It does motivate and control much human interaction. One can observe this reality in operation constantly and everywhere. It is the irreplaceable reality serving as the foundation of humanity's ethical existence.

Rights* is: The product of an implicit agreement among rational beings, made and held by virtue of their rationality, not to obtain actions nor the products or conditions of action from one another, except through voluntary consent objectively gained.

---

* As the reader proceeds through the text, the necessity of regarding "rights" as a singular concept, denoting a single, noncomplex agreement, will become obvious.

Rights is an agreement that they will not force one another to take action, nor unjustly deprive another of any value his effort has produced, nor place another in any circumstance without the voluntary consent of that other - a consent that is gained with full awareness. This agreement establishes the practice of acting together only on the basis of the informed and voluntary consent of everyone involved—a consent that is obtained without force or deception.

Rights pertains to an individual's freedom of action. An individual has a right to make free choices among alternatives and act on these choices based on his or her own desires, purposes, and values so long as these choices and actions do not interfere with the rightful choices and actions, or violate the rights of another.

The first great creation of ethics—the creation that made all the rest possible—is the creation of individual rights. The scope of ethics then expanded from this. It began by making trust between rational beings their natural state. Individual rights and explicit agreements make productive interaction between ethical agents possible.

Solitude and Society

In a state of solitude, a person has a right to do whatever he or she is capable of doing. An individual has this right in the sense that no one else is relevantly involved and there is no possibility of violating the rights of others.

When ethical agents live and interact together, the benefit of the rights agreement is so great and so obvious, the detriment of not having this agreement is so manifestly ruinous, that the agreement literally "goes without saying." It is, in various ways, the basis of all benevolence, justice, and cooperation among people.

As cavemen became more and more rational, someone began to give some thought to this. The idea caught on. They began to form this agreement among themselves. Eventually, it was formed, without words, naturally and spontaneously, simply as a matter of course. It is an agreement to forego aggression in favor of communication, agreement, and interaction.

As reason began to enlighten their lives, cavemen realized that aggression is dysfunctional and that nothing produces human progress and well-being more perfectly than free and spontaneous cooperation. The practice of recognizing rights spread. The process still continues. It is often inconvenient but always alluring. In the long run, nothing else makes sense. When this agreement is put aside, there is nothing whatsoever to protect people against each other's brutal irrationality or to assure good faith and justice in their interactions. Individual rights is a reality that we see surrounding us everyday.

> When this agreement is put aside, there is nothing whatsoever to protect people against each other's brutal irrationality or to assure good faith and justice in their interactions.

The recognition of rights is an essential element of the ethical interaction between agents. It is an original and implicit agreement that shapes every future agreement. It is an agreement that agreements will be kept.

The recognition of rights is an essential element of the ethical interaction between agents. It is an original and implicit agreement that shapes every future agreement.

The violation of rights produces aggression and coercion. The recognition of rights produces justice and trust. It is easy to see that without the recognition of rights, trust is a fatal illusion. Justified trust, in its turn, produces ethical interaction. As ethical agents become aware of the benefits of trading values that they possess or can produce for values they do not possess or cannot produce, the existence of a justified trust makes trade and interaction their most significant asset.

Next time you are sharing a bottle of champagne propose a toast to the caveman who first "gave some thought to this." The world is a far better place for his having been here. We are indebted to him.

Ethical Anthropology

Suppose an "anthropologist" from another planet came to earth to study humankind. If he were to understand humans, he would have to be capable of understanding an animal organism with the power of reason. He would have to understand the demands for action and the vulnerability that humans face. Otherwise, he could not understand human motivations or actions. This would mean that he would be unable to understand human beings. This would apply to extraterrestrial anthropologists, but it applies no less to health care professionals. The first demand placed on health care professionals is that they recognize the nature of human beings.

The first demand placed on health care professionals is that they recognize the nature of human beings.

In order to make his study, our visiting anthropologist might decide to study the nature of the health care setting. He would discover that, if certain conditions are in place, the health care setting is both intelligible and predictable. But if these conditions are not in place, it is neither. Considerations must be examined. Choices must be made. Ethics applies to all and only things that must examine considerations and make choices and decisions, that is, all and only to individual women and men.

Through the nature and purpose of the health care setting, the anthropologist would discover that humans enjoy benefits and suffer harms through unforeseeable events. Then he would discover that human beings and human life are enhanced if the following conditions are in place:

These are the human character traits that make the establishment of a health care setting possible. They are produced by well-structured ethical values. So long as these character traits direct events in the health care setting, it is intelligible. When they do not, the health care setting becomes an unintelligible, causal, and morally catastrophic shared state of unawareness.

These character traits are expected when the health care setting is established. However, awareness of their necessity is often lost. As in many spheres

2.1 Enhancement of Human Life

Cooperation is possible and human action is predictable.

There is a natural benevolence among humans, and trust in the goodwill of others is reasonable.

Integrity, reason, and respect for the rights of a reasoning being supports interaction.

Foresightful and purposeful interaction based on an exchange of values is possible.

People can foresee the probable consequences of their actions.

of human action, the real world is abandoned and another world is created out of cultural pressures, vague feelings, and empty words. Ethical agents become disoriented through the repetition of meaningless sounds and motions. This unreal world displaces reality. In this new world failure is common. No clear differentiation between ethical and nonethical aspects can be made. The second demand placed on health care professionals is that they recognize the ethical nature, demands, and purpose of the health care setting. Everything else follows from this.

This recognition is a precondition to all ethically justifiable interactions in the health care setting (Table 2.1). Empathy and benevolence are preconditional to this recognition. There is no genuine recognition between nurse and patient without a consciousness of this wider context.

> The second demand placed on health care professionals is that they recognize the ethical nature, demands, and purpose of the health care setting.

Ethical Approach of Professional and Patient

The philosopher Lao Tzu (604 BC) (Brown, 1938) has told us "The longest journey begins with the first step." This is so obvious that we can see it for ourselves. We can hardly avoid seeing it. But it is so obvious that, without Lao Tzu, we might never have noticed the importance of it.

It is also obvious that we can take the first step of a journey in confusion. We may have brought the patient along. When we take the first step in confusion, or from an unthinking and arrogant certainty, it is often in the wrong direction. If it is taken in the wrong direction, at the end of our journey we may find ourselves very far from our destination. If it is an ethical journey, we will probably be unaware of this and remain unaware of it. Our patient may not.

A series of actions taken in the pursuit of vital and fundamental goals may be regarded as an ethical journey. The possibility of arriving at an undesirable destination is very real for an ethical journey.

Preparing for the Ethical Journey

To get the direction of any journey precisely right, the initial preparations are very important.

To get the direction of any journey precisely right, the initial preparations are very important. The same is true of the direction of professional practice. These preparations are pivotal in the ethical decision making of any professional. In order to be certain of its discovery, a number of conditions of the search, if practical, are desirable:

1. The world outside the health care setting should not be considered. The world outside the health care setting is an invitation to confusion. The ethical aspects of a situation are usually so snarled in irrelevant memories, logistic and administrative concerns, and the demands of hands-on care that they are obscured unless outside factors are carefully ignored.

2. The details of the health care setting should be clearly perceived. It is also necessary to be aware of the authentically ethical aspects of a situation. These aspects are an integral part of the health care setting. They are not random occurrences. They are to be dealt with calmly, competently, and sequentially, not off-handedly and not inflexibly.

3. The essential qualities of the ethical situation should be visualized. For instance, it is commonly agreed that bioethics calls for a patient's right to self-determination to be respected. A patient's right to self-determination can be a fuzzy abstraction. Its outline may become visible only in the most obvious circumstances.

   A patient is on her way to have a hysterectomy. She tells you as you are taking her to the operating room that she hopes that after the operation she can get pregnant. She very much wants to have a child. This situation beckons to the nurse to stop the surgery until this can be resolved. However, very few situations are as simple as this.

   A cloudy understanding of a patient's right to self-assertion—his right to control his own situation—is better than no ethical understanding at all. But it is better, and far more useful, if a nurse understands that a patient has a right to be protected against undesired or undesirable interaction of any sort. This illustrates self-assertion.

4. The essential qualities of a situation are those qualities that can, properly, guide the nurse's ethical actions. They are like landmarks on a trip, guiding the traveler to her destination. The ethical aspects of a situation should be isolated. One should be able to draw general, but tentative, conclusions that apply to very similar situations. No situation will be precisely the same but, without these general conclusions, a nurse has to face similar situations, one by one, without a basic understanding.

5. It is important to make decisions that have a beneficial effect into the future. It is of no importance to make decisions whose benefits cease the moment the actions are taken. Ethical actions do not have to occur in disjointed series. They can be taken in ongoing integrated sequences.

6. Her decisions should be based on stable and permanent values, not on values that are impermanent and changing. They should be relevant values,

appropriate to a human being in the health care setting. These values, certainly, should be the patient's values and appropriate to the patient at this time. It is better, therefore, to see where these stable and permanent values are than to identify transitory ones.

The Nature of Ethical Aspects

Take the sparsest situation imaginable. Imagine two lost people meeting in the middle of a wasteland. Not even in this situation is every aspect an ethical aspect. One person plans to follow the North Star and walk out of the wasteland. The other intends to build a fire and lay down debris spelling out "Help" in the hope that a passing airplane will sight him.

Each person has come from different states of life. Each has different motivations. Each has different ways of going about things and each will return to different conditions of life. Each has a unique set of abilities, strengths, and weaknesses. The way each has chosen to escape the wasteland is not an ethical aspect of the situation. Neither is the background from which each has come, nor the conditions of life to which they hope to return. Their state of health is not an ethical aspect and neither is their knowledge or lack of knowledge.

Every ethical aspect of a situation arises in relation to aspects that are not, in themselves, ethical. The nonethical aspects of a situation determine what can be done. The ethical aspects—in relation to a purpose—determine what ought to be done, given what can be done.

Jane sees a young girl, Nancy, drowning. Jane cannot swim. There is a life preserver at hand. This establishes what Jane can do, but not what Jane ought to do. Jane's ethical character, her natural empathy for other human beings, and her sense of beneficence determines what she ought to do.

> The nonethical aspects of a situation determine what can be done. The ethical aspects—in relation to a purpose—determine what ought to be done, given what can be done.

Since ethics has to do with actions taken in the pursuit of vital (essentially related to the preservation or enhancement of life) and fundamental (essential to making a person's life what she wants her life to be) goals, to rescue Nancy is, at that time, Jane's only vital and fundamental goal—to act in honor of her own life by preserving Nancy's. Sharing an affirmation of the value of life that their awareness implies, highlights the ethical aspects of the situation for Jane and Nancy. Nancy's desire and efforts to survive are ethical aspects.

Suppose, when Nancy's peril arose, Jane had not been present, and Nancy saved her own life by grabbing onto a log that came floating by. In doing this, she achieved a vital and fundamental goal. She saved her life. The floating log is obviously not an ethical aspect of this situation. Nancy's action is its only ethical aspect. Only those aspects of a situation that relate to human purposes and human virtues are ethical aspects of a situation.

To put it another way, the ethical aspects of a situation are determined by the human intentions that are set to operate in the situation. What is ethically relevant in any situation is determined by the purposes of the agents who can act in it. That something is relevant, of necessity, implies that it is important to some person in relation to a purpose. This is not to say that what one ought to do in any situation is simply relative to one's desires. To go from "I want X" to "Therefore it is good (or right) that I do Y" is neither ethical nor rational. Justifiability is radically important to ethical decision making. To be the source of justifiable actions, one's desires must be justifiable in terms of their foreseeable consequences.

The third, and most crucial, step of the journey is for the nurse to discover the mapmaker, the authority that will guide the ethical journey, the authority that will guide their interactions to its justifiable destination.

Trial and Error

Because no two human beings are entirely different, every nurse can feel a certain empathy with the human hopes and fears of all persons. She has the basic resources necessary to learn through experience. She can master ethical action through trial and error.

But this is the slowest possible way. While she is learning in this way, she may make many blunders. She may do many things that eventually will bring about harm. She may fail to do many things that would have brought about much good. She may never learn which principles or guidelines are right for ethical action. She may never master the art of applying these principles well in specific cases. Many ethical agents never do.

Formalism

Certain authorities advise a health care professional to adopt formalistic principles. These are principles that are to be applied indiscriminately without regard to consequences.

If a professional is to act benevolently, she will be able to justify only those actions that bring about a preponderance of benefit over harm. Actions taken ritualistically without concern for the nature of their effects are not actions that are intended to avoid harm and bring about good. Actions can be taken without a prior and specific process of ethical analysis. However, these actions, properly speaking, do not have an ethical motivation in the sense that they do not have an objective and, consequently, not a beneficial motivation.

> Actions taken ritualistically without concern for the nature of their effects are not actions that are intended to avoid harm and bring about good.

Animals without the power of reason never reach the level of the ethical. This is true whether they lack the power of reason by nature (as is the case with non-human animals) or by choice (as is the case with humans). If the actions they take avoid harm and bring about good, this is by accident not design.

So, for a professional ethic, authorities who offer formalistic rules are not reliable.

Convenience

Other authorities would advise a health care professional to hold the convenience of others as her principle of ethical judgment. This principle is, at best, the principle of etiquette. Taken beyond the level of etiquette, it ignores the fact that a health care professional has knowledge and specific functions to perform.

It seems apparent that this is inappropriate if a professional has a specific role. This principle would make it impossible to fill her professional role. She cannot hold the convenience of others as the principle of her professional or her ethical judgment.

Jake, recovering from open heart surgery, is attached to a number of confining apparatuses. Jake is becoming increasingly agitated from inactivity. His family has asked his nurse not to get him out of bed until they arrive. This would be very pleasant and convenient for both the nurse and his family. However, his agitation is causing a fluctuation in his vital signs. Proper nursing practice requires Jake's nurse to set aside convenience as a principle of judgment. All rational bioethical decision making requires precisely the same thing.

If the principle of convenience were appropriate, robots would make ideal nurses because robots are specifically designed for convenience. A nurse is not a robot, and there is little reason to leap to the conclusion that the betrayal of her knowledge and the sacrifice of her mind is her best answer to the problem of ethical decision making. Still, less is a wild vanity that tells a nurse that she is automatically right in her evaluation of a patient's situation because it is impossible for her to be wrong and it is unnecessary for her to exert effort to be right. In order to practice ethically, a nurse's understanding must be complete enough to make her able to do good while she avoids doing harm. She must exercise the use of her judgment in the practice of her profession. In fact, this exercise of judgment is the first demand of beneficence. So there is still a need to find an authority who understands the requirements of a justifiable bioethical decision making process.

The Final Authority

The only other possibility is for a nurse as the agent of her patient to learn the requirements of right action from a reliable authority on the subject. This leaves the problem of discovering an authority that is reliable.

There is an authority who would advise a health care professional to begin from an objective awareness of what is going on in the health care setting. He would ask the professional to exercise her time and effort in acting to help her patient to achieve a passage from his current state of well-being to a more perfect state. He would advise her to justify her actions on the basis of her professional agreement.

This authority, of course, is the patient.

Musings

No one ever did or said more to establish intelligible causal sequences in human relationships than the caveman "who gave it some thought."

There is a group of facts naturally tending to form a unique and intelligible context when nurse and patient come together. These facts establish a relationship between them through an interweaving of purposes and a meeting of the minds. A patient needs a nurse to provide him with the benefit of her professional skills. A nurse needs a patient in order to live her professional role. Their shared purposes takes the form of an implicit agreement to interact and has this as its purpose – their self-directed interaction – the control by each of his or her time and effort into productive interactions in filling their needs.

The most basic link between people dictates that the first step of interaction shall be an agreement "not to obtain action . . . except through voluntary consent, objectively gained."

A nurse is the agent of her patient, doing for her patient what he would do for himself if he were able. That which nurses profess (i.e., that to which they agree) is beneficence. Their education, training, and experience fit them to exercise beneficence in the health care setting. The first ethical demand placed on nurses is that they accept the nature of human beings. The next ethical demand placed on them is that they recognize the nature, demands, and purposes of the health care setting. If a nurse is to act beneficently, she must know why she is doing what she is doing. These are the first steps of her ethical professional action. A nurse cannot act, let alone act beneficently, without this awareness. In order to know why she is doing what she is doing, a nurse must exercise judgment. Judgment is a precondition of beneficence. If a nurse does not know why her actions are beneficent, they are not beneficent. Beneficence begins in judgment.

> A nurse is the agent of her patient, doing for her patient what he would do for himself if he were able.

This implies that it is impossible to function under a professional ethic without recognizing the patient as the center of ethical decision making and, therefore, as the final authority as to the direction of his ethical interactions. It requires the nurse to act as the agent of her patient until such time as he regains his own agency.

A health care professional helps the patient in navigating through myriad facts by means of appropriate actions. However, a health care professional must never forget, and may, now and again, remind her patient that the patient's life, health, and well-being set the destination.

Study Guide

1. Does the fact that the patient is the final authority mean that any patient has a right to do anything and to make any type of demands on the nurse and other health care professionals? Support your answer.
2. Why must rights be a singular term and how does this implicit agreement foster understanding?
3. What does the following statement mean: "Ethics pervades the practice of everyday life"?
4. Why is justification so important to bioethical decision making?
5. How does the rights agreement, the agreement not to aggress, foster interaction with patients?

6. What does it mean to be the agent of a patient?
7. What is the purpose of symphonology?

References

Brown, B. (Ed.). (1938). *The wisdom of the Chinese*. Garden City, NY: Doubleday.

Churchill, L. R. (1989). Reviving a distinctive medical ethic. *Hastings Center Report, 19*(3), 28–30.

Stanislavski, C. (1963). *An actor's handbook*. New York: Theatre Arts Books.

van Hooft, S. (1990). Moral education for nursing decisions. *Journal of Advanced Nursing, 15*, 210–215.

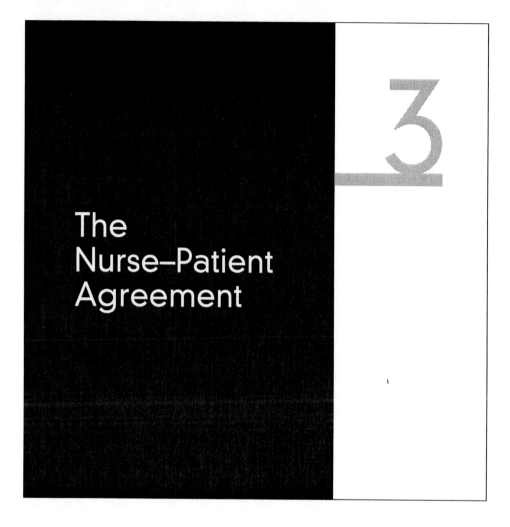

The Nurse–Patient Agreement

An agreement is a shared state of awareness on the basis of which interaction occurs. Imagine two people engaged together in some behavior: They are playing volleyball, carrying a plank, going out to dinner, holding hands at the movies, or taking a rocket to the moon. There are four possible sources of their behavior:

- Their behavior is directed by coercion. One person is compelling another to interact or both are being compelled by a third person.
- Their behavior is directed by deception. One person is aware of what he or she is doing while the other has been deceived into cooperating, or both have been deceived by a third person.
- Their behavior is determined by evasion. Whatever they are doing there is information available to them that would reveal a better course of action. They are carefully keeping themselves unaware of this information.
- Neither is forced or deceived. They are not blocking their awareness of any relevant factor. They are acting together by agreement. The terms of their agreement are understood by both.

Only the fourth source of their interaction, only that which is directed by objective agreement, can be justifiable ethical interaction. Coercion or deception violates the rights of the person who is forced or deceived. There is no way to justify violating a person's rights. *Rights* is: *The product of an implicit agreement among rational beings, made and held by virtue of their rationality, not to obtain actions nor the products or conditions of action - except through voluntary consent, objectively gained.* It is the rock bottom, fundamental interpersonal ethical concept. It is not possible to violate another person's rights and effectively fill the role of nurse or of a reasoning human individual.

But Is There a Nurse/Patient Agreement?

A question suggests itself as to whether the professional–patient relationship is based on an actual agreement. For a moment, let us entertain the idea that there is no form of agreement between them. A nurse is motivated to be a nurse. A patient is compelled to be a patient. But their motivations produce no agreement. This is impossible to conceive. *Nurse* and *patient* are defined—one in terms of the other. Their understanding of their common purpose—to interact—is, in itself, an agreement to be a nurse and a patient. Their state of mind when they initiate interaction, the inferred passivity and suffering of the patient, and the nurse's inferred commitment to her profession combine to shape an implicit agreement between them.

> Their understanding of their common purpose— to interact—is, in itself, an agreement to be a nurse and a patient.

If there is no form of agreement between them, there can be no fidelity between them. And the professional–patient relationship requires fidelity. The professionalism of the professional necessarily involves fidelity. The condition of the patient calls for fidelity on the part of the patient as long as their relationship lasts. There is no fidelity between two people who pass each other on the street simply because there is no common purpose between them. Consequently, there is no motivation to form an agreement. Between professional and patient the case is very different.

Fidelity is made specific by the terms of an agreement. Without the terms of an agreement:

- Their interaction is not based on a purpose.
- There is no solid basis for interaction between them.
- There is nothing to establish the parameters of fidelity.
- A nurse has no basis for a stable commitment to her patient.
- A patient has no objective reason to feel confident under a nurse's care.

Without an agreement between them, professional and patient can have no explicit understanding of their roles. Professional and patient cannot begin to understand their functioning in the relationship unless an agreement exists between them. Reliably effective communication cannot take place. Their agreement is, of necessity, prior to their understanding. It is what is understood.

The agreement makes each agent stronger. What one agent might not notice, the other can see, or discussion leads them to what otherwise might have been missed by each.

To the extent that there is no explicit understanding of the roles established by their agreement, there is no foundation for their interaction. There is no way for them to structure their interaction. What action could a nurse take if she had no idea what the response of a patient would be? What actions could a patient expect a nurse to take if he had no certain knowledge that she was acting in her capacity as his nurse?

Without a prior agreement, a nurse cannot be certain that her patient regarded himself as her patient. Without this agreement, a patient cannot be sure that his nurse regarded herself as his nurse. Nurses do what they do by agreement. An agreement produces expectations and commitments justifying those expectations.

Therefore, these problems do not arise between professional and patient. These problems do not arise, simply because there is an agreement between them. They do not think about it in these terms—and they do not have to think about it—because their agreement solves these problems before they arise.

Their agreement makes it possible for each to function. It also makes it necessary for each to apply ethical reasoning to his or her actions. Their agreement is the beginning and the principle of their ethical reasoning. Even when "a patient is not able to take part in the forming of an agreement or actively participate in it, it is an implicit agreement based on a high probability that, if the patient were able, it would be formed" (Husted & Husted, in press).

> Their agreement is the beginning and the principle of their ethical reasoning.

Dilemma 3.1

Mrs. B. is an 86-year-old widow who lives in a California retirement home. She is a gentle, sociable lady and likes to reminisce about her work doing make-up for movie stars. She has no family locally but does have one good friend nearby and a 101-year-old sister on the East Coast. She is in the hospital for treatment of an infection, from which she is recovering. She also has chronic kidney failure and has been on dialysis for about 8 months. For at least the past 3 months, Mrs. B. has told her doctors, her nurses, and her friend that she wants to stop the dialysis. She understands that her life depends on receiving it, but she declares that she hates the process and does not want to live this way. Yet she continues to board the van that takes her to the dialysis center three times each week. She claims that every time she tells her doctor she wants to stop, he describes the risks of falls, fractures, and a miserable end. This frightens her (Colter, Ganzimi, & Cohen, 2000, p. 24). What is the nurse's responsibility in this case?

Motivations

A most intimate ethical relationship emerges between a nurse and a patient. This relationship is formed on the side of the patient by the desire to regain a state of agency. The loss of agency is a frightening experience. It can involve, to a degree, the loss of the patient's self-image. It can be a very painful experience. It makes a patient dependent on others.

> A most intimate ethical relationship emerges between a nurse and a patient. This relationship is formed on the side of the patient by the desire to regain a state of agency.

On a nurse's side, the relationship is formed by her response to her patient. Ideally, it will not be formed by any value of the patient's dependency on her, but by her emotional intolerance of her patient's misfortune. This is the attitude that leads most into a health care career.

At the same time, it is to be hoped that a nurse will be strong enough not to wallow in her emotions and allow them to inhibit her actions. She must not allow herself to be burned out by her emotions. And she must not allow herself to resent her patient for being disabled. It would not do for both of them to be disabled.

> On a nurse's side, the relationship is formed by her response to her patient.

But not every relationship between nurse and patient is structured in this way. The motivations of each are sometimes deflected from their appropriate course. He may handle his loss of agency and self-image—his state of dependence—in a way that a nurse finds burdensome. Her response to her patient may be resentment. She may be motivated by an emotional intolerance, not of her patient's misfortune but of her patient himself.

When this occurs, it arises from the breaking of an agreement—an agreement a professional originally made with herself when she began her career in health care.

> A well-ordered nurse–patient relationship involves implied expectations and obligations accepted and agreed to by each. In every case, the expectations and obligations arise somewhat differently.

A well-ordered nurse–patient relationship involves implied expectations and obligations accepted and agreed to by each. In every case, the expectations and obligations arise somewhat differently. These differences are determined by a number of contextual factors. Chief among them are the condition of the patient and the way in which the ethical character-structures of nurse and patient mesh or fail to mesh in their relationship. The quality of their relationship sets the outline of their interaction.

How Is This Agreement Formed?

A health care professional does not sit on the patient's bed with pen and paper and say "Now we have to form our agreement." But an agreement is formed nonetheless.

A health care professional walks into a patient's room or a patient's home. The patient is lying in a bed or sitting in a chair. Right there, the agreement is set up: "You are my patient. I will be your nurse." "You are my nurse. I will be your patient." Without being spoken, this agreement implicitly arises between them.

The ethical aspects of the agreement are implied by this. "You are my patient. I will support your virtues—the strength of your character." (Every virtue is a form of strength). My strength—the strength my knowledge can give you—will be here to support your recovery. The response is: "You are my nurse. My virtues will interact with yours." Their discovery of each other is sufficient to produce the agreement. They immediately recognize the facts that have brought them together. The agreement arises when a nurse, in effect, accepts a patient's invitation to be his nurse and a patient accepts a nurse's offer to be his nurse.

Their agreement is structured by the expectations and commitments of each. Each agrees to satisfy the reasonable expectations of the other. Both agree to live up to their commitment to the other. The nurse is a professional. The patient is an amateur; therefore, the nurse's agreement is of a different sort and necessarily stronger. It ought to be, in the words of Aristotle, "fixed and stable."

> *Their expectations and commitments establish the nature of the agreement between a professional and her patient. This agreement formulates the expectations and the commitments of each. It establishes the boundaries of the successful and unsuccessful in ethical interaction.*

It establishes what each has a right to expect from the other—within their interactions. To live up to the agreement is right. To fail to live up to the agreement cannot, in any objective sense, be right. It defines the wrong.

Now and then a nurse or a patient will establish their relationship on the basis of bullying or sadism. This makes the existence of an agreement impossible. Such an arrangement is ethically intolerable. Whatever can be done to rectify it, such as making a different arrangement, ought to be done. One ought to not tell oneself: "This is the way it has to be done." It is not.

> To live up to the agreement is right. To fail to live up to the agreement cannot, in any objective sense, be right. It defines the wrong.

Agreement and Interaction

Interactions are complementary actions—actions and reactions—arising between agents on the basis of an agreement. No interaction is possible without an agreement. No interaction between people is possible until they agree upon what each is going to do.

Agreement between nurse and patient is a form of recognition between them. It involves, for instance, recognition of the factual as well as the ethical dimensions of their interaction. An agreement sets up a causal chain of actions between nurse and patient and the purposes they desire to achieve. An agreement creates a context for their interaction. Wherever there is a connectable gap between the causal chain and the desired end, the gap is nearly always the result of a failure of someone to recognize some aspect of the context created by their agreement. Once this recognition is achieved, the links of the chain can be reconnected.

3.1

The agreement.

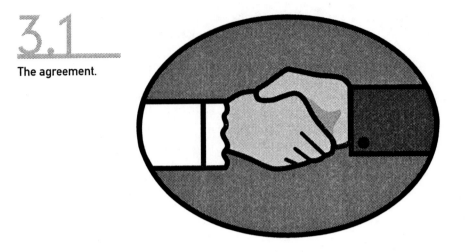

> Their agreement requires that a nurse be willing to support her patient in any purpose to which he has a right and which is appropriate to his state.

There is no question as to whether an agreement can exist or ought to exist (Figure 3.1). Without an agreement, professional interaction cannot begin. Their agreement requires that a nurse be willing to support her patient in any purpose to which he has a right and which is appropriate to his state. A failure to do this is a failure to act as the agent of her patient.

The Role of Benevolence

Benevolence is a psychological inclination to do good.

Whatever raises an agent or a patient from a certain state of perfection (a condition appropriate to survival and flourishing) to a state of greater perfection is good in relation to this person. Whatever reduces an agent from a certain state of perfection to a lesser state is evil. Whatever brings an agent to the condition of a patient is evil in relation to this agent. *(A patient is an agent whose power of agency is diminished.)* Benevolence motivates a nurse to act effectively as the agent of her patient—to guide and assist him in achieving a state of greater perfection. It generates caring and justice. Caring and justice are grounded in benevolence. Caring is benevolence expressed through the emotions. Justice is benevolence expressed through reason.

To act with beneficence, a nurse must be able to act on the basis of understanding. Understanding between a nurse and her patient depends on an agreement on what is to be understood. This understanding is held in that meeting of the minds, which is the dynamic basis of a professional, practice-based ethic. If a nurse is to do nothing that will bring about harm and everything possible that will bring about good—if she is to act on the basis of beneficence—she must know *why she is doing what she is doing*. She must be capable of acting on the basis of ethical understanding. To have ethical understanding, it is necessary to gain understanding.

Communication

The Biblical story of the Tower of Babel illustrates both the desirability and the necessity of communication and agreement to the success of interactions.

At one time, there was a universal language. A group of Babylonians, discontent with the way God was managing human affairs, decided to build a tower up to heaven, throw him out, and run things the way they ought to be run. When God observed this waste of time, he became perturbed, but, also being amused, he took pity on them.

In order to frustrate the intentions of the builders of the Tower of Babel, God changed the language of each, creating a multitude of languages. This made it impossible for them to communicate, agree, and interact with one another. Work on the tower stopped and eventually it collapsed (Gen 11:1–9).

The Bible asks this question: "How can two walk together lest they agree?" (Amos 3:3). If you think about this, you will see that two cannot walk *together* without agreeing that they will.

Builders cannot build a tower and two cannot walk together without communication and agreement between them. Two cannot interact to enhance each other's lives and overcome conflict when it arises without an agreement. The more closely this agreement is woven into the present context, the more effective the resulting interaction can be expected to be.

An unspoken but formal agreement is absolutely necessary between a health care professional and a patient. Health care is not an intelligible activity without it. No more than walking together is an intelligible activity if people cannot or do not agree. If an activity is not intelligible, if people cannot understand what they are doing, the activity is ineffective, if not impossible.

> An unspoken but formal agreement is absolutely necessary between a health care professional and a patient. Health care is not an intelligible activity without it.

The Wax Tablet (Tabula Rasa)

If people cannot understand what they are doing and why they are doing it, an ethically well-ordered health care system is impossible. When understanding another person is important and seems very difficult, there is a technique that will make understanding possible, if anything at all will make understanding possible. This technique might be called "The Wax Tablet."

Since the Golden Age of Greece there have been at least two views on the condition of the mind at birth. One is that of Plato: the mind possesses knowledge at birth—innate ideas. The other is that of Aristotle: the mind possesses no knowledge prior to experience, but is rather like a shaved wax tablet, a tabula rasa, upon which experience will write—all knowledge begins with experience.

Isolate yourself: Make your mind as nearly like a wax tablet as possible. Now, take a razor and shave away everything that makes you who you are. Shave away any ideas you have picked up from your culture, any religious attitudes, any attitudes that you hold because of your gender. Shave away your family circle—everything and anything that is familiar to you. Now adopt your patients' cultural background, religion, gender, health condition, family background and whatever peculiarities you have noted in him or her. Then ask yourself: being him, what is your attitude and motivation in your present circumstance. Almost invariably you will understand him.

Purpose and Understanding

A hundred times in a lifetime one—everyone—will utter this plaint, "I just cannot understand other people." And every time they come to this painful realization either they have come together with others with whom they share no purpose in common or with whom they no longer share a purpose. Or, they, themselves, have no purpose. People without a purpose cannot understand themselves.

People who have not come together for years enjoy reminding each other about purposes of the past. Through each other they reexperience times when they were most understandable to themselves.

People who form an agreement to work together on a purpose almost immediately understand one another better than people trying to "figure each other out" while they carry on a conversation.

The implications of how and why they form an agreement—what agreements and purposes mean to them—the strength and weakness of their motivating ideas reveal who they are while they are not thinking about it and trying to disguise it.

Dilemma 3.2

Dee, a social worker, is assigned to Anna, an elderly immigrant lady from Eastern Europe who is suffering from emphysema. She is almost destitute and very proud. She will not accept charity. Dee cannot persuade Anna to accept food stamps and Anna is frequently hungry. What can Dee do?

Agreement and Understanding

The motivating power of a firm agreement is well illustrated in the most famous ethical parable in the Western world, the story of Solomon and two mothers. King Solomon is proverbially thought of as the wisest man who ever lived. He was the king of Israel and served as judge in all disputes between the citizens of Israel.

One night, two women who shared a house each bore a baby. The child of one woman died; the child of the other survived. When the mother who bore the living child slept, the other woman stole the living child and gave the mother her dead child. Needless to say, a conflict arose between the two women. They were brought before King Solomon. When Solomon heard the case, he ordered that a sword be brought to him and commanded one of his guards to cut the child in half, giving each woman one half of the child. The woman whose child had died quickly agreed to this arrangement, but the living child's mother instantly asked that the child be given to the other woman (1 Kings, 3:16-28). Solomon gave the child to its mother.

Solomon made his famous decision on the basis of the nature of an ethical agreement. Solomon knew that the agreement between a woman and a child that is not her own is not so strong, but that she might, out of envy and spite, agree to the death of the child. On the other hand, the agreement between a woman and a child that is her own will never permit her to agree to the death of her child in order to satisfy her resentment.

Solomon's task was to achieve awareness of the true mother's identity. He was able to do this by discovering the power of the contextual interweavings that motivate an agreement.

The Fallacy of Assumptions

The resolution of an ethical dilemma cannot be justified by the fact that the decision maker *assumes, with no adequate reason to believe*, that it will produce the most desirable short-term or long-term consequences. If it can be justified by an assumption that it will, then it can as easily be defeated by an assumption that it will not. One assumption is as good as another. An assumption is a conclusion that is not based on the examination of considerations. Nothing can be justified by an assumption. An assumption cannot guide analysis. It is an appeal to ignorance.

Communication and Understanding

One day, two inhabitants of a jungle village passed a coconut tree. As they passed, a coconut fell from the tree to the ground. An argument arose between them as to who had a right to possession of the coconut. Finally, in despair, they decided to do what seemed to be the only fair thing to do. They split the coconut in half. Each islander took one half of the coconut. They shook hands. Each departed and went on his way.

Could any arrangement be more perfect than this? Surely, this is the ideal resolution to this dilemma. This is the way ethical decisions ought to be made— (?)—the way ethical interaction ought to take place—(??).

In solving their dilemma, they faced a choice between fairness, which is an obvious standard of choice, and a calm and reasoned dialogue that might have led to a better understanding and a more perfect arrangement given their circumstances. They concentrated their attention and discussion entirely upon the context of the situation—that lovely coconut laying on the ground. They communicated nothing to each other about the context of their personal knowledge or awareness of their needs and desires.

When they reached their destinations, one villager scooped the fruit out of his coconut and threw it away. He needed a cup and his only interest in his half was the shell that he could use to hold water. The other villager scooped out the fruit and threw away the shell. His family was hungry and he only wanted the fruit.

Had they communicated and come to an agreement based on mutual under-standing, one villager would have had twice the number of cups and the other twice as much fruit. They had served their ethical principle—fairness—perfectly and their own human needs very badly. So it is, all too often, in the health care setting. The more often actions are based on immediate, unquestioned *assumptions*, the more often the resulting action fails human welfare. *The more time that is devoted to generalized ethical theorizing, the less time there is devoted to valuable human concerns.*

Every agreement, to be effective, must be aimed toward a final value to be attained through understanding and interaction. The more important this value and the clearer the perception of it, the more powerful will be its motivational pull. Nurses often complain that they do not have enough time to achieve an understanding of their patients. This may be true. Time is rigid and difficult to stretch. But time does not give understanding. Awareness gives understanding. When one knows what to look for, awareness can easily be stretched.

> When one knows what to look for, awareness can easily be stretched.

Imagination and distant memories without atten-tion to the present context serve as windows so dirty it is not possible to see outside. The only productive solutions are solutions suggested to awareness by the present reality. If they had lifted their awareness to a higher plane, the villagers would have discovered that understanding what we want is a function of desire. Understanding why we want what we want is a function of reason and a far better way of understanding.

A precondition to understanding a person is:

> Imagination and distant mem-ories without attention to the present context serve as win-dows so dirtied it is not possi-ble to see outside.

- Understanding a person's background and his-tory, and whether he accepted or rebelled against these.
- Understanding the person's purposes.
- Understanding the person's agreements and his unwillingness to form certain agreements.
- Understanding what the person is communicat-ing.

Agreement—The Foundation of Interaction

The actions that a health care professional takes in her role as a professional always have an ethical aspect. They are always concerned with vital and funda-mental goals. In her role as a professional, she acts as an agent for her patient. The ethical aspects of this relationship are complex and not always easy to grasp.

Every human relationship—pitcher and catcher on a softball team, two peo-ple dancing, trapeze artists, drivers getting directions—arises from an explicit or implicit agreement. The relationship that arises between a professional and patient is one instance of this. The principles by which a professional makes a decision ought to be derived from the actual dynamics of this agreement. The dynamics of the agreement are formed by the values a patient seeks to attain, maintain, or regain in the relationship. On the professional's part, they are the values that she agrees to help her patient realize. On their part it is by the ways they can interact to achieve their purposes.

A patient, in becoming a patient, has a specific purpose and is forced by circumstances to take on a specific role. A professional, in becoming a professional, has a specific purpose and takes on a specific role—to act for those who cannot act for themselves. Their purposes interface by design. The purpose of a patient (regaining or maintaining the power of agency) determines the role of a professional.

> Every human relationship - pitcher and catcher on a softball team—two people dancing, trapeze artists, drivers getting directions—arises from an explicit or implicit agreement. The relationship that arises between a professional and patient is one instance of this.

A professional, in becoming a professional, becomes the agent of her patient. A professional does for her patient what the patient would do for himself had he not lost his power of agency. She assists him in regaining the ability to take independent actions. The interrelationship between them is formed by the nature of an agent (one who acts for a patient) and the nature of a patient (one who lacks the power to act for himself). In the interaction of professional and patient, their roles structure the implicit agreement between them. They agree, in effect, that, since the patient is a patient, the professional agent will act as an agent for the patient. *The entire area of a professional's ethical action lies within these contours of responsibility established by their agreement.*

That there is objective and voluntary consent between a health care professional and patient means that there is an interweaving of their purposes. Objective and voluntary consent never occurs outside of this interweaving. This shared state of mind—this agreement—makes their relationship intelligible and, thereby, governs their interaction. Their effective interaction produces intelligible causal

> A professional does for her patient what the patient would do for himself had he not lost his power of agency.

sequences. It implies that a patient should not make any arbitrary demands on a health care professional and a health care professional any arbitrary demands on a patient. Arbitrary demands, as well as coercion, do not arise within a shared state of awareness.

All interaction begins with this "voluntary consent, objectively gained." Voluntary consent, objectively gained, can only be established by agreement. Interaction according to agreement and according to coercion are not simply two means to the same objec-

> Objective and voluntary consent never occurs outside of this interweaving.

tive. Every step is different. They reflect two utterly diverse perspectives on human relationships and interaction. The means are so different that they change the character of the objectives. One is a value agents achieve through reciprocity. The other is a value one extorts by coercion. There are two bases for coercion: One holds the beneficiary of action, the patient, as an end in himself. The other holds the (apparent) beneficiary as a means to the ends of the nurse.

The expectations, such as reciprocity and coercion, established by an agreement, establish the nature of the context and the meaning of every motivation and every action.

This most basic link between people dictates that the first step of interaction shall be an agreement "not to gain action . . . except through voluntary consent, objectively gained," which is reciprocity.

For effective nursing interventions, as well as ethical interactions to take place between nurse and patient, each must be open to the other. The best way for this to be achieved and sustained is through the establishment of mutually caused intelligible sequences. The professional–patient agreement is a sort of schedule of these sequences.

Dilemma 3.3

Lori is an RN who works in a clinic where they treat many people who are indigent; many are homeless. One day during her lunch break when she is taking her walk she encounters Paul. They greet each other and continue walking. Paul was one of her patients at the clinic. He is homeless and has confided in Lori that his lifestyle was not one of which he is proud. He was at the clinic being treated for a number of STDs in addition to a heart condition and other chronic illnesses. His lifestyle made his heart condition worse and the clinic was trying to get him placed in low-income housing, which he refused. Suddenly, Lori heard a commotion behind her and saw that Paul had collapsed. She quickly went over to him and realized that he was in cardiac arrest. What is her responsibility to Paul? What is her responsibility to herself?

Relationship of a Nurse and Patient

The relationship between nurse and patient is codified in the implicit agreement that establishes the relationship between nurse and patient. In light of this agreement, there is only one authority to whom a professional can turn for advice on the purpose motivating their relationship—her patient. Nurses can enhance their ability to be agents of their patients by examining their own agency and what it would mean to lose it (Houck & Bongiorno, 2006).

A health care professional practicing responsibly, practices according to the purposes of her profession. If one is a responsible health care professional, then:

- One conscientiously acts as an agent. One acts with as keen an awareness and as firm a determination as one's patient would if he were able.
- One makes one's patient the reason for one's being as an agent and a professional. Therefore, he is the center of one's attention and activity. This is defined by her professional agreement and it defines her agency as a nurse.
- Interaction is guided by two objective standards—the skilled professional action of a nurse and the benefit of a patient. This is the justification for every change in action and interaction.

▧ Interaction is based on voluntary consent, objectively gained. This assures that neither party to the agreement will suffer a rights violation. It
assures that the agreement will be an agreement.

Purpose and Probability

In order to act purposefully and ethically, a nurse must always act according to
the evidence she has of the array of values held by a patient. Let us examine
this process through a thought experiment:

Suppose a nurse, Sylvia, stranded on a deserted island, has to make an ethical decision concerning a stranger who washed up on shore. The stranger is
both naked and comatose. He has a hemorrhaging wound to the head and neck.
Sylvia has no way of discovering the name of the stranger, let alone his specific
desires, purposes, or values. Nonetheless, it is quite possible for Sylvia's action
in regard to this stranger to be determined according to a proper ethical standard. In this situation, she can use the element of purpose to arrive at perfectly
justifiable decisions and actions.

Every nurse, in every situation of this type, with little difficulty can come up
with an answer to these interrelated questions:

▧ What would the maximum number of persons most desire in this circumstance?
▧ What would be the purpose of the maximum number of persons in this
circumstance if they could act for themselves?

Any decision that a nurse will make on the basis of a reasoned answer to
these questions is ethically justifiable. There will, in fact, be no other ethically
justifiable way of arriving at a decision. If a health care professional has virtually
no evidence to go on, he or she must go on what little evidence is available. This
is how decisions should be made for those who cannot participate and for whom
a nurse has no prior knowledge of what they would want.

Sylvia has evidence of the sex and approximate age of the stranger. This tells
her almost nothing. She can see that the stranger is a human person. This tells
her all that she needs to know. It is perfectly reasonable for Sylvia to form her
conclusion according to the purposes that most persons would hold. Whatever
purposes the maximum number of persons would hold in this circumstance,
this stranger would probably hold. When probability and reason is all you have,
then you must act on the basis of what you have.

A fireman leaving a burning house might see a
packet of letters and a scrapbook on a table. If he can
only save one, he has a perplexing problem. He has no
way of knowing which the homeowners would prefer
he save. Sylvia has no such problem.

Suppose that the stranger in our thought experiment were conscious. Sylvia can see that he is bleeding from the cut on his head and neck. Under these
circumstances, Sylvia would probably act automatically and without stopping to
ask permission. But Sylvia might ask him if he wants her to stop the bleeding.
The odds are overwhelming that the stranger would reply that he did. Then she
would know exactly what the context requires.

> When probability and reason
> is all you have, then you must
> act on the basis of what you
> have.

Sylvia does not have all this evidence. She does, however, have all the evidence that she needs. She has enough evidence on which to make a reasoned judgment. *In a circumstance of this type, the fact that it is reasoned is sufficient to justify the judgment.*

In an emergency, a health care professional will almost automatically act for the purpose of saving lives. What other justification could the health care professional have for this except that the maximum number of people in the maximum number of circumstances would want their lives to be saved? Sylvia is justified by the fact that any individual person in the emergency would almost certainly want to be saved.

It is not necessary to be a tea leaf reader to be an effective ethical agent. That she will act according to her best judgment forms part of a nurse's implicit agreement with her patient. It forms part of her relationship to the rest of the world. It is a fundamental part of her role.

However, some people are very strange. Suppose that the stranger for whom Sylvia acted were to claim that the decision she made was a wrong decision. Suppose, for want of a better supposition, that he believes that a woman touching his head on a Tuesday defiles him. He declares that he would have preferred bleeding to death to being defiled.

Let us examine the implications of this. Under the circumstances, Sylvia made her decision on the basis of all the evidence available to her—the evidence she had of the stranger being a person. If the decision she made and the action she took, based on her analysis of the evidence, were a wrong decision and action, then either:

A. It is a fact that the majority of people washed onto the shore of a deserted island, with head and neck lacerations, would want to bleed to death and Sylvia should have known this; or

B. Sylvia made a mistake when she reasoned from the evidence that was presented to her. An ethical agent should not make decisions by reasoning from evidence.

If the stranger attempts to justify his claim on alternative A, he attempts to justify it on an absurdity. Imagine a group of people with profusely bleeding scalp wounds sitting on a beach and replying to offers of help with, "No thanks, don't bother. I would just as soon enjoy the sound of the waves and bleed to death." Try to imagine this.

If the stranger attempts to justify his claim by alternative B, that Sylvia ought not to have acted on a reasoned conclusion based on her evidence, then his position is even more absurd.

If she ought not to have decided according to her recognition of the evidence, then she ought to have acted without thinking. But, if she ought to have acted without thinking, then anything she did would be right. If a person ought to act without thinking, then there is no way that what she does can be wrong. In this case, his claim that she should not have taken the actions she did contradicts itself. There will be nothing to limit the number of actions that she might have taken.

Let us assume that Sylvia ought to have decided on what to do without thinking, without reasoning according to the evidence available to her. If a person's action is based on thinking then, within limits, that action will be predictable. Thinking will limit the number of actions that might be taken. If a person acts without thinking, then her ensuing action will be unpredictable. If Sylvia ought to have acted without thinking, she might have done anything at all. If she would have been right to do anything at all, then any action she took would be justified. If any action she took would be justified, then the decision and action that she actually did take would be justified and could not be condemned.

In the nature of things, a nurse can justify her ethical decisions and actions through the element of purpose. Purpose is, or ought to be, a principle and a standard of, just as it is the motivation of, all bioethical decision making.

Every person is unique, but every person is a person, and in being a person, is the same as every other person and ethically equal to every other person. Sometimes, as in this case, a decision must be made on the basis of a person's "sameness." Every human being, and his every virtue, is purposive. It is always safe to assume that if what you are dealing with is a human being, then what you are dealing with has purpose. This, in itself, when necessary, justifies ethical action.

Dilemma 3.4

A certain patient is in a persistent vegetative state. There is no predictable chance that he will recover from his condition. He has requested that if he were in this state he be allowed to die. Do beneficence and respect for his autonomy require that he be kept alive? Or that he be allowed to die?

It can be argued that:

- He must be allowed to die. The unique individual that he once was no longer exists. The recognition of his right to autonomy includes recognition of the fact that there is no autonomous being to be kept alive.
- He must be allowed to die on the basis of beneficence. Biological survival in the sense of the preservation of electrochemical processes is in no way the equivalent of a human life. If there were any foreseeable possibility of his attaining even the lowest level of a human life, the demands of beneficence might be entirely different. There is no hope for a worthwhile and human life, and respect for his once human dignity requires that he be allowed to die.

The agent has an exclusive right to decide. His decision is authoritative.

On the other hand:

- He must be kept alive. One possesses life only once and life is precious above everything else. Without life, nothing whatever is of any value. The patient's staying alive is a tribute he pays to himself and to his life. Beneficence demands that he be assisted in staying alive.
- He must be kept alive since no one has a right to terminate the life of an autonomous individual. What the patient was in the past is no longer relevant. His autonomy now is the unique nature of his present existence—even if it is only these electrochemical processes. Recognition of his present autonomy demands that his life be preserved.

The recognition of a patient's autonomy and the motivation of a nurse's beneficence do not necessarily lead to one exclusive and justifiable decision. This is because no rule, principle, or standard, as we shall see, should by itself inspire a feeling of perfect confidence in any decision. One can be "certain" of the perfection of one's decision only if one ignores the context and makes a formalistic decision irrelevant to the situation. Whenever one makes a relevant judgment, not having absolute knowledge, one may make an imperfect decision.

> One can be "certain" of the perfection one's decision only if one ignores the context and makes a formalistic decision irrelevant to the situation.

There is no context in which one has absolute knowledge. This is not a reason to ignore the context. It is, rather, a reason to develop the ability to function within a context, to content oneself with achieving what is objectively possible and desirable, and to ignore an ethical "perfection" that can only be achieved by going outside of the agreement and discarding professional relevance.

It is not the perfection of a decision, but the reasoning that motivated it that justifies a decision. When the reasoning for a decision and the reasoning against it are equally valid either is justifiable. But the reason must not be tainted by personal assumptions. No argument should be offered unless there is a distinct possibility that it is an argument that the patient might make.

> No argument should be offered unless there is a distinct possibility that it is an argument that the patient might make.

The Agreement One Has With Oneself

Every nurse ought to examine her life, at least to the point where she comes to an agreement with herself that she will be a nurse. To the extent that a nurse has not made this agreement with herself—a commitment to be a nurse—she resembles a patient more than she resembles what she would be if she were a nurse.

> *A nurse who directs her long-term actions guided by her awareness of what is needed in order for her to keep that agreement, embraces her profession. A nurse who is inspired by it, and who is dedicated to it, is far less likely to experience burn-out.*
>
> *A nurse [who] tries to avoid taking those long-term actions that constitute her professional life breaks the agreement she made with herself to be a professional. She becomes indifferent. She undermines herself as a professional and as a person. If she has replaced her confidence and pride with indifference, she has done this because she abandoned **herself** when she abandoned her profession.*
>
> *If one is a nurse and is likely to continue to be a nurse, one ought to take the actions called for by the health care professions. At worst, this will make life far less boring. At best, it may restore one to the confident expectations and the pride that she began with at the beginning of her career.*

> *Dedication to what one professes—acting on that which one affirms and believes—is sometimes difficult to do. Adversities and frustrations arise. And these attack one's desire and one's sense of self. (Husted & Husted, 1999, p. 17)*

But overcoming them through dedication produces pride in oneself as a professional. A patient could not reasonably ask for more and should not find less.

An objective agreement is any agreement in which both parties to the agreement are aware of the:

- Reason for the agreement.
- Terms of the agreement.
- The intentions of the other party to the agreement.

A nonobjective agreement is any agreement in which one or both parties lack awareness of these aspects of the agreement. A nonobjective agreement is a splintered, ineffective agreement. If it is a professional agreement, it will, predictably, fail the needs of the professional and her patient and the responsibilities of the profession.

What Would Happen If...?

Few bioethics texts make the human values of those engaged in health care interaction the central focus of their concern. All give some attention to the values and well-being of patients. None hold the health care professional as the primary beneficiary of bioethical interaction. "Respect for the dignity of others is a familiar professional prescription and has a robust theoretical basis. Respect for one's own dignity is given less attention" (Gallagher, 2004, p. 587). This would be the focus of a rational self-interest ethic.

Rational Self-Interest

A rational self-interest ethic is practiced by an ethical agent with a view to enhance her life through interaction based on objective agreements—a trade of values—from which she benefits by achieving what she desires to achieve.

An agent's rational self-interest is defined in terms of her understanding of her individual nature against the background of what is needed for her personal development. It also requires a complete acceptance of the nature, motivations, and the self-interest of her "trading partners." Irrational self-interest is a contradiction in terms. Whatever is irrational cannot be to one's self-interest. Whatever decisions and actions truly serve one's self-interest cannot be irrational. Rational self-interest must begin in reason. The rationality of a nurse's choice of professions can be measured by the degree of satisfaction and fulfillment she finds in it.

> An agent's rational self-interest is defined in terms of her understanding of her individual nature against the background of what is needed for her personal development.

A patient's rational self-interest is defined in terms of his understanding of his individual nature against the background of what is needed for his personal development. It also requires a complete acceptance of the nature and needs of his survival and flourishing.

> A patient's rational self-interest is defined in terms of his understanding of his individual nature against the background of what is needed for his personal development.

The rationality of a rational self-interest ethic begins in its rejection of self-abandonment as the only possible approach to a profession. It equally rejects evasion, deception, or coercion as the basis of interaction. Rational interaction is conducted on the basis of objective understanding, self-respect, agreement, and fidelity. It cannot be conducted on the basis of unexamined emotions, self-doubt, or the desire to evade responsibility.

The functioning of a rational self-interest ethics is well formulated by William Shakespeare in these famous words:

This above all: to thine own self be true,
And it must follow, as the night the day,
Thou canst not then be false to any man. (Hamlet, Act I, Scene I)

In this, as in a multitude of things, Shakespeare seems to go too far—but he does not. He is right on the money. To be true to oneself one must know oneself and respect oneself.

Let us conduct a little experiment in thought and examine the foreseeable consequences of a nurse practicing according to a rational self-interest ethic.

A nurse's rational self-interest is achieved through the competence of her professional activity. It is expressed by satisfaction in the practice of her profession, by confidence in her competence to act, in the pride she takes in herself and her professional activities, in her feelings of contentment, and, above all, in her pride in her ethical habits. All of this grows out of her professional actions and her assurance that these actions are appropriate to her profession. It arises from her skill at the practice—and the spirit—of her profession. Every nurse begins her career with the decision that she will be a nurse. When she reaches this decision, she assumes that, in some way, her self-interest will be achieved in nursing.

If a hospital administrator wished to demonstrate the ethical attitude of a nurse untainted by rational self-interest he would simply have to find one who:

- Hates every minute of her life.
- Believes she is destroying herself by pursuing the profession of nursing.
- Feels a quiet contempt and resentment toward her patient.
- Puts on a cheerful air that is the contrary of what she feels.

The contrary view is that a nurse's first ethical task is the struggle to abandon who she is and become a cheerful nobody. The proper term for this position is irrational self-disinterest. It gets all the favorable press. Yet, it benefits no one. It benefits neither nurse nor patient. Rational self-interest, that is, reciprocity, is not the scourge that its critics claim. The idea that either an ethic counsels self-abandonment and beneficence or self-interest and malificence is fallacious. It is the fallacy of a false alternative. The rational self-interest ethic described by Benedict Spinoza is a third alternative. It is the only alternative of the three that will produce an enduring beneficence. Self-abandonment will ultimately produce resentment toward patients. An irrational self-interest will produce a brutal unconcern. A rational self-interest ethic will reveal itself in a commitment to the patient, sincere concern, benevolence, and pride. Give it a try.

> *The more each man seeks his own profit and endeavors to preserve himself, the more power does he possess to live according to the guidance of reason. But men most agree in nature when they live according to the guidance of reason. Therefore, men will be most profitable to one another when each man seeks most what is profitable to himself (Spinoza, Pt. 4, Prop. 35, Coro. 2).*

A nurse's true self-interest is not served—it is lost the day she decides that her self-interest conflicts with that of her patients.

A nurse is the agent of a patient doing for a patient what he would do for himself if he were able. A patient needs a rational agent to do for him what he would do for himself, simply because what he would do for himself needs to be rational. A patient needs a self-interested nurse (a nurse whose self-interest is fulfilled in nursing) because what he would do for himself needs to be self-interested.

Dilemma 3.5

Consider this simple but telling case: You are taking care of a 5-year-old child, Jeffrey, with a seizure disorder of unknown origin. He asked you to stay with him until his parents arrive from work. You know that this will be about 2 hours or so beyond your shift for which you will not get paid, but you agree to stay with him because he is so very frightened. As you are giving report your friends arrive from various floors to tell you that they have an early birthday surprise for you. They have purchased tickets to a concert that you desperately want to see. What should you do? How did you arrive at your decision?

Musings

Ethical realities are common experiences for all persons. They are not something accepted by mere convention. Nor are they something brought into being by legislation. Everyone has desires and purposes. Everyone must act to achieve her desires and purposes.

Everyone faces the need to think before he or she takes actions. There is an alternative to the need to think. But it is most undesirable. The alternative is that someone will suffer. These factors cannot exist without bringing the need for ethical thought—for "practical reason"—into existence.

That purpose and value are ethical phenomena pertaining to all people, that all people possess rights, and that all people possess ethical agency are not matters on which one decides. They are ethical realities already there for one to discover. Ethical realities are human realities, not because people have the power to choose them, but because they are part of human nature and part of the human situation. The supreme interpersonal reality is the network of agreements that makes human interaction possible.

> *For a nurse, as a professional, far and away the most important agreement—the agreement that must precede any agreement she can have with her patient—is the agreement she has made with herself. A nurse who practices her profession without dedicating herself to it, practices her profession without dedicating herself to herself. (Husted & Husted, 1999, pp.16–17)*

The nurse–patient agreement is the court of last resort for justifying professional decisions. The more effectively a nurse meets the ethical agreement, the more effective she is as an ethical agent and as a professional. On the other hand, it is possible for her to fulfill the agreement so ineffectively that she will hardly be a professional or an ethical agent at all.

The evolution and traditions of health care have produced certain definite expectations. These expectations form a bridge joining together the professional and patient. When a patient enters the health care system, these expectations create an implicit agreement between them. The terms of the agreement are precisely the expectations defining the health care professions and the health care professional's commitment to her profession.

The appropriateness of the terms of their agreement depends upon their human nature. More narrowly, it depends on the purpose of their interaction. Through necessity, nurse and patient interact under the terms of this agreement. Either the terms of their agreement guide their interaction or their behaviors are unintelligible. The agreement becomes a process in which two conscious beings create a resolution between them that then becomes their strategy for action. The agreement is foundational.

Agreement is shown in interaction. When the agreement is objective and sound, the nurse and patient benefit. When it is not, one or both suffer through it. When an agreement causes suffering, it is a flawed agreement. When it brings objective benefit, it is a sound agreement. An agreement can be analyzed by reference to the bioethical standards. The bioethical standards are in conflict with the forming of an irrational agreement.

If the desire behind an agreement is a rational, objective, noncoercive, and non-self-destructive desire, then the agreement, given the context, is the final "court of appeal" concerning interpersonal actions. The purposes of the patient and the nurse, as a nurse, are codified in the agreement. The ethical status of any decision, choice, or action is a function of the relationship of that decision, choice, or action to these purposes. The agreement, then, is the beginning of a nurse's ethical journey—and its principle. All, immediate and contextual, ethical understanding arises in the context of this agreement.

Study Guide

1. Think about agreements that exist in physical things that enable you to function in your everyday life, such as wheels on a car, pen to paper, a needle

to skin. Now try to think about things in your nursing world that agree and enable you to function. These are not agreements involving people, but they are agreements nonetheless.

2. Now think about how your function as a nurse or as a student nurse (or any health care professional) within the context of an agreement. Does this agreement obligate you to perform in a certain way? Think about some of these ways.

3. What if there was not an agreement? Would the health care environment take on a different function? What would happen?

4. What does it mean to have an agreement with yourself?

5. How does rational self-interest benefit you and your patient?

References

Colter, M., Ganzimi, L., & Cohen, L., M. (2000). Resolution and ambivalence/Commentaries. *The Hasting Center Report, 30*(6), 24–25. Retrieved July 4, 2006, from Proquest database.

Gallagher, A. (2004). Dignity and respect for dignity—two key health professional values: Implications for nursing practice. *Nursing Ethics, 11*, 587–599.

Houck, N. M., & Bongiorno, A. W. (2006). Innovations in the public policy education of nursing students. *Journal of the New York State Nurses Association*, Fall/Winter, 4–9.

Husted, J. H., & Husted, G. L. (1999). Agreement: The origin of ethical action. *Critical Care Nursing, 22*(3), 12–18.

Husted, G. L., & Husted, J. H. (in press). The ethical experience of caring for vulnerable populations: The symphonological approach. In M. de Chesnay (Ed.), *Caring for the vulnerable: Perspectives in nursing theory, practice, and research*. Boston: Jones and Bartlett.

Spinoza's ethics. (Original work published 1675). (Any publication of the work is sufficient).

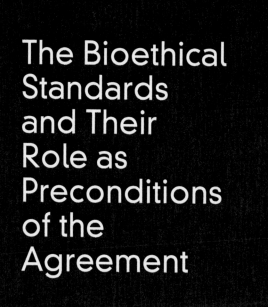

The Bioethical Standards and Their Role as Preconditions of the Agreement

The bioethical standards—the principles that generate and structure the professional–patient agreement—are:

- Autonomy–independent uniqueness
- Freedom
- Objectivity
- Self-assertion
- Beneficence
- Fidelity

The Bioethical Standards and the Professional–Patient Agreement

The health care system has arisen by virtue of specific human needs and desires. These desires, needs, and the purposes they inspire structure the role of everyone in the health care system. They determine the nature of the role filled by nurses. They are the need and desire for life, health, and well-being—the human need to escape suffering and to regain agency when agency has been impaired or lost. One need remains – the patient's need to recover the emotional optimism and psychic stability that were internal parts of his autonomy before the ordeal that brought him into the health care setting.

A nurse in a health care setting knows why she is there. A patient knows, or comes to know, why he is there. His nurse also knows why he is there. Each comes to know on the most basic level. He is there to regain his power to take purposeful actions.

> A person's power of agency is his power or capacity to initiate and carry out actions directed toward goals.

A person's power of agency is his power or capacity to initiate and carry out actions directed toward goals. It is his awareness of control over himself—his actions and his circumstances—when this can be translated into actual action and control. A patient comes into the health care setting in order to overcome a physical or psychological disability. He is there to regain his power to act. But no patient regards agency as his final purpose. His final purpose is the goals toward which he directs purposeful action. Agency is a value in that it enables an agent to realize purposes beyond itself. For the health care system, agency is a goal in itself. But a patient is in the health care setting so that he will be able to return to the football field, the concert stage, or the factory floor. He is there in order to return to his family and to his life.

If the nurse understands this agency from the patient's perspective, their attitude toward each other is that of friends with a purpose, making progress together.

The Bioethical Standards as Virtues and Rights

An agreement can be analyzed by reference to the bioethical standards. The bioethical standards are in conflict with the forming of an irrational agreement. Given the volitional and rational nature of the parties to the agreement, the bioethical standards are, as will become obvious, intricately bound up with it. To a large extent they will determine its outcome.

Autonomy

Autonomy as Independent Uniqueness

Every ethical agent is autonomous. An autonomous agent is one with the right and the power to take actions and pursue goals according to personal desire and without obtaining prior permission. One cannot make an agreement without being an autonomous agent. And every autonomous agent has the right to enter into agreements and to refuse to enter into agreements.

By nature, every human is autonomous. Everyone is, at least potentially, independent, self-directed, and unique. Every individual has a right to independence, self-direction, and uniqueness.

If it is an easy matter to affirm this, it is also an easy matter to deny it. It is a truth that is fashionable today. Tomorrow it may come to be thought of as unfashionable and, therefore, untrue. This would radically undermine the welfare of patients. It would be a setback for the ethical quality of medical and nursing practice.

So we have taken the liberty of contextually redefining the term *autonomy* in order to make it signify a visible and undeniable character structure. That is, each unique independent and self-directed individual's differences serve as the basis on which autonomy and its constituent character-structures are identified. This epitomized the conditions of character analysis. The term *autonomy* will signify individual uniqueness. This makes it more useful analytically without losing its connotations of independence and self-directedness.

> *Certain terms used in the book are redefined for the sake of maximum useful-ness. Autonomy is one of these terms. The way a person exercises his or her self-governance and right to take independent action is not determined by the mere fact that the person is independent and self-governing. It is determined by that person's unique desires and values—his or her unique character structure. A nurse understands her patient, or anyone else, better if she makes herself aware of the ways in which he is unique than she does if she simply makes herself aware of his independence and right to self-governance alone. And, by far, the most effective way she can ethically interact with his independence and right to self-governance is by ethically interacting with his uniqueness. (For the technical sense in which terms are used in this text, the reader is referred to the Glossary.)*

An ethical agent directs his efforts in ways determined by the way he has developed his unique individual nature. He is independently capable of expressing his character in unique actions, directed in highly personal directions.

Autonomy, as a bioethical standard, refers to the uniqueness of an individual person. This uniqueness is the specific nature—the interwoven character structures—of that person.

> Autonomy, as a bioethical standard, refers to the uniqueness of an individual person. This uniqueness is the specific nature—the interwoven character structures—of that person.

Autonomy as *Ethical Equality*

Rational animality is the fundamental nature of every human. We are all part of the same species—reasoning animals. It is our nature as living beings to be capable of thinking things over and moving about from place to place. This defines us. The needs of our animal nature determine us to the pursuit of life-sustaining goals. Our rationality assists, and also determines us to the pursuit of life-serving and fulfilling goals. Our autonomy, that is, our uniqueness, determines that for every individual these goals will be different. Our ability to reason, to choose, and to decide makes us free but responsible. This is how our uniqueness develops.

Our ethical nature arises from our identity as members of the species. Everyone of this species, by nature, enjoys an ethical dignity equal to every other.

No ethical agent is both identical in ethical dignity and superior (and, therefore, not identical) by nature to others of the same species.

Every human being has an individual right to act on his unique and independent purposes and desires. No human being is less or more independent than another. None has a right to override the purposes and desires of others. No one human being, and no collection of human beings, has a right to alienate the self-directedness of another. This is so vital to bioethics that we will subject it to a rigorous analysis—an analysis conducted via introspection.

> Everyone of this species, by nature, enjoys an ethical dignity equal to every other.

Reflect on your self-experience and this is what you will find: You, as a human individual, are an organism that moves about from place to place under your own power. You guide your movements through thought—the ability to relate yourself to reality through the power of reason—and the inescapable need to choose and decide.

The choices you must make are, in many cases, the choices every animal organism must make—survival choices. But there are many choices other animal organisms cannot make—choices made via meanings and reason. Many choices you make are highly individualized—choices you make according to your purposes and the meanings you find in your lived world. The rational-animal nature of a human individual endows every person from birth with a striking potential.

A nurse's patients, in all but the most extreme cases, enjoy this potential. So do nurses. This potential is a matchless capacity for growth and development. This fact is the biological foundation of ethics.

Let us wander over to the Ethicist Island. Now, on this island we find everything that is or could be, everything except a living being with the power of reason. Only a living being with the power of reason can concern itself with vital and fundamental choices and decisions. A vital decision being one essentially related to the preservation or enhancement of life. A fundamental decision being one that begins a chain of causes and effects whose nature will be determined by the nature of this most basic choice.

Prior to this being entering onto the scene, no such thing as ethics is either possible or imaginable. But, when this being enters on the scene, the absence of a need for ethics is not possible and cannot even be imagined.

Throughout the whole species of humankind, each person is different. Our differences begin to emerge when our development begins. This continues through the accumulation of our experiences and the mental and physical actions we take in relation to these experiences. Through the flourishing of our potential for development, we become what our nature and choices allow us to become. For each of us, who we become is unique. Throughout our lifetime, this uniqueness becomes more and more a part of us and, as we mature and become more active, we become more and more unique and complex. This is the experience and history of every human individual. Every person begins life as an individual different from all others, as each leaf in the forest is different from all others. Uniqueness increases throughout maturation and development.

The fact that each member of our species undergoes growth and development implies three facts. These facts are vital to bioethical understanding.

1. You, and every other person, have a right to growth, development, and the pursuit of a destiny. Given your nature and the nature of all the people around you, it is an absurdity to believe that someone else has a right to determine your development or destiny, or that you have a right to determine the development or destiny of another (Husted & Husted, 1997). When the cavemen formed the rights agreement many thousands of years ago, they made no special arrangements for you and someone else who would be superior or inferior to you.
2. No two individuals will develop identically. You will be different from everyone else in the world. You, and every other person, will develop in your own time and circumstances and according to your own experiences, decisions, and actions.
3. There is no rational, ethical basis for any person to refuse to accept the fact that another is unique in particular (nonaggressive) ways. There is no justification for you to refuse to accept the unique character structure of another—a patient most especially.

In the right to be unique and to act from that uniqueness, every individual is the absolute ethical equal of every other. It cannot be otherwise.

In the right to be unique and to act from that uniqueness, every individual is the absolute ethical equal of every other. It cannot be otherwise.

The Right to Autonomy

For these reasons, we define *autonomy* as independent uniqueness. An individual's right to autonomy is his or her right to be the unique rational being he or she is. This obviously includes the right to take independent and self-directed actions. This is the right to self-assertion. The right to self-assertion is derived from the right to autonomy. But then, every bioethical standard is derived from the standard of autonomy. If the standard of autonomy—the fact that each individual is, by absolute right, unique and independent—cannot be defended, no standard can be defended. No ethical judgment would be possible. Nothing would be good or bad, right or wrong. Or every ethical agent would be good or bad, right or wrong, together.

In the context of the bioethical standards, autonomy is the ultimate standard of the rightness or wrongness of a nurse's ethical decisions. If a nurse is to be able to justify her decisions and actions, she must take account of the autonomy of her patient because she is the agent of her patient doing for her patient what he would do for himself if he were able.

But then, every bioethical standard is derived from the standard of autonomy.

Unlike an abstract right to self-determination and independence, this right does not depend upon political fashions. The right to be a unique person is nothing more than the right to be what one is. For any individual person, the right to be what one is, is, very simply, the right to exist. Quite often, a person's right to self-determination and independence, which is an implicit part of his right to be who he is, can be rationalized away by others. But his right to exist and to be who he is ethically in the nature of things is absolute and cannot be set aside. Ultimately, his right to self-determination and independence arises from his right to be who he is. His right to act as who he is, is an aspect of his right to be what he is.

> For any individual person, the right to be what one is, is, very simply, the right to exist.

The reason why individuals make an agreement and the terms of the agreement they make arise from who they are.

Autonomy as a Precondition of Agreement

The fact that people have different needs and values logically motivates their interaction. If they did not, they would have no reason to interact.

Autonomy—the uniqueness of every person—is a precondition of the health care professional–patient agreement. That each individual is unique and independent is, itself, an agreement that is implied and structures every other agreement. As an agreement, it is a bioethical standard.

> *For either professional or patient to violate the autonomy of the other is to act as if no agreement exists between them. For this is, implicitly, to deny a necessary precondition of the existence of an agreement. If no agreement exists, then no stable and intelligible relationship can exist between them. Their differences do not, as often is assumed, produce a basis for fear and distrust between them. Their differences extend into their goals and values and make trade desirable. The differences among people are the only reason they can be of benefit to one another.*

Recognition of the right to autonomy involves a willingness not to interfere with actions toward goals that are not one's own. It involves recognition of the fact that a patient's purposes cannot be abridged on the grounds that the patient or his purposes are different from some personal or societal norm. A nurse has no right to attempt to frustrate a patient's purposes, no matter how much they differ from or clash with her own. Nor does any health care professional have a right to enforce or interfere with an obligation that a patient has chosen for himself.

Dilemma 4.1

Mabel has been diagnosed with cancer of the liver. She is 3 months pregnant with her first child. She and her husband, Mark, have been trying for a long time to have a child. Mabel's physician tells them that in order to treat her effectively, he will need to use radiation and chemotherapy. This will cause severe defects in the child, or more likely, an abortion. The physician recommends that treatment begin before the baby's due date. He suggests aborting the fetus and starting immediately. In his opinion, to wait until delivery would be detrimental, perhaps fatal to Mabel. But Mabel wants to wait until the child is delivered. How can her nurse, Sharen, best help Mabel?

The notion of an enforced obligation that a patient has to herself is ethically unintelligible. Health care professionals are not, nor ought they be, enforcers of anything. A patient's autonomy is recognized through the recognition of his right to decide for himself.

A patient does not make a choice or decision in a vacuum. However, it is the health care professional's responsibility to remove as much coercion or undue influence as possible. With Mabel's life at stake, indirection is not undue influence.

> A patient does not make a choice or decision in a vacuum. However, it is the health care professional's responsibility to remove as much coercion or undue influence as possible.

Freedom

Freedom as a bioethical standard is self-directedness — an agent's capacity and consequent right to take long-term actions based on the agent's own values and motivations.

The standard of freedom involves an extended sequence of events, especially a sequence extended over a lifetime. One can possess freedom without making a long-term agreement, but one cannot make a long-term agreement without possessing freedom.

> Freedom as a bioethical standard is self-directedness — an agent's capacity and consequent right to take long-term actions based on the agent's own values and motivations.

Susan is walking down the street. Suddenly she is confronted by college posters and placards on the one side and Air Force posters and placards on the other. She stops to contemplate them. She believed that she had made her decision, but again she finds that she is unsure. So far, Susan is passive. The posters and placards are, so to speak, coming out and influencing Susan. Susan is taking no external action in relation to them. In the context of this experience, she remains passive.

Susan exercises her capacity for freedom and decides to enroll in college. She enters the admission's office and talks with a secretary there. She decides to fill out an application for admission. In these experiences, Susan is active. She has become an agent taking action toward a long-term goal.

Susan might very well have decided not to enroll in college. This would also have been an action and exercise of her freedom. But it would have been an exercise of her freedom, not involving any agreement with any other person. It would have been a decision involving only an agreement with herself.

Suppose Susan was unable to decide about going to college. Her subsequent actions, including her agreement with the secretary, would never have occurred. She would have been passive throughout the whole event. Throughout this entire event, Susan had the power and right to exercise agency or to refrain from engaging in positive action.

Without the power and right to make a voluntary choice, there can be no "meeting of the minds." But she did have this power and right.

Without a meeting of the minds, there can be no agreement. Without agreement, there can be no ethical interaction. Freedom is presupposed in any decision involving action with long-term consequences.

Dilemma 4.2

Edgar has been in the hospital for almost 12 weeks. His prognosis is very poor, but the family remains insistent on the patient's remaining a full code, despite the physician's opinions on the poor prognosis and his present and future quality of life. Edgar has multiple medical problems, including metastatic cancer. He has been heard to say on a number of occasions, "I do not want to live." He now is semicomatose and cannot make his wants known. The family remains unrealistically optimistic.

When one person refuses to respect the rights of another, a meeting of the minds between them is impossible. The conflict between them leaves no room for an agreement. In the absence of an agreement, there is no basis between them for trust and ethically guided interaction.

The Interweaving of Autonomy and Freedom

An agent possesses freedom in two senses:

1. In a biological sense, every agent possesses freedom in that he has the potential for taking independent actions determining the future course of his life.
2. In an ethical sense, every agent possesses freedom since there is nothing in human nature to justify one agent's right to interfere with the independent action of another. Whatever rights an individual possesses, he possesses by virtue of his human nature.

Every ethical agent possesses an identical human nature. Therefore, every ethical agent possesses identical rights. That one human is more human than another and, by this fact, possessed of "superior" rights is an absurdity. It is the same type of absurdity the pigs in George Orwell's *Animal Farm* (1945) were guilty of when they declared that, "Some animals are more equal than others."

All ethical agents possess freedom equal to that of all other ethical agents and nothing more. An agent's existential freedom is enormously increased by her possession of rights. But it is limited by the fact that others also possess rights. Ethically, no agent has a right to violate the rights of others. In complaining against fraud or coercion, she assumes rights for herself. In assuming rights for herself, she assumes that others also possess rights (Gewirth, 1978).

Autonomy accrues to a patient by virtue of the fact that he has the power to pursue goals peculiar to his own unique desires. Freedom accrues to a patient by virtue of the fact that reasoning agents can and must plan and take actions directed toward future goals.

> Ethically, no agent has a right to violate the rights of others.

One implication of freedom is the doctrine that nothing should be done to a patient without the patient's consent. It is a direct implication of the standard of autonomy.

Autonomy permits a patient to be what he is. Freedom permits him to act for that which he perceives as his own benefit—to act on what he is. Under the standard of freedom, one may not interfere with a patient's purposes. One may not compel a patient to act, or to submit to the actions of others, against his will.

Freedom is established by the very same line of reasoning as autonomy. To violate the standard of freedom is to violate the nature of an agent. It is particularly incongruous in a biomedical setting. The whole purpose of a biomedical setting is to enable a patient to regain agency, not to assist him in losing it. To work for a patient's agency, and, at the same time, to violate it reveals a contradiction in one's actions. There is no such thing as an ethically justifiable contradiction. The agreement does not call for a patient to deliver whatever power of agency he possesses to a health care professional. A person's right to freedom is his right to the privacy of his will.

Suppose someone wrote a biography of Paul McCartney. Someone else wrote a biography of John Lennon. A third biographer wrote about the life of George Harrison, and a fourth, the life of Ringo Starr. Suppose further that each biography discussed the life of its subject without ever mentioning the existence of the other three. These biographies would miss that which was of historic significance in the life of the Beatles. None would be a complete, or even a relevant, account of the life of its subject.

> The whole purpose of a biomedical setting is to enable a patient to regain agency, not to assist him in losing it.

The case is very much the same with autonomy and freedom. Neither can be understood without the other. They are intrinsically intertwined.

That an agent is autonomous, that he possesses desires, values, and purposes peculiar to himself, is the sole reason he requires a right to freedom. It is the reason why rational agents implicitly agree to respect these rights. At the same time, that an agent has a right to freedom means that he has a right to autonomy. Freedom is the freedom to take unique and independent actions.

> A person's right to freedom is his right to the privacy of his will.

One can develop one's autonomy only if one enjoys the freedom provided by rights. Rights allows one to plan in terms of a lifetime. Rights allows one to relate oneself to reality abstractly, objectively, and proactively. One can devote one's time and effort to self-controlled actions if one need not be reactive. One can strive for growth and flourishing only if survival is not one's only concern. One can enjoy the advantages of fidelity if agents exercise goodwill. Rights turns aggression and coercion inside out, and produces a demand for "voluntary consent, objectively gained."

> That an agent is autonomous, that he possesses desires, values, and purposes peculiar to himself, is the sole reason he requires a right to freedom.

Freedom as a Precondition of Agreement

Whenever two people reach an agreement, each implicitly assumes that the other possesses freedom—the power and the right to act toward his own goals, guided by his own awareness. This is a necessary precondition and a principle of their agreement.

> If there was no nurse–patient agreement, there would be no nurse–patient relationship. If there was no nurse–patient relationship, the nurse would have no right to take any action whatever in regard to the patient.

If a nurse remembers the necessary preconditions of an agreement, she has a powerful ethical resource. For, in the very nature of health care, every nurse has an agreement with every patient. Freedom is one of the necessary preconditions and principles of the nurse–patient agreement, as it is of every agreement.

A nurse should never forget that a patient has the right to free decision, choice, and action. To forget that a patient rights include this, is to forget that there is a nurse–patient agreement. If there was no nurse–patient agreement, there would be no nurse–patient relationship. If there was no nurse–patient relationship, the nurse would have no right to take any action in regard to the patient.

Dilemma 4.3

A patient exercises his freedom by bringing himself into a health care setting. He comes into the hospital with a cardiac condition. While he is in the health care setting, he becomes quite friendly with his nurse. One day, he swears his nurse to secrecy. Then he informs her of a certain fact regarding his condition. During the course of his treatment, the patient becomes incapable of making a decision. This poses a dilemma for his nurse around the standard of freedom. She has promised to maintain confidentiality in the matter he related to her. But the information the patient gave her is now needed by the physician to treat him effectively. What does she do?

Objectivity

As an intellectual capacity, objectivity is a person's ability to be aware of things as they are in themselves apart from his awareness and evaluations. As a physical capacity, objectivity is a person's ability to act on this awareness.

As a bioethical standard, objectivity is a nurse's or patient's ability to achieve and sustain the exercise of his objective awareness. In relation to the standard of autonomy, it is a patient's right to be supported in the act of exercising and acting on objective awareness.

It is logically impossible to have confidence in an agreement if one cannot have confidence in the understanding of the people making the agreement. For then, one could not achieve certainty concerning the terms or even the existence of an agreement. An uncertain agreement—one in which no one can have any confidence—is, in fact, no agreement at all.

People can understand each other without entering into an agreement. The sun is bright. Paul reports to Marcy that the sun is bright. Paul has brought understanding to Marcy. But no agreement has been entered into between Paul and Marcy.

On the other hand, no one can enter into an agreement unless the parties to the agreement have reached a meeting of the minds. Harry and Bill agree to share the driving on a trip to Fort Lauderdale. Harry does not know how to drive. There cannot be a meeting of the minds. The agreement that Bill assumes to exist really does not exist. One can achieve objective awareness without entering into an agreement. But one cannot enter into an agreement unless one has achieved objective awareness.

> As a bioethical standard, objectivity is a nurse's or patient's ability to achieve and sustain the exercise of his objective awareness.

Long ago, people began to communicate with each other on an abstract level. Early on, some genius of our species noted that, if people are going to communicate and interact on this level, objective awareness is of the highest importance. Without an objective awareness established upon objective facts, no person could trust herself or her own judgment. A fortiori, there could not be trust among humans. Without trust, there cannot be communication and interaction. If people do not communicate with each other objectively, their only recourse will be to give up communication and, therefore, interaction.

All the bioethical standards, in one way or another, involve objectivity. The standard of objectivity requires that a nurse accepts the truth concerning the unique nature of her patient and her patient's inalienable right to direct the course of his life. The standard of freedom implies the need of objective awareness. It also implies an emotional level wherein the ability to act on objective awareness is not undermined.

> All the bioethical standards, in one way or another, involve objectivity.

Dilemma 4.4

Luke is a young man who is dying from a severely debilitating disease. He has been ill for a long time. Betty, a dietitian, is called in as a dietary consult by the physician. The physician wants to begin total parenteral nutrition on this patient to prevent further debilitation. Luke is no longer able to communicate his wishes and he has no immediate family to consult. Betty believes that this method of treatment is inappropriate for a person in Luke's situation. Betty discusses this with Luke's nurse, Flo. What, if anything, should Betty and Flo do in this situation?

Objectivity as the Precondition of Agreement

One person cannot make an agreement with another person unless he rightly expects objectivity from that other person. There cannot be objectivity without a meeting of the minds. Each party to the agreement must have an informed knowledge of its terms. Without this knowledge, a person obviously cannot be party to an agreement. Each party to an agreement must be certain of the terms of the agreement. He can be certain of the terms of the agreement only if he has an assurance that he has access to its objective terms—the terms as they relate to reality. Therefore, objectivity is a standard—an ethical measure of an agreement. As a necessary precondition of an agreement, it is a bioethical principle.

Self-Assertion

The standard of self-assertion involves one event or a very short series of events. Self-assertion as a bioethical standard is the power and right of an agent to control his time and effort. It implies a person's self-governance. As a general rule, freedom is the right to pursue long-term courses of action without being interfered with, self-assertion, in its broadest sense, is the right to control one's time and effort—one's right not to be deceived or coerced into taking or refraining from taking short-term actions.

An agent's self-assertion is his right to determine for himself the meaning and importance of a context. It is also his right to:

- Form purposes.
- Pursue his goals.
- Bring about changes.
- Act from, and on the basis of, his awareness of who he is; his awareness of his autonomy.

Every other ethical agent (and every patient is an ethical agent) has precisely the same rights. This last right does not imply a right to violate the rights of any other ethical agent.

> Self-assertion as a bioethical standard is the power and right of an agent to control his time and effort. It implies a person's self-governance.

> At any specific stage during which one is exercising freedom to pursue a long-term goal, one is also exercising self-assertion.

One can be a self-assertive person and never make agreements. Making an agreement may involve giving up part of one's control of one's time and effort. But the practical benefits of making agreements would not be possible to one who did not possess this right. Many of the benefits of long-term planning, when this involves agreements with others, would be lost to a person who could not control his time and effort. Freedom involves relatively long-term actions. Self-assertion involves relatively short-term actions. At any specific stage during which one is exercising freedom to pursue a long-term goal, one is also exercising self-assertion.

A patient voluntarily gives up a part of his self-assertion to a health care professional. This much is obvious. There is, however, no reason for a health care professional to assume that her patient gives up all right to self-assertion.

Self-assertion, as a standard, is a health care professional's obligation to protect her patient from coerced action or undesired interaction. The whole world does not have a right to determine a patient's actions and nor does an individual. This is also implied by a patient's right to freedom. No one has a right to violate a patient's rights. Nor does any health care professional have a right to violate a third person's rights for the benefit of a patient.

A patient's right to self-assertion is one right that a health care professional ought to be especially careful to protect. A violation of this right involves the unsupportable implication that the patient has no human rights. But the worth and dignity of a health care professional rests in the fact that she deals with those who possess rights and human dignity.

Self-assertion is the virtue that makes a patient's most basic actions possible. It is the source of those actions that a patient can carry to a successful conclusion. Therefore, it is the first action that a nurse ought to reinforce.

Demeaning the status of the patient involves demeaning the status of the health care professional herself. Protecting the self-assertion of a patient is precisely a recognition of his worth and human dignity. Protecting the worth and dignity of the patient is a professional's tribute to her own worth and dignity. "Personal control and autonomy [self-assertion] are powerful components in terms of life satisfaction, survival, and how one defines one's role" (Rice, Beck, & Stevenson, 1997, p. 32). There can be no justification for denying this to a patient.

Dilemma 4.5

Sarah, a 36-year-old, married woman with five young children, was dying of ovarian cancer. Through a philanthropic organization an all-expense-paid trip was arranged for Sarah's family. Sarah and her family were elated. To go on the vacation, Sarah would have to discontinue her treatments. The physician was adamant about her not doing this; saying that without her treatments she would have no chance to live. The treatments left her too weak and sick to travel. Sarah wanted to take the trip, but her oncologist was adamant about her not going, insisting that she would have time for the trip later. Was this an example of paternalism? How should Sarah's situation be resolved? (Hospice of the Bluegrass, 2006)

Self-Assertion as a Precondition of Agreement

Individuals must enjoy some degree of self-control and isolation from one another. Without the freedom from distraction provided by this isolation, an individual could not maintain his integrity or function effectively. Nurses must be sensitive to the many ways that patients seek to gain control of the context of their lives (Volker, Kahn, & Penticuff, 2004).

Everyone has a need for the power of self-assertion. This requires a certain degree of isolation. This isolation is essential for a person's self-awareness. It is also essential for the exercise of a person's freedom. This isolation—this moral defense against coercion—is the value that the standard of self-assertion offers a patient.

To make an agreement with one who lacked the power of self-assertion would be as useless as trying to iron a blouse with an ice cube. Every professional must be, at least implicitly, aware of the power of self-assertion in a patient with whom she makes an agreement. She has no right, thereafter, to act as if she lacked this knowledge.

> He cannot agree to exert effort if he does not own and control his effort.

If a person has no right to self-assertion, then there is no such thing as self-governance. If one has no right to self-governance, he has no right to make an agreement. One cannot make an agreement for the disposition of that which he does not own. He cannot agree to exert effort if he does not own and control his effort. He cannot agree to devote time if he does not own his time. Only a person who has a secure hold on his time and effort, can exercise the virtue of self-assertion. An agreement could not be formed without the exercise of this virtue. Therefore, it is a principle of agreement.

Thought and Action

Actions can suffer from vices:

- The action of inertia—the absence of action where action is called for. Opportunities and responsibilities come and go, but the agent is passive in regard to them.
- Disoriented actions. The agent may anticipate the need for actions to be taken to meet future circumstances. And either these circumstances never arise, which was foreseeable, or he responds to circumstances which do arise without understanding what benefits they offer or what harms are latent in them.
- Compulsive actions—actions taken in response to pent-up nervous energy. The agent's actions provide no possible benefit other than a momentary release of feelings of anxiety.
- Compliant actions—actions spontaneously following any suggestion made by anyone for any reason are essentially flawed. No process of thought and analysis has gone into their motivation. These are vicious actions, that is, passions.
- Actions of an obstinate agent. This brings us full circle—the actions of one who will not be dissuaded from a course of action that is non-productive nor who can be persuaded, or persuade herself, to engage in a course of action that in her context promises to be productive.

There are two virtues that directly involve action and these vices can characterize each of the two. The first type of action is self-assertive action.

Self-assertive action is action taken here and now. The motivation for these actions is benefits chosen by an agent for the here and now. To seek a more comfortable position or location, a more pleasant temperature, conversation, or a period of quiet thought—benefits that are not vital, but of some importance here and now.

The next type of action is long-term action—action made possible by the virtue of freedom. Where self-assertion involves control of time and effort, freedom involves an agent's independent uniqueness, values that are vital to an agent, values beyond the animal level and appropriate to a unique value seeking human being. Through freedom an agent chooses, not momentary comforts, but chooses according to his own motivations, his life plans, and the fulfillment of his autonomy.

> Self-assertive action is action taken here and now. The motivation for these actions is benefits chosen by an agent for the here and now.

Self-assertion and freedom are each, for different functions in the life of a human being, the virtues of a patient's actions. They are also the virtues of a nurse's actions. And finally, of course, they are the virtues of a nurse's actions when she is acting for a patient. But, in regard to her immediate interactions with patients, her most important virtues are the virtues of her self-assertion.

The standards of self-assertion and freedom involve not only physical actions but also mental actions. In a hierarchy of mental, cognitive actions, simpler and more basic actions are actions that come under the standard of self-assertion.

> The standards of self-assertion and freedom involve not only physical actions but also mental actions.

To illustrate the differences between self-assertion and freedom we will step out of the ethical realm into the realm of epistemology—the study of the acquisition and nature of knowledge.

For self-assertion, the process would begin with:

- Awareness of a state of affairs that is congruent or incongruent with one's present knowledge.
- A switch of purposeful attention to this state of affairs.
- Realization of one's uncertainty.
- Attention to the context of knowledge, of the situation, and/or of awareness.
- Analysis and a search for insight into a present dilemma.
- Discovery.
- Insight and the initiation of action.

This is, in effect, the epistemological hierarchy of ethics in the health care setting. For freedom applied to the acquisition of knowledge, the process would begin at attention to the context.

It would then continue with:

- Logical ordering.
- Inclusion and exclusion of variables.
- Choices among alternatives.
- Decisions.
- Establishment of contextual certainty.
- Retention of knowledge.
- Acquisition of further knowledge.

That is, in effect, the epistemological hierarchy of the formation of an ethical system on the part of an ethicist or an individual in the lifetime, trial-and-error task of forming his character.

Beneficence

As to diseases, make a habit of two things — to help, or at least to do no harm. (Hippocrates [460–377 BC], Epidemics, Book I, Sec. XI)

The concept of beneficence refers to the fact that every agent acts to achieve benefits and to avoid harm.

As a bioethical standard, beneficence is the power of an agent, and the necessity he faces, to act to acquire the benefits he desires and the needs his life requires.

In February 1985, [the] New Jersey appellate court ruled that a hospital had the right to dismiss a nurse who refused, for "moral, medical and philosophic" reasons, to administer kidney dialysis treatments to a terminally ill double amputee.

Mrs. Warthen [the nurse] asked to be replaced, arguing that she could not submit the man to dialysis because he was dying and the procedure was causing additional complications. She ... was fired. ... The three-judge appellate panel agreed with the hospital ... (Humphry & Wickett, 1986, p. 122)

> As a bioethical standard, beneficence is the power of an agent, and the necessity he faces, to act to acquire the benefits he desires and the needs his life requires.

Mrs. Warthen was motivated to take her position by her understanding of beneficence and objectivity. Most health care professionals would agree that her stand was beneficent and objective. No doubt the hospital where Mrs. Warthen worked held the value of beneficence in high esteem. But the value of its beneficence was not very influential in this instance. Health care professionals sometimes appeal to a concern for objectivity (reduced to truth-telling) in order to violate the requirements of beneficence. This is one instance of an apparent conflict between the bioethical standards.

Dilemma 4.6

Sixteen-year-old Robin is dying from lupus erythematosus. She is very fearful. Toward the end, she screams, over and over, "Don't let me die!" Robin's parents are called to the hospital, but before they arrive, Robin dies. They ask Robin's nurse if their daughter's death was peaceful. Robin's nurse dutifully relates all the details of Robin's death. Empathy would have made Robin's nurse weak. For Robin's nurse to share the human feelings of Robin's parents might have made her relating the truth unbearably painful. She is strengthened in her duty by apathy. She finds, in the absence of feeling, a sort of strength. If empathy among persons is a virtue, then this context does not call for truth. But if submission to the duty to tell the truth is a virtue, then empathy is a vice. There is no benevolent purpose served by Robin's parents hearing the truth. The consequences of the nurse's truth-telling are entirely evil.

It is conceivable, but not very likely, that a person could act beneficently without making agreements. Under most circumstances, it is inconceivable that people without a sense of beneficence would make agreements. Under no circumstances should we make an agreement with this person. What possible purpose could be served by making an agreement with someone who had no intention of helping us to attain a benefit that we desire.

Once a nurse's analysis has progressed from the stage of self-assertion to the stage of beneficence (benefit seeking), the time has come for a nurse to reinforce, through praise and gentle assistance, his efforts to achieve benefits. All along, the attitude of a nurse toward a patient's objective judgment should reinforce the patient's objective judgment. When a nurse develops a close relationship with a patient, she can greatly benefit him by reinforcing his long-term plans—his freedom.

Beneficence is, among other things, a quality of actions. It characterizes actions that are motivated by benevolence. Benevolence is a frame of mind. It is a consistent attitude of goodwill toward another or toward oneself. Beneficence is the practice of acting on the prompting of goodwill—the desire to benefit one with whom one empathizes.

Patients do not always find beneficence in a health care setting. The situation is far from perfect today. It is infinitely better than it once was. But it is cyclic and it is slipping backward. Conditions during her time led Florence Nightingale (1991) to declare that it is strange but necessary to enunciate as the very first requirement in a hospital that it should do the sick no harm. Nightingale was right. Whatever becomes fashionable, beneficence is, of necessity, an integral part of the nurse–patient agreement. A beneficent nurse acts with empathy for her patient—and without resentment or malice.

Although a patient, on entering a hospital, makes a commitment to let the hospital function as a hospital, a patient has an absolute right to decline treatment or any form of abuse. "To force a patient to undergo treatment against his or her wishes . . . constitutes both a violation of autonomy, and the infliction of harm.

> A beneficent nurse acts with empathy for her patient—and without resentment or malice.

In cases such as these, the autonomous patient determines what constitutes unwarranted suffering" (Fowler & Levine-Ariff, 1987, p. 193). Conflicts can arise concerning the demands of beneficence and the natural function of a health care setting. These are, in fact, the most common bioethical dilemmas. But, in the final analysis, none are genuine dilemmas.

Beneficence as a Precondition of Agreement

Each individual person has a need to achieve good and avoid harm. Beneficence is a bioethical standard (and, more generally, a standard of ethical action) because humans are beings who can impede and injure one another. This is proved by the fact that they do impede and injure one another. They can also agree on and exercise beneficence toward one another. This is proved by the fact that they do agree on and exercise beneficence toward one another. The standard of beneficence arises when ethical agents have attained a sufficient degree of rationality to recognize the advantages of acting from benevolence. Beneficence is a precondition and principle of agreement.

Symphonology does not recognize nonmaleficence as a bioethical standard. The reasons are twofold: First, it is implied by beneficence. If one does harm one has failed to act beneficently. If one acts beneficently, ipso facto, one will do no harm. Second, if 150 years after Florence Nightingale, a nurse must be counseled not to bring about harm or other evil consequences, it is futile to offer this person any ethical advice. This nurse has given up her profession and lost her pride and with it her fidelity.

Fidelity

Fidelity, as a bioethical standard, is an individual's faithfulness to his autonomy. For a nurse, fidelity is commitment to the obligation she has accepted in her professional role. A nurse lives her profession through fidelity. Fidelity is commitment to a promise. This is the promise, in her agreement, to honor her agreement with her patient. But a nurse's fidelity is not fidelity to an agreement. It is a commitment to her patient. More precisely, it is fidelity to her patient's life, health, and well-being. "Fidelity also implies an active concern for the well-being of those to whom a commitment exists" (Shirey, 2005, p. 61).

> Fidelity, as a bioethical standard, is an individual's faithfulness to his autonomy. For a nurse, fidelity is commitment to the obligation she has accepted in her professional role.

A nurse has an obligation to attend to her patient in the sense of providing care for him. She also has an obligation to attend to him in the sense of listening to him and counseling him. At the very least, she has an obligation to protect him from preventable harm.

Any person, including a nurse, has a right to speak out to protect any other person, including a patient, from harm. This is an aspect of beneficence. When a nurse "blows the whistle" to protect a patient, she relies on something more central to their agreement than mere benevolence. Whistle blowing is an aspect of fidelity.

For a patient, the demands of fidelity are quite different from those for the nurse. This is because the roles of nurse and patient are very different. A nurse's role, by definition, is much more active than a patient's.

> *If a patient fails to exercise fidelity to the agreement (e.g., if he fails to give the health professional information she needs in order to give him optimum treatment), he makes it impossible for his nurse to act effectively as his agent. Yet, she is unaware that she does not have this information. She is unaware that, to this extent, she is unable to act as the agent of her patient. Some part of her context is intelligible to her. She is able to act more or less effectively in this. But a great deal of her context is not available—and intelligible—to her. This is particularly harmful because she is not aware of this lack of intelligibility in her context.*

This certainly does not mean that a patient has no moral obligation to exercise fidelity. If a nurse is to be the agent of a patient, the patient must cooperate in the exercise of this agency. This is an exercise of his responsibility to be faithful to his life, health, and well-being. Fidelity to himself and to his nurse is simply a recognition of what a nurse is. This includes the avoidance of behavior that makes contradictory demands on her. For example:

- After surgery, a patient expects a nurse to protect him from pneumonia. But he refuses to cough and practice deep breathing postoperatively.
- A patient expects a physical therapist to help him become more mobile after a stroke. But he refuses to go to physical therapy.
- A patient expects a nurse to protect him from injury. But he refuses to get assistance before getting out of bed.

If a patient does not honor the terms implied by his agreement with his nurse, he violates this agreement. Worse still, he violates his own purposes. If a nurse does not honor the terms implied by her agreement with herself, she violates her purposes—she disconnects from her life.

Fidelity always involves an agreement. So, of course, it is not possible to practice fidelity without making agreements. It is also not possible to keep an agreement without practicing fidelity. An agreement made without the anticipation of fidelity is a logical impossibility. An agreement made without the anticipation of fidelity is to ethics what a square circle is to geometry.

However, in expecting fidelity from her patient, a nurse must always bear in mind the incapacities that his condition forces upon him. When she does not receive the cooperation of a patient, she must remember her commitment to her profession. Even when things cannot be done perfectly, she must do the best she can. This is her obligation to her profession, her employer, and to herself.

> An agreement made without the anticipation of fidelity is a logical impossibility.

Fidelity as a Precondition of Agreement

Agreements serve a purpose in human lives. This purpose is the benefit that people gain through cooperation. Through cooperation, ethical agents are able to achieve good and to avoid harm. It contradicts the nature of an agreement, then, that people would form an agreement and, within the confines of that agreement, refuse to do good or at least do no harm to one another.

> Agreements serve a purpose in human lives. This purpose is the benefit that people gain through cooperation.

It is a very easy matter to see that no agreement between two people can be maintained if the standard of fidelity is not maintained. Fidelity is an outgrowth of the recognition of the other standards. To gain the benefits of interaction, individuals must be able to rely on each other. This reliance is made possible by the implicit and explicit understandings upon which their interaction is based. Fidelity is fidelity to these understandings. It is an essential principle of agreement. Agreement would not be possible to imagine without fidelity.

> Fidelity is an outgrowth of the recognition of the other standards.

A denial of the relevance of any of the bioethical standards to the agreement cannot be logically justified. In one way or another, the denial would make a claim that, if it were true, would undermine all possibility of an agreement. To greatly simplify the matter, it is rather like someone declaring, "I don't speak a word of English," where the very fact that this claim is made in English falsifies it.

If a nurse makes an agreement with a patient, she makes an agreement with a being who is autonomous, free, and so forth. If she interacts as if he were not autonomous, free, and so forth, to this extent she violates her agreement. To the extent that she violates her agreement she refuses to act as a nurse. Her agreement and actions contradict each other. This is important. A nurse does not make any new ethical agreement after the nurse–patient agreement. Every ethical agreement is implied in this agreement.

Dilemma 4.7

Martha has bone cancer and is suffering excruciating pain. Treatment has been unsuccessful. She is dying. She is heavily medicated but is still in terrible pain. The question of withdrawing food and fluids has been raised by Debbie, her nurse, who suggests that Martha be allowed to die. This is met with outrage from her colleagues. The only benefit the nurse's colleagues can envision is Martha's sacrifice to "ethical" ideals essentially irrelevant to Martha's situation. If ethical ideals do demand this, it is unfortunate because this idea certainly debases the concept of benevolence.

The Aspects of Fidelity

The first virtue of a nurse, as a nurse, is fidelity to her patient. The first virtue of a patient, as a patient, is fidelity to himself.

The classic virtues—wisdom, courage, reciprocity, integrity, pride, and justice—are not disregarded by bioethics. They are implied by the principle of fidelity to the nurse–patient agreement. Every virtue and every value involves fidelity, and without fidelity, nothing holds together. Fidelity is essential to a professional ethic. The contemporary ethical systems make fidelity impossible.

The virtue of wisdom requires a nurse to counsel and interact with her patient on the basis of a well-grounded knowledge. It calls on her to communicate with her patient. It requires her not to interact with her patient on the basis of unexamined beliefs, a lazy reliance on emotions, self-righteous rationalizations, or an unrealistic opinion of her ethical hunches.

The virtue of courage calls on a nurse to defend her own rights and never to violate the rights of her patient. It requires her to accept her own humanity and the humanity of her patient. It requires her to accept the uniqueness and the independence of the patient whose agent she is. Courage inspires independent action for the benefit of a patient. It is shown in her acceptance of a patient's desire even when this desire is not in line with social mores and customs (McFadden, 1996). "If [a nurse] chooses for her patient, she chooses for her profession.... This decision requires a certain kind of courage—a courage that... is indispensable to the development of a great nurse" (Husted & Husted, 1998, p. 53).

Reciprocity is a spontaneous exchange of values, especially when this practice is sustained over a period of time without any formal arrangements. The factor of surprise creates on both sides the most luxurious of the virtues—gratitude. Gratitude is the virtue that is the capstone of fidelity and all its aspects. The other aspects of fidelity are in different ways forms of reciprocity. As far as we know, it has never been said, but it ought to have been said—so we are going to say it: An ounce of reciprocity is worth a pound of any other aspect of fidelity. When a patient has expectations of the nurse and a nurse tacitly commits to a patient and the patient gives trust to the nurse, this is a stellar example of reciprocity.

> When a patient has expectations of the nurse and a nurse tacitly commits to a patient and the patient gives trust to the nurse, this is a stellar example of reciprocity. The expectations of a patient are a value to a dedicated nurse. If the nurse returns this value with the value of a tacit commitment—expressed in her attitude and in her actions—this begins a process of reciprocity. If the patient responds to his nurse with trust this is the confirmation of reciprocity.

Reciprocity and Self-Interest

The possibilities for establishing a series of reciprocal-like trades perfectly illustrates the ethical nature and location of rational self-interest.

Irrational self-interest: A receives several values from B who hopes to set up a reciprocal relationship with A. A retains the values he has received from B and does not respond in kind. The predictable effect of this will be that no one knowing of A's character will enter in a relationship of reciprocity with him.

Self abandonment: C receives an insignificant value from D. He reciprocates with a very significant value. D continues to send C insignificant values and C continues to send D desirable values in return. The predictable outcome is that C has a substantial number of "trading partners" sending him, what are, in effect, baubles and geegaws. C responds with worthwhile benefits. E sends a value of significant worth to C hoping to set up a reciprocal relationship. C's selfless generosity has impoverished him to the point where he cannot respond to E.

Rational self-interest: F sends a value of significant worth to G. Sometime later G provides something of equal worth. Out of gratitude, F responds to this. Quite soon G responds in kind and a pattern of activity and a relationship of trust is set up between the two. Over time, each is able to provide the other with benefits the other would not have been unable to acquire on his own. The process of reciprocity over time enriches both and each becomes known as a trustworthy trading partner.

F and G were motivated by what they perceive as their self-interest. Their perception was clear and their self-interest was rational. Their fellow townspeople—both those who had abandoned their self-interest and those who practice an irrational form of self-interest—would sit in the town square and try to solve the mystery of how F and G were so successful when they were so purely motivated or so clever and, yet, were not successful.

In a bioethical context, integrity is a synonym for fidelity. Integrity is the name of the virtue that an agent practices when she is faithful to herself, the external world, and the relationship between them. One way of describing this that should make it clear is this: When intelligible causal sequences accurately describe the process from an agent's experience to his belief, to his body of knowledge, to his communication with others, the decision he makes and, finally, to his action, then he is practicing integrity.

Pride, as a virtue, inspires a nurse's commitment to herself to strive for professional excellence—to exercise fidelity toward her patient. Pride becomes a virtue when it motivates a nurse, through an agreement she has made with herself, to do nothing of which she need be ashamed, whatever others might think or do (Husted & Husted, 1999). It arises from the expectation she has of herself that she will not fail to act on her professional agreement, and do this as efficiently—as beneficently—as she can.

Very few health care professionals, as patients, would want to be cared for by someone who took no pride in herself as a professional. If a nurse would not want this for herself, it follows that she ought not offer it to her patients.

The virtue of justice calls on a professional and patient to exchange values—to take meaning from and give meaning to their relationship. This makes justice, in a health care context, a type of friendship.

To be a friend one must know how to suspend voluntarily his own perspective with its attendant needs and interests; he must know how to discover the principle that is the innermost being of the other; he must know how to use this principle to explore the personal world of the other; he must possess the discretion to will his friend's fulfillment without abrogating his friend's self-responsibility; and he must himself be capable of profound self-disclosure. . . . The will to

4.1

Husteds'
Symphonological
Bioethical Decision
Making Model I.

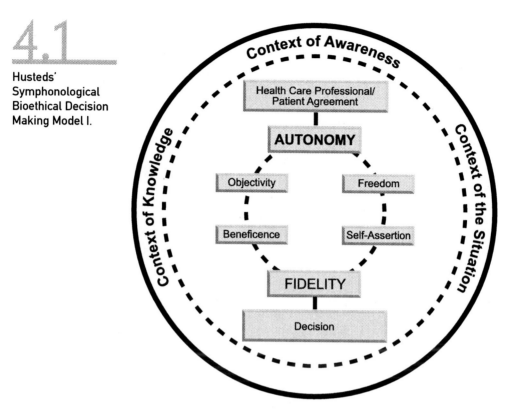

friendship expresses the recognition that one is in oneself not the totality of goodness but rather an aspect—an aspect that in its actualization summons complementary aspects, willing their actualization together with its own. (Norton, 1976, p. 304)

In the context of professional nursing, the principle that Norton speaks of, "the principle that is the innermost being of the other," is a patient's fidelity to his health, well-being, and happiness.

In the matter of the villagers and the coconut from chapter 3, the principle was the needs and desires of each villager. By failing to "suspend voluntarily his own [narrow] perspective with its attendant needs and interests . . . to explore the personal world of the other" each, in being fair to himself and to the other, committed an unseen injustice against himself and the other.

The function of a professional ethic is to move the implicit professional–patient agreement from a necessary formality to a state of mutual trust—as would befit a state of friendship (Figure 4.1). A professional "wills her patient's fulfillment without abrogating his self-responsibility." A patient appropriately responds with some level of gratitude. Gratitude is an incentive to friendship. Friendship is an incentive to achieve understanding, concern, and support. A professional appropriately acts with concern. Without this motivation, one cannot act as a professional. Without concern, one cannot be, in its true sense, a professional. Gratitude is the most reasonable response to friendship and concern. Gratitude is a form of justice and, for nurse and patient alike, the most pleasant of the virtues. A patient's freely given gratitude is health care's Olympic gold medal.

Musings

Whenever an agreement exists between two people, each has expectations and responsibilities as a result of that agreement. This is true of the professional–patient agreement, as it is true of every agreement. It is the expectations of a benefit that she will receive that motivates a person to take on the responsibilities of an agreement.

Every agreement is formed by the human character structures signified by bioethical standards. They are preconditions shaping any agreement. "Just as the bioethical standards are not to be considered as concrete directives, so too, they are not distinct entities. Each standard blends with the others as representative of the unique character of the individual" (Scotto, 2005, p. 591).

It consists in the specific terms of that agreement and a commitment by each party to the agreement that he will be faithful to it. Fidelity to this commitment requires that each be aware of and respect the nature of the other. Without this awareness and respect, there is no reliable interaction. Fidelity to one's awareness is basic to agreement and interaction.

> *Figure 4.1 is meant to be a guide for those using the theory of a practice-based, symphonological ethic. It gives a visual picture of the concepts and their approximate relationships. However, no diagram can convey the meanings, relationships, and use of the theory without an understanding of the theory itself.*

Study Guide

1. Define and discuss all the bioethical standards.
2. Think of ways in which you could assess your patient according to the bioethical standards. What is the meaning of these standards as preconditions?
3. Does the agreement include them all or could one or more be absent and there still be an agreement? Explain.

References

Fowler, M. D. M., & Levine-Ariff, J. (1987). *Ethics at the bedside*. Philadelphia, PA: J. B. Lippincott.

Gewirth, A. (1978). *Reason and morality*. Chicago: The University of Chicago Press.

Hospice of the Bluegrass. (2006). *Sarah: Autonomy and medical paternalism*. Retrieved October 24, 2006, from www.hospicefoundation.org

Humphry, D., & Wickett, A. (1986). *The right to die: Understanding euthanasia*. New York: Harper and Row.

Husted, G. L., & Husted, J. H. (1997). Is cloning moral? *Nursing and Health Care, 18*, 168–169.

Husted, G. L., & Husted, J. H. (1998). The nurse as cynic—etiology and Rx. *Advanced Practice Nursing Quarterly, 4*(3), 51–53.

Husted, J. H., & Husted, G. L. (1999). Agreement: The origin of ethical action. *Critical Care Nursing, 22*(3), 12–18.

McFadden, E. A. (1996). Moral development and reproductive health decisions. *JOGNN, 25,* 507–512.

Nightingale, F. (1991). *As Miss Nightingale said. . . : Florence Nightingale through her sayings: A Victorian perspective.* (M. Baly, Ed.). London: Scutari Press.

Norton, D. L. (1976). *Personal destinies: A philosophy of ethical individualism.* Princeton, NJ: Princeton University Press.

Orwell, G. (1945). *Animal farm.* London: Secker & Warburg.

Rice, V. H., Beck, C., & Stevenson, J. S. (1997). Ethical issues relative to autonomy and personal control in independent and cognitively impaired elders. *Nursing Outlook, 45,* 27–34.

Scotto, C. (2005). Symphonological bioethical theory. In A. M. Tomey & M. R. Alligood (Eds.), *Nursing theorists and their work* (6th ed., pp. 584–601). St Louis, MI: Mosby.

Shirey, M. R. (2005). Ethical climate in nursing practice: The leader's role. *Healthcare Law, Ethics, and Regulation, 7,* 59–67.

Volker, D. L., Kahn, D., & Penticuff, J. H. (2004). Patient control and end-of-life care. Part II: The patient perspective. *Oncology Nursing Forum, 31,* 954–960.

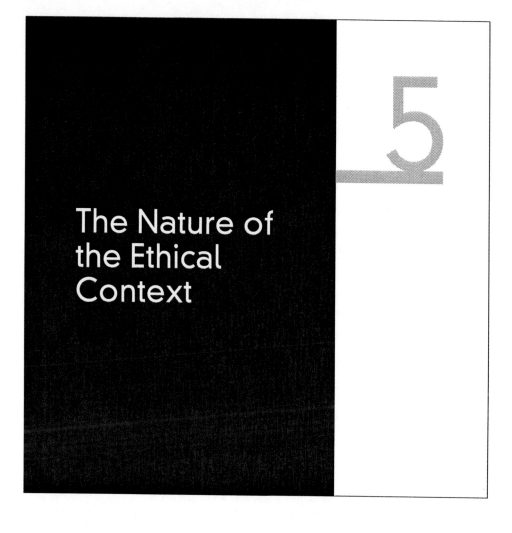

The Nature of
the Ethical
Context

5

Imagine this scene: Your name is Alice. You are the Alice in Lewis Carroll's Wonderland. You work in a kitchen in Wonderland.

The ethic of the kitchen is harsh, badly proportioned, and unjust.

If you drop an egg, and fail to report having dropped it, an unhappy child will go to bed hungry.

So, if you drop an egg and want to prevent a child's unhappiness, you ought to report that you have dropped it.

Last time one of the kitchen workers dropped an egg and reported it, the Queen of Hearts had her beheaded.

You are in a perilous situation—one where you ought to think very carefully before reporting the loss of an egg.

Very seldom is the context of an ethical situation as clear-cut as this. But, in a very basic way, the context is relevant to every ethical decision and action.

If you decide to report the fact that you dropped the egg, this will be an ethical decision. It may make a child very happy. It may also be the last ethical decision you will ever make.

Imagine the character of a child who would be happy about your decision if he or she knew the particulars (the context) of it.

If you decide not to report the fact that you dropped the egg, this will also be an ethical decision. Unlike many ethical decisions, it would be a contextual, well proportioned, and rational decision.

The Scope of the Context

In ethics everything is contextual; and the context of every action is unique and unduplicable, with the result that even a small difference between two situations may yield a difference in our moral verdict. (Hospers, 1972, p. 63)

Driving 55 miles per hour in a 55-mile per hour zone is ordinarily quite justifiable. It is not justifiable if the road is covered with ice. What is and what is not justifiable entirely depends upon the context. If one wants to drive safely from point A to point B, the condition of the road is a central factor one must consider in referring to the context to justify one's speed.

> What is and what is not justifiable entirely depends upon the context.

Dilemma 5.1

Martin is a home health nurse for the Visiting Nurses' Association. He has been caring for Frank for 9 months. Frank has severe chronic obstructive pulmonary disease (COPD). He is rushed into the hospital every 4 to 6 weeks for severe respiratory distress. Frank is a heavy smoker despite his condition. He is also nonadherent in other aspects of his care, such as diet. Martin is considering asking the physician to discontinue home visits since he has been unable to influence Frank's habits. What are the bioethical ramifications of stopping treatment in this case?

The Context of Practice

No noncontextual system is relevant to practice, nor is any noncontextual system objectively justifiable. A decision not justified by the context, one based on assumptions unrelated to the values or genuine well-being of a patient, cannot be an objectively justifiable decision for a specific patient in a specific context (Husted & Husted, 2004). This is equally true in an ethical context as it is in the context of a nursing intervention.

> No noncontextual system is relevant to practice, nor is any noncontextual system objectively justifiable.

If a system is to inspire relevant and justifiable actions, it must be adaptable to the context in which the action is to take place. Ethical actions are justified by reference to ethical purposes, just as nursing actions are justified by reference to nursing purposes. Each is justified by goals that serve life, health, and well-being. The context provides two resources. The first is a cognitive resource—it increases understanding. It reveals what is to be done. The second is an ethical resource. It reveals why this is to be done, if there is anything that needs to be done. Without the context there would be no way of knowing that there is something to be done.

Ethical purposes are justified by reference to a patient's vital, fundamental, and, personal values. A patient's purposes are brought to the situation by the patient.

The interweaving of a patient's purposes, a situation, a nurse's awareness of these purposes and the situation, and her knowledge gained from past experiences forms her context. The facts that are relevant to a purpose—to a nurse's decisions and actions—will be found in the situation. These facts, the considerations found in the context, this knowledge, and the nurse's purposive awareness are interwoven in order to bring the context into existence.

> These facts, the considerations found in the context, this knowledge, and the nurse's purposive awareness are interwoven in order to bring the context into existence.

This concept was suggested to us by Megan Mraz, a PhD student, in our bioethics class in 2007.

By the same token, any change of mind, any "differences in our moral verdict" ought to be traceable to changes in what one has previously identified as part of the context. Unless the new factor can be clearly identified as being contextually relevant, it is certain that the moral verdict has been reached through subjective and whimsical reasons.

Ethical actions are actions taken in the pursuit of vital and fundamental goals. They are actions intended to make an important difference in a person's life. Ethical action involves a purpose and an interplay between a person and a situation. This situation must either offer the person the possibility of achieving some value or it must threaten the loss of some value (Husted & Husted, 1993).

Dilemma 5.2

Mrs. Allison, a 46-year-old Australian woman, was admitted to Outback Hospital in critical condition. On report, Ron, Mrs. Allison's nurse, takes note of the fact that she has gotten worse on the 3–11 shift. He decides to make her the first patient he visits after report. He assesses Mrs. Allison and decides that, in his opinion (he considers himself an expert practitioner), she is extremely critical and needs to have more aggressive treatment done quickly. He is aware that his hospital does not have the means to give her the treatment she needs but that another urban hospital about 30 miles away does.

The policy at Outback is that an attending physician must sign a transfer order. The attending physician cannot be reached. Since Outback is a small, rural hospital, there are no interns or residents and no physicians at the hospital. It is around midnight. Ron would have tried to convince another physician to break policy and sign the transfer order since Mrs. Allison's condition is worsening, but this is not an option. Ron cannot convince anyone in nursing administration to risk going against the policy. What should he do?

The Three Elements of Context

A context is the interweaving of the relevant facts of a situation—the facts that are necessary to act upon to bring about a desired result, an agent's awareness of these facts, and the knowledge an agent has of how to deal most effectively with these facts. A context consists of these three distinct but dynamically interrelated elements.

The context of the situation is the aspects of a situation that are helpful in understanding the situation and to acting effectively in it. The variables that a health care professional finds within her patient's situation form the context of the situation. Every time a health care professional takes on the care of a patient, this action places her in a context. Factors such as the patient's history and physical findings, the physician's diagnosis, the patient's family situation, laboratory results, the emotional state of the patient, and the age and sex of the patient form the context of a health care situation. A nurse deals with this context every time she engages with a patient.

> A context is the interweaving of the relevant facts of a situation—the facts that are necessary to act upon to bring about a desired result, an agent's awareness of these facts, and the knowledge an agent has of how to deal most effectively with these facts.

The interrelations among the patient's medical condition, his individual circumstances, plans for the future, present motivations, and the resources of his character are aspects of his individual situation. How these relate to his fundamental desires, his purposes, and his need to regain a state of agency are part of the context of the ethical situation.

In an ethical context, agency is the power to initiate action and to sustain the actions necessary to successful living. Generally, in any ethical relationship between two people, each functions as an ethical agent. In the relationship between a nurse and her patient, the situation is entirely different. To a greater or lesser extent, a nurse becomes the agent of her patient insofar as he cannot act for himself. She takes on a greater ethical agency and responsibility. She does this until he regains his agency.

The context of knowledge is an agent's preexisting knowledge relevant to the situation.

> The context of knowledge is an agent's preexisting knowledge relevant to the situation.

A nurse brings with her a body of knowledge that enables her to approach each situation appropriately and effectively. This includes knowledge of factors that are usually found in a situation of this type, knowledge of the forms that individual peculiarities might take, and knowledge of factors that serve as clues indicating that this situation may have peculiar twists and turns.

The context of awareness is her present awareness of the relevant aspects of the situation. These are the aspects that are necessary to understanding the situation and to acting effectively in it. The context of her awareness forms a bridge between the situation and the knowledge that enables her to deal effectively with it. The forming of a context of awareness is the purpose of an assessment. A health care professional needs to become aware of the relevant aspects of her patient's situation. She needs this awareness so that she can give care based on a specific patient's actual situation. She uses her knowledge to group and prioritize the relevant aspects (the context) of the situation. In order to formulate an individualized plan of care, a nurse calls on her context of knowledge in order to achieve an objective awareness of the situation.

This is not a nurse's entire context. The context of her awareness also includes awareness of this patient as an ethical being, his virtues (the strength in his character that will help him oppose his disability), and how he relates to the ethical (the vital and fundamental aspects of his life). Her awareness of his ethical relation to himself—the physical, cognitive, and emotional resources he can bring to bear to achieve benefit and avoid harm—forms the contextual ethical knowledge that enables her to effectively interact with her patient.

> The context of awareness is her present awareness of the relevant aspects of the situation. These are the aspects that are necessary to understanding the situation and to acting effectively in it.

To have objective awareness is to bring what is already known to bear on the problem of what needs to be known and what can be known of a situation in order to determine the possibilities for gain and loss in regard to a patient's human values. Solving a problem requires that the elements of the problem be understandable. If they are not understandable, then some way must be found to make them understandable. Facts need to be identified, collected, and sorted in order to be put into a meaningful pattern (Polanyi, 1948).

The Interweaving of Contexts

The context of the situation is a context of discovery. Through the context of the situation, an agent discovers whether something ought to be done, what ought to be done, and for whom it ought to be done. The context of knowledge is a context of justification. Through the context of knowledge, an agent discovers why it should be done and how it should be done. The context of awareness is a context of engagement—when an agent actively enters a dilemma or situation in order to resolve it.

A context is the interweaving of three things: knowledge, situation, and awareness.

An agent's preexisting knowledge is the general knowledge she brings to the situation as opposed to the information she gains from her experience of the specific factors of the situation. Thus, a nurse's recognition of a patient's right to make and act on decisions is part of her preexisting knowledge. Preexisting contextual knowledge is applicable to an ethical context but possessed by an ethical agent prior to her experience of the specific context.

A context is very much like a sweater. All the strands making up a sweater are interwoven. Likewise, all the facts, realities, ideas, and beliefs making up a context are interwoven. The interweaving of a sweater is what keeps the strands together and makes it a sweater. Likewise, the interweaving of the strands of

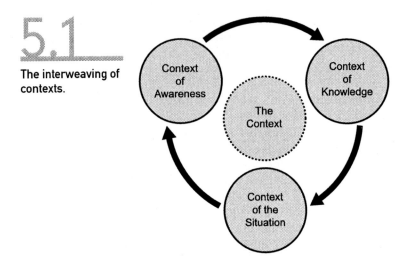

5.1

The interweaving of contexts.

a context is what keeps it together and makes it a context. Efficient ethical decision making requires an interweaving of the context of the situation and the context of knowledge through the context of awareness in a way that leads to an appropriate insight (Figure 5.1).

On any given day, in order for a person to decide whether she ought to wear a coat to go outside, she must have a preexisting context of knowledge. She ought to know, in general, which weather conditions call for a coat. She ought to discover the context of the situation. She must determine what the actual weather conditions are outside at this time. This she does through her context of awareness. It is desirable for her to determine what changes in the weather are in store. Whether she will wear a coat is her dilemma. Knowing what weather conditions, in general, mandate the wearing of a coat is in her context of knowledge. It is that part that she brings to the situation. The weather conditions, as they are outside right now, is the context of this specific situation. Her awareness of these conditions is that part of her knowledge that she acquires directly from the situation. She accomplishes this through the context of her awareness.

Weaving the elements of the context together, the decision would be made like this:

- It is now below 40°F (context of the situation).
- Whenever it is below 40°F, I ought to wear a coat outdoors (context of knowledge; what she brings to the situation).
- Now I ought to wear a coat (context of awareness; what she finds in the situation).

This process of ethical decision making is given in syllogistic form only for the purpose of illustrating it. It is not suggested that ethical analysis ought to be put in syllogistic form. A syllogism, in a real case, may narrow the context to the point where crucially relevant points are left out of consideration leading to a flawed decision.

This decision is based on an interweaving of the context of the situation into the context of the agent's knowledge, by means of the context of awareness. It is a logically justifiable decision.

5.1	Interweaving of the Three Elements of Context
Element	**Description**
The context of the situation.	The situation as it is related to an agent's purposes and actions. Those facts that can assist or hinder her purposes and actions
The context of knowledge (brought to the situation).	The knowledge relevant to a situation that an agent brings to the situation.
The context of awareness (of what is discovered in the situation and her knowledge).	The ideas that form the agent's awareness of the situation. This is awareness of the actions she might take and how the situation will assist or hinder her purposes and actions.

The Context of the Situation

The agent's context of knowledge, including her awareness of relevant principles of judgment, enables her to recognize the context of the situation (Table 5.1). Attention to the aspects of the situation that are relevant to her purposes through the context of her awareness makes it possible for an agent to relate her ethical actions to her ethical purposes.

If an ethical agent were to take actions without reference to the context of the situation, the situation would be irrelevant to her actions. Her actions would also be irrelevant in relation to the situation. Her actions would be unintelligible and purposeless.

For this reason, a discussion of ethical issues in isolation from a context can never lead to a meaningful ethical insight. Issues are, of necessity, disjointed and unrelated to real-life situations or to one another. Outside of the context there is no way to differentiate between the relevant and the irrelevant.

When issues in isolation form a context (rather a pseudo context), the context is sufficient only to lead a nurse to a predetermined conclusion. For this reason, discussions of ethical issues often serve not to strengthen and expand a nurse's knowledge but to harden her prejudices. She is thrown back on the nebulous ethical notions that she has acquired, without analysis, through random cultural influences.

> If an ethical agent were to take actions without reference to the context of the situation, the situation would be irrelevant to her actions.

It is very easy to discuss issues such as organ transplantation, abortion, cloning, euthanasia, the use of fetal tissue, genetic engineering, treatment of anencephalic infants, and human experimentation and come away fundamentally uninfluenced by the discussion and with nothing to apply to a real-life dilemma.

The context of a situation is those aspects of the situation that enable a health care professional to identify its nature—what the situation is and what it is not. The aspects of the situation relate to the purposes of the people acting in it. To act according to the context of the situation means to act with awareness of the human purposes that make the situation important as an object of attention. This requires awareness of the ethical resources that can be brought to bear to serve life, health, and well-being. Purposes produce causal processes, and the stronger the purposes, the stronger the causal processes. The more obvious it is that events are the result of the causal actions of interacting agents and the effects of their actions, the more intelligible the context. The more difficult it is to perceive the purposes that motivate actions and the relationship between causes and effects, the less intelligible the context will be. Overall, strong causal processes make for an intelligible context.

Her awareness of causal processes in the context makes it possible for a professional to guide her actions according to what is implied by the situation in relation to her professional and ethical purposes. Without an awareness of the context of the situation, she has no reason to act and she cannot act on the basis of reason.

The Context of Knowledge

The context of the situation provides a nurse with an awareness that there is something to be done. In conjunction with her knowledge of her patient's purposes, it provides her with an awareness of what is to be done. *Keeping the context* is the state of maintaining an awareness of the factors relevant to her ethical actions and changes in these factors. Keeping the context is the first order of ethical action. The context must shape a person's actions if she is to act effectively.

Keeping the context is the state of maintaining an awareness of the factors relevant to her ethical actions and changes in these factors.

The fact that there is a situation accessible to the purposes of an agent is not enough for the existence of a context. There must be an agent whose knowledge enables her to recognize the nature of the situation. In addition, she must have a desire to act within the situation. She must see it as either requiring action to prevent some undesirable consequence or possessing aspects necessary to the accomplishment of a desirable goal.

In reference to ethical decision making, a context of knowledge is a body of previously acquired knowledge. The value of that knowledge is achieved through a context of the situation and a state of present awareness.

In reference to ethical decision making, a context of knowledge is a body of previously acquired knowledge. The value of that knowledge is achieved through a context of the situation and a state of present awareness.

The Context of Awareness

This awareness (knowledge) on the part of an agent presupposes that she is able to put the relevant aspects of the situation together into an intelligible form. This is what a nurse does, for instance, each time she makes a nursing diagnosis.

For a nurse to maintain awareness of the context of the situation while she is acting requires her to maintain an awareness of the agreements and responsibilities that structure her ethical situation. It also means she needs to maintain an awareness of changes in those contextual factors that must shape her actions if she is to act effectively. A nurse maintaining these attitudes and abilities in relation to the ethical aspects of her practice is holding to the standards of her practice.

An agent's context of awareness includes her awareness of those aspects of the situation that invite action. Her awareness of the possibilities for success in alternative courses of action is also part of her context of awareness. Here awareness of the context is her context of awareness.

> This awareness (knowledge) on the part of an agent presupposes that she is able to put the relevant aspects of the situation together into an intelligible form.

An agent's keeping the context of her knowledge involves an awareness of changes in what is known of changes in her context of knowledge and an awareness of the emergence of new factors that threaten the realization of her purposes that offer new ways of realizing them or that offer new values worthy of pursuit.

> For a nurse to maintain awareness of the context of the situation while she is acting requires her to maintain an awareness of the agreements and responsibilities that structure her ethical situation.

Tina has promised to take a group of chronically ill pediatric patients to the zoo. Her purpose is to share their enjoyment. The children—their desires and their handicaps—form the essential context of the situation. While Tina is preparing for the trip, she discovers that Brucie, the sickest of the children, is scheduled for surgery the next day and will not be able to go on the trip. This change in the situation causes Tina to cancel the trip. She would not enjoy the trip knowing that Brucie could not come with them. She hopes the children would not want to go without Brucie and will be content to wait until later for the trip.

Tina maintained an awareness of the context. This enabled her to be aware of a change in the context and the influence this change had on her purpose. Then, however, Tina discovered another fact in the situation—a fact that changed the context for her again. She discovered that Brucie was afraid of animals and really did not want to go to the zoo. So Tina explained the situation (less than the entire truth) to the children. Brucie was spared an embarrassing moment, and everyone had a wonderful time at the zoo.

Every decision that an agent makes, if she acts in (or according to) the context must be made according to:

- Her knowledge.
- That which is relevant in the situation.
- Her awareness of what is relevant in the situation.

Her knowledge enables her to recognize what is relevant in the situation. That which is relevant in the situation enables her to apply her knowledge. Both enable her to act to accomplish her purposes.

Reasoning To and Reasoning From a Decision

There is a habitual way of thinking that keeps a person from changing her ethical decisions and her actions. This always causes chaos and misery. The worst part is that when we form this habit, we are very seldom aware of adopting it. But many people, too late, have discovered that their personal tragedy was caused by this way of thinking. And many never discover it, especially when it causes a patient's personal tragedy.

This way of thinking involves the difference between reasoning to a decision and reasoning from a decision. If you reason to a decision, you start with objective reality (what is out there in the health care setting), that is, your patient's world. If you reason from a decision, you start from you own subjectivity (from your present unquestioned beliefs) and from your feelings.

Two examples of reasoning to a decision are: "As a nurse, what should my ethical attitude toward my profession be?" and "What can I learn from my patients?" Two examples of reasoning from a decision are: "As a nurse, how am I going to go about forcing my beliefs onto the health care setting?" and "What can my patients learn from me?"

The difference is in where you begin. If you begin with facts out there in the world, you can make a decision based on what you discover out in the world. If you begin with the fact that the efficient practice of your profession calls for a specific and consistent ethical attitude—and that it is your task to create it—you will be reasoning from the objective facts to a decision. This is beginning from an objective perspective.

If you begin with your feelings, or the way things seem to you, or decisions that you made in the past, and you neglect to look at facts here and now, you will be reasoning from a decision that is already made and trying to rationalize that decision. This is beginning from a subjective perspective: "I am indifferent to the ethical foundation of my profession. I will think of excuses on the spur of the moment." The worst part of this is, if you do begin here, you may never get out of the subjective perspective into the realities of your profession.

If you begin and end with what others call to your attention, you will never get to your knowledge, and you will never know anything. If you begin and end with considerations, you will end by integrating what you learn of each ethical dilemma into your present knowledge (Table 5.2).

The Abandoned Context

Imagine that you live on an island. This island is ruled by a disoriented and ill-directed king. The king of the island is passionately interested in increasing the happiness and contentment of his subjects. This poses a serious threat to them. At this time, there are exactly 100 inhabitants on the island. A panel of experts has informed the king that 10 of his subjects are the happiest and most contented 10% on the island. Another 10 are in the 90th percentile, and so on down to the unhappiest and most discontented 10% of the population.

The king reasons that without this unhappiest 10% of the population, the society he rules would be happier. Accordingly, the king has the 10 least happy citizens of his island kingdom drowned.

5.2 Aspects of Consideration

Aspects	Descriptions
Purposes	The end the agent intends to bring about.
Context	Those facts that will assist or conflict with their purposes.
Situation	Facts in the physical world and the knowledge of the other agent(s).
Awareness	The facts of the situation of which the agent are aware.
Knowledge	Relevant knowledge brought to the situation.
Causal progression	The present force and direction of events.

Now, assuming you were not one of the unhappy 10, let us continue. When this statistically unhappy 10% is disposed of, the island society, on a mathematical basis, is about 5.5% happier and more content. At the same time, you will notice, your mood is entirely unchanged. It is the same with everyone on the island. Not one individual is happier or more content by an eyelash. A disinterested observer might discover a number of flaws in the king's decision-making process:

1. A context can enable a person to begin to solve an ethical dilemma. It cannot, by itself, serve to solve the dilemma. The king assumed that the dilemma, in effect, solved itself. He applied no ethical analysis to the context. He simply observed the context and applied a mathematical equation.

2. The king was not aware of the difference between the nature of a group of 100 women and men and the nature of a single individual woman or man. This is the central reason why he failed to solve the dilemma he perceived. He failed to maintain, or possess, a context of knowledge. Before a person becomes a king— or an ethical agent—he should know the difference between a percentage and a person. The king did not maintain an awareness of the difference between concrete realities (the individual women and men who lived on the island) and mental abstractions (the percentages studied by his panel of experts).

3. He failed to maintain the context of the situation. If there are two people on an island and one dies, the sum of his happiness will not accrue to the other. His death may very well diminish the happiness of the other. What holds true of two people, in this context, holds true of a hundred. The king's action was entirely irrational. In order to maintain the context, a person must differentiate between the rational and the irrational. The king did not.

4. The king did not maintain an awareness of simple causal factors. There are values that make people happy and content, and losses that make them unhappy and discontent. Other people on the island had died without their deaths influencing the happiness or unhappiness of the entire citizenry. There is nothing in the nature of individual people or happiness or death such that the death of the unhappy increases the happiness of the living.

5. The king kept himself unaware of the nature of a fundamental, interpersonal, ethical concept. He maintained an unawareness of the rights of his subjects. The right, for instance, to act for one's survival or to strive for one's

happiness cannot be the rights of a percentage. All rights are the rights of individuals.

The king kept himself unaware of the fact that rights accrue to people because of their human nature. The belief that a person loses his right to life when he becomes unhappy is absurd. There is nothing in the nature of individual people, of rights, or of happiness to justify this belief.

The king would not have made a good biomedical professional. For him, 100 people as a group is a reality no different from an individual man or woman. No one who cannot differentiate between an individual and a group can make a good king or a good biomedical professional.

> Ethics, and especially bioethics, has to do with individuals.

Ethics, and especially bioethics, has to do with individuals. The context is interpersonal and individual—a context involving interacting individuals. It is not a solitary context. But neither is it a group or a statistical context.

Dilemma 5.3

A John Doe came in with a massive subdural hematoma. He had surgery and was not doing well. The police helped to identify him but were unable to locate next of kin. The following night, he progressed to brain death. Donor network was notified per protocol. The patient could not express his wishes and there was no family, not even a friend or girlfriend, to tell the team what he would want. In the morning the donor coordinator had a meeting with the MDs and the hospital attorney to document that everything had been done to try to locate his family and that the patient was an excellent candidate for organ donation. They proceeded to take him to the OR and harvest his organs. Were there any rights violations involved in doing this? (Personal communication from a graduate nursing student, 2006).

Ethical Individualism and the Law

Every patient who enters the health care system, concerned for his survival and well-being, enters as an ethical individualist. Many lawsuits have originated over the failure of the health care system to recognize this. Virtually every law that relates to these issues sanctions the patient's ethical individualism. The law recognizes (among other things):

> Every patient who enters the health care system, concerned for his survival and well-being, enters as an ethical individualist.

- A patient's legal right to give an informed consent. No one has a legal right to treat a patient without his consent. No one has a legal right to obtain a patient's consent without the patient's knowing to what he is giving his consent.
- A patient's legal right to refuse treatment.
- A patient's legal right, postmortem, to be protected against the "harvesting" of organs.

- The legal right of children to medical attention regardless of the wishes of their parents.
- A patient's legal right to confidentiality.
- An individual's legal right to refuse to donate organs (e.g., bone marrow) to a relative.
- A patient's legal right not to participate in research against his wishes.
- A patient's legal right to be protected against malpractice or wrongful death.

This is not to suggest that ethical individualism is desirable and proper because it is sanctioned by the law. Individual rights are not produced by law. Rather, laws are purposeless and unintelligible if they are not derived from individual rights (Guido, 2006). Contemporary medical law is desirable and proper because it is sanctioned by ethical individualism.

Each of these rights had to be recognized as an ethical right before it was enacted as a legal right. At the same time, the legal system is not always consistent.

Dilemma 5.4

Harold has a gangrenous leg. Harold's physician wants to perform an amputation in order to save Harold's life. Harold refuses the surgery. His physician tells him, "No one could possibly want this." She gets a court order declaring Harold incompetent. The court order permits her to perform the surgery. Harold's physician tells herself that she has acted benevolently. Has she?

The Necessary, the Sufficient, and the Ethical

Let us pause to examine a crucial aspect of ethical reality through a thought experiment.

Your son shows the symptoms of a physical disorder leading you to take him to a pediatrician. The pediatrician examines him and tells you, "Your son will have to have a nephrectomy." Stunned, you leave the pediatrician's office and stop in a nearby coffee shop. In a few moments, the pediatrician comes in and you beckon him over. A remarkable conversation takes place.

> Each of these rights had to be recognized as an ethical right before it was enacted as a legal right. At the same time, the legal system is not always consistent.

You ask the pediatrician, "If my son undergoes a nephrectomy, will this be sufficient for his recovery?" The pediatrician replies, "No, in all honesty, I cannot say that the operation alone will bring about his recovery. The operation, in itself, will not be sufficient to bring your son back to good health."

You continue to question the pediatrician by asking him, "Is this operation a necessary part of my son's recovery? Would it be possible to bring him back to health without the operation?" The pediatrician replies, "Well, yes. There are other ways to treat him that will bring about an optimum recovery. The nephrectomy is not a necessary mode of treatment. In fact, the nephrectomy is neither sufficient in itself to return your son to health, nor is it necessary for his recovery."

You smile and rise. You express your pleasure at having met the pediatrician. You turn, breathe a sigh of relief, herd your son through the door, and, needless to say, you never visit this pediatrician again.

If one thing is neither necessary nor sufficient to bring about a second thing, it has no significant causal relation to the second thing (Mill, 1843). If a nephrectomy is neither necessary nor sufficient to the recovery of your son, it is entirely useless and irrelevant in relation to your son's treatment and recovery.

Let us examine how the necessary and the sufficient plays out in bioethics.

If an ethical approach provides what is necessary and an agent wants to succeed at ethical interaction, then she should follow this approach. It is necessary to her ethical action, which means that her ethical interactions cannot succeed without it.

If it is sufficient, it is more desirable (it alone will bring about the desired outcome). It includes all that is necessary, so the necessary is no longer a relevant consideration. It is superior to any other way of directing her actions, therefore, she ought to adopt it in preference to a different approach.

If it is both necessary and sufficient then, by all means, an agent ought to adopt it. Since it is necessary, she cannot succeed without it. Since it is sufficient, nothing else is necessary. If an ethical approach is neither necessary nor sufficient, if it will not enable an agent to succeed at ethical interaction, and whether or not her ethical interaction can succeed without it, it is of no use to her. There is no reason for her to adopt it.

Dilemma 5.5

Cal and Art are homosexual partners and have been living together for 10 years. Cal is in the final stages of AIDS. He has not made out a living will or durable power of attorney for health care. The family has said that they want everything possible done to keep him alive. Cal is now in a coma and cannot speak for himself. Art has told the physician and the family that this is not what Cal wanted. He told Art that he did not want heroic measures at the end. The family will not listen to Art and are trying to forbid him to come into the room. What is necessary and what is sufficient to make a justifiable ethical decision in this context?

The Bioethical Categories

I am a man. Nothing human is alien to me. (Terence, 163 BC, Heauton Timo-roumenos (The Self Tormentor), Act I.)

Under most circumstances it is impossible to attain perfect certainty. However, in order to justify her decisions and actions, a nurse must attain at least

5.3 The Bioethical Categories

Doing the Right Thing	How to Do the Right Thing
At the right time:	When it is known to be the right thing and when the action will be most effective.
For the right reason:	With the knowledge of why this is the right thing to do.
In the right way:	Knowing that not only is it the right thing to do but that it is being done in a way designed to produce the greatest foreseeable benefit.
With the right person:	When the person with whom one is interacting is the person one ought to be interacting with and in relation to whom ethical actions can be known to be relevant and appropriate.
To the right extent:	With the appropriate expenditure of time and effort—neither deficiently nor excessively.

one level of certainty. She must attain the certainty that her decisions and actions have relevance to her patient's situation. To deal with the choices she must make, a nurse must develop a sensitivity to what is happening, and she must allow herself to discover that the ideas that pass through her mind are not automatically and infallibly correct: "Any ethical analysis that does not take account of uncertainty will be inadequate to the concrete realities of clinical practice" (Beresford, 1991, p. 9).

It interweaves like this: For Aristotle (McKeon, 1941), every virtue is a form of excellence at a basic function. A virtuous person is one who acts well on the basis of efficient thinking. A virtuous nurse is a nurse who is competent at nursing practice as a result of efficient thinking.

The actions of a competent nurse can be justified, the competence behind them being the standard of their justification. Through the bioethical categories, the nurse's practice can be justified five times over.

The right thing to do is that which one has agreed to do when one has agreed to do that which one's profession consists in and what this implies.

"Context is complex and comprehensive, dynamic, and interactive. Despite how tempting and how much easier it is to resort to the general, the abstract, and the theoretical, any form of bioethics that does not put moral [ethical] problems in their myriad contexts is, in many senses of the word, unreal" (Hoffmaster, 2004, p. 40).

A practice-based ethic must be different: It cannot assume that knowledge of the right thing to do is possible without the supporting knowledge of the other categories (Table 5.3). Without this knowledge of, why, how, with whom, and how far action is to be taken, the right thing to do is isolated, out of context, and uncertain. It is this knowledge that forms knowledge of the right thing to do. And, without this knowledge there is no knowledge of the right thing to do.

Contextual Certainty

While persons seek certainty in their decisions, "... moral [ethical] certainty can provide [unwarranted] comfort for the ethical decision maker...and stifle dialogue and in-depth discussion of the [situation]" (Wurzbach, 1999, p. 287). Wurzbach goes on to say that when nurses "feel" too certain of their decisions, they tend not to question their own beliefs and actions, do not dialogue with themselves, and do not look for possible alternatives to their actions so mistakes can be avoided. They may overlook the possibilities of *gentle coercion*—dialogue with a view to persuade by means of activating a patient's understanding and self-ownership, an appeal to a patient's reasoning power.

The only possible ethical certainty a person can have in a biomedical setting is contextual certainty, which is possible to a limited time and a specific circumstance. Certainty is only possible to the extent that:

- One has relevant facts available as evidence pointing toward a decision—the context of the situation.
- One has relevant knowledge to apply to these facts—a context of knowledge.
- One is presently aware of these facts, and this knowledge—a context of awareness.

An attempt to escape awareness of the situation, to evade one's knowledge, or to escape into the blissful self-righteousness of a contemporary ethical system can replace the effort to understand and to change this. Irrelevance and evasion are not solutions to the problem of certainty.

> The only possible ethical certainty a person can have in a biomedical setting is contextual certainty, which is possible to a limited time and a specific circumstance.

Certainty, like every cognitive state, should be arrived at contextually and objectively. Take the case of a certain state of affairs; we can call it X. Either X is the case or X is not the case. In respect of our knowledge, there are three possibilities:

1. We are certain that X is the case.
2. We are in doubt (uncertain) as to whether X is the case.
3. We are certain that X is not the case.

In order for our state of mind to be objective, it must be shaped by the state of affairs of which we are aware. It cannot be shaped by subjective factors, for example, desires. In order for it to be contextual, the state of mind must be determined by the factors relating to X of which we are aware—all of these factors and nothing but these factors.

If all our objective and contextual knowledge and awareness points to the fact that X is the case, then, in the context of our knowledge and awareness, we are objectively certain that X is the case.

If all our objective and contextual knowledge and awareness points to the fact that X is not the case, then, in the context of our knowledge and awareness, we are objectively certain that X is not the case.

If one part of our knowledge and awareness points to the fact that X is the case and another part points to the fact that X is not the case, then, in the context of our knowledge and awareness, we are objectively and contextually in a state of doubt.

Dilemma 5.6

Mrs. L. had cancer of the throat and needed extensive surgery, radiation, and chemotherapy to possibly cure her. The surgery would require a temporary, and possibly permanent, tracheotomy that the woman adamantly refused. Though the tracheotomy was thought to be a temporary airway solution to get her through the immediate post-op period, it was also needed to lessen or prevent complications resulting with the radiation that would follow. She could not be convinced. This woman was young with school-age children and her husband and surgeon were very concerned about the probable outcomes as a result of her decision. Therefore, they decided to go against Mrs. L.'s wished and perform the tracheotomy. (Personal communication, graduate nursing student, 2007).

Agreement, the Categories, and Justification

If you have a patient, you have an agreement with your patient. This agreement does more than simply establish your relationship. It will also enable you to fix your attention on what is relevant. The agreement is what makes him your patient. It specifies what "being your patient" and "being his nurse" mean. If you keep the agreement you act to do all of these things—all woven together. The agreement answers all the questions.

1. What is the right thing to do?

    The right thing to do is what you have agreed to do. Otherwise you have agreed to do the wrong thing, which is absurd. What you have agreed to do is your responsibility. The responsibility to do what you have agreed to do is the strongest obligation you can possibly have. It is the only responsibility you have. This is your self-evident justification.

2. When is the right time to take action?

    The right time is when action is relevant, and it is relevant when the terms of the agreement call for action. If the agreement did not call for action, it would not be relevant. This is your only way of knowing when you ought to take action. The existence of the agreement justifies the timing of action. This establishes sequentiality.

    However, there is the problem of whether time will be available when the ideal time arises. Time is extended by the practice-based ethic. Dilemmas are analyzed and resolved as they are forming, not after. Crises are avoided. Time, is saved, stress is avoided.

3. What is the right reason for taking actions?

    The reason is that one is a health care professional who has agreed to take these actions. Being a health care professional, acting as the agent of a patient, is doing for the patient what the patient would do for himself if he were able. This defines your profession. This is your reason to take action. It is a perfect justification for taking action. This tends to establish intelligibility.

4. What is the right extent of action?

The right extent is the extent your agreement calls for, given the context; the extent implied by your agreement insofar as you agreement is structured by your patient's needs and your abilities. The agreement is your justification; it is the reason for action. It is the driving force, the "nerve" of what you are doing. This establishes causality.

5. Who is the right person?

The right person is your patient. Who you are as a health care professional is defined in terms of your patient. As a health care professional, your first responsibility is to your patient—to do what you have agreed to do. And your professional agreement, all things being equal, is with your patient. This is the reason-for-being of your profession.

6. What is the right way to take action?

The right way to take action is through actions appropriate to your agreement and the patient with whom you have an agreement.

The right way is shaped by that which is implicit behind the agreement. The right way is the way appropriate to your reading of the character structures of your patient. Your agreement is based on the objective standards that are behind, and implicit in, the agreement. These outline the nature and needs of your patient and, therefore, the proper forms of interaction.

Justification and Purpose

It is logically impossible for a nurse to be able to justify her thinking and yet be blameworthy for her actions. If she has done the best she can, given the context of her knowledge, this is all that can be asked of her.

It is also impossible for a nurse to be praiseworthy for her actions while she is unable to justify the thinking that produced those actions. If the good results that came from her actions were accidental, there is nothing in this for which she can be praised. Both intention and effect are relevant to the quality of an ethical action.

A nurse justifies her actions by describing how these actions would, foreseeably, accomplish an ethical purpose. The purpose that justifies her actions is the subject of the agreement. Along with the purpose, there may also be an agreement on the actions that may or may not be taken.

For a decision or action to be justified, four conditions are necessary:

- The goal of the decision or action must be this predetermined purpose.
- There must be reason to believe that this decision or action will tend to bring about the accomplishment of its purpose.
- It must not be an action prohibited by the agreement.
- It must not be an action that would interfere with actions specified in the agreement.

In a health care setting, the bioethical agreement is an instrument by which both professional and patient can maximize the benefits of their relationship. Without the agreement, there would be no professional criteria on which to base ethical judgments. Each party to the agreement has ethical responsibilities according to the terms of the agreement and only according to these terms.

The nature and terms of the agreement between nurse and patient are usually not made explicit for the participants. However, the terms of this agreement are generally known and accepted.

> *A surgical group was consulted to see a patient with an ascending thoracic aneurysm. One of the older surgeons in the group went to see the patient. As the surgeon was very pleasant and informative, the patient and the family immediately built a rapport with her. Because she was so helpful and inspired such a feeling of trust, the patient and family believed that they could trust her and asked her to perform the surgery. The surgeon agreed. The patient's nurse was very surprised to hear that this particular surgeon was performing the surgery. She knew that this surgeon was semiretired and had not done this type of complicated surgery for many years. Should she give the patient and family this information?*

Agreement and Context

The center of a nurse's ethical context cannot be posterity, the environment, cultural values, or anything but herself and her individual patient. Her professional agreement cannot be with anyone but with her patient. The ethical limits of her professional context lie entirely within her professional agreement.

Without the nurse–patient agreement, no bioethical context would ever arise. The nurse and the patient's situation and interactions would be unintelligible. Only in the context of the agreement do they become intelligible. Only through an agreement does a nursing situation become a context. Only in proportion to the nurse and patient's dedication to the agreement is the nurse–patient situation an intelligible context. A nurse's professional practice is based on this agreement. When her ethical practice is based on this agreement and its practice, her ethical interactions are practice-based. The ideas, attitudes, and motivations of her ethical and her professional practice are in lockstep.

Nursing, as an activity, has a nature entirely its own. It is different from all other types of activity. It is an activity oriented toward specific purposes. It is characterized by specific interpersonal interactions. The nature of these interactions is determined by the nature and purpose of nursing.

Within the interpersonal relationship of nurse and patient there is an interweaving of expectations and commitments. These expectations and commitments shape the nature of the relationship for both nurse and patient. This complex of expectations and commitments between nurse and patient forms an agreement between them. Each agrees to satisfy, to one extent or another, the expectations of the other. Both agree to live up to the commitments each has made to the other. Their agreement is the recognition by each of the expectations and commitments existing between them.

Only in proportion to the nurse and patient's dedication to the agreement is the nurse–patient situation an intelligible context.

This complex of expectations and commitments between nurse and patient forms an agreement between them. Each agrees to satisfy, to one extent or another, the expectations of the other.

Interactions between people must be based on expectations and responsibilities that are known by each. The interweaving of their purposes and obligations forms the agreement that makes their interaction possible. When this agreement is abandoned, there is no pattern to their interactions. Without fidelity and intelligible patterns of interaction between nurse and patient, nursing is not a specific activity. Ethically, and in practice generally, it is nothing but unpredictable episodes of an embarrassing caricature of nursing.

> The interweaving of their purposes and obligations forms the agreement that makes their interaction possible.

Dilemma 5.7

John and Peggy were married for several years and were not able to conceive. They visited a fertility clinic where Peggy was induced to produce several eggs. The eggs were then fertilized with John's sperm and several 8-cell embryos were artificially produced in a glass test tube. Peggy then underwent surgery and was implanted with the embryos five different times. None of the attempts to have a child were successful.

John and Peggy began to have marital problems after a few years. The clinic had frozen 10 of the embryos made by John and Peggy during a happier time in their marriage. Peggy decided to keep the embryos to use in future procedures to try and have a baby. She felt that the embryos were her last chance at being a mother. John, however, decided to never have children with his ex-wife and wished to donate the embryos to research. Who owns the embryos? (The case of the embryos without parents, 2000)

The Self-Creation of the Ego

Context may or may not be the most important topic in ethics. But, no ethical concept is of any use without the concept of context. I was discussing this with my friend Tom. I see him all too seldom. When we get together it is always with our crowd. He lives a long way from town. So, sometimes we communicate by writing.

We were discussing this topic when he asked me about the earliest context I remember forming. Tom has an unbelievable memory. I could not understand how he would know the nature of his earliest context. I could not see how he would know the nature of mine. But something about his attitude suggested that he believed he could. The rest of our crowd began to arrive and Tom promised to write me. Day after day I waited for the letter. Thoughts of the letter became an obsession. I could think of nothing else. I knew that Tom's letter would be momentous. Was he putting a number of early contexts in their temporal order? None of the thoughts I conjured up were a vague echo of Tom's letter. It revealed so much. It is thought provoking. I will share it with you just as it came.

Dear Fellow Reminiscer:

You may not remember, but this is almost exactly the way it happened. It was your very first context. I know that now you are glad you formed it. If you had not we would not be reminiscing like this.

There was nothing. Ok the throbbing. But the throbbing only highlighted the rest of nothing.

When you emerged into the noisy cold, you were overwhelmed by a kaleidoscope of lights, temperatures, aromas, sounds, colors, pressures. . . . This is the "what-is"—the overwhelming, oceanic, noisy, cold. You were not observing it. You were just there, although you did not know it. There was no you to know it. There was just the cold moving noise. You were a neonate surrounded by people for whom the world is meaningful. They were there for your sake—to nurture you. But they were there in a very different way—in context. The contrasting colors and sounds structure a meaningful, intelligible world for those who have achieved the power of awareness and formed a context. They can structure their awareness and form purposes.

For the neonate they do not even produce confusion.

Only an object can produce confusion, and since you were not a fully aware, consciously oriented subject, for you there was no object. For you, there was no "you". That which was there before you, whatever it was, was not even a "something". That which was to become you had no way to experience anything. You had no experience of yourself. There was no yourself. Think of it: You had no suspicion that someone was coming.

You were not conscious—not even of not being conscious. Therefore, there was no basis for a judgment by you that the big cold place was an external reality surrounding an internal reality. You were not a subject who was conscious of objects. This is why it is so hard to remember.

Well, eventually, you started to respond to stimuli from the unbelievable 'Where' you had bumbled into, and events in your organism, hunger, for instance. Gradually you began to identify these responses as responses. You found that there was something else, apart from the stimuli—something being stimulated—something ready to be discovered, something ready to be created. It was the first glimmerings of you—a producer's production of himself. In this way the self-creation of your Ego—your unique and independent Self began. Your 'I'—you—began to respond to this stimuli.

Your 'I' created itself by means of your responses to these responses. Through its responses, your 'I' discovered desire. Through its desire it discovered its powers. It discovered the independence of the world and your dependent isolation through the objects of your consciousness and the actions of your mind. You drew what had previously been your unawareness back onto and into yourself—your Ego. You completed yourself when the action of your mind and its nature became conscious of each other. The action of your mind and its response to the object that is your mind. And the discriminating return of your new found awareness onto the new found external world.

You created your Ego when you discovered it. You created it by discovering it. That which you discovered did not exist before you discovered it.

After your Ego created itself, your final task was to return to the outer world without losing the Self you had created.

In this way you established your existence and its context. This is the first context you were ever in. And you are still in it. When you first entered into it, it was infinity. Then it became much—very much smaller. Then, slowly it began to expand. We never leave this context (as long as we live). We are in numerous contexts at any time. The first context is the background context of every other. We imagine that we enter various contexts from no context. Not so.

In the Self creation of your Ego—that part of you that you know as "I". You formed your very first context.

Warmest congratulations,

Tom.

Musings

Achieving awareness of the context means integrating that which is present in one's awareness of the circumstances into all the relevant knowledge that one possesses. Achieving awareness of the context is a process of assimilating the context of the situation into a context of knowledge. Losing awareness of the context means ignoring relevant items of knowledge or relevant aspects of the situation. Failing to achieve awareness of the context is the worst possible way to begin a decision-making process. Not having awareness of the context makes it impossible to justify a decision or to act effectively.

When a nurse retains awareness of the bioethical context, she and her patient are most apt to gain the maximum benefit of ethical action. Success follows effective action. Effective action follows active awareness.

"The nurse functions both as a professional and as a human being within a variety of contexts. These contexts influence directly or indirectly the way in which the nurse performs caring tasks" (Gastmans, 1998, p.236).

There is a group of facts naturally tending to form a unique and intelligible context when nurse and patient come together. A patient needs a nurse to provide him with the benefit of her professional skills. A nurse needs a patient in order to live her professional role. These facts establish a relationship between them through a meeting of the minds. This meeting is a tacit agreement to interact and has this as its purpose—their interactive self-directedness—the control by each of their time and effort into intelligible causal sequences.

Study Guide

1. Give an example of how you have used context today in making a decision - it may have not been an ethical decision, but context is something we use everyday and throughout our day.
2. Imagine to yourself a health care system devoid of any attention to the context. What would you see? Try to imagine, further, functioning in this system.
3. How do the three elements of the context help to guide you when collecting data on which to make decisions?

4. Explain the difference between the necessary and the sufficient. Give an example of when something could be necessary but not sufficient or when something is sufficient in itself.
5. What is the relationship of the agreement to the context?

References

Beresford, E. B. (1991). Uncertainty and the shaping of medical decision. *Hastings Center Report, 21*(4), 6–11.

The case of the embryos without parents. (2000). *Bioethics Case Study.* Retrieved October 24, 2006, from http://www.mhhe.com/biosci/genbio/olc_linkedcontent/bioethics_cases/g-bioe-04.htm

Gastmans, C. (1998). Challenges to nursing values in a changing nursing environment. *Nursing Ethics, 4,* 236–244.

Guido, G. W. (2006). *Legal and ethical issues in nursing* (4th ed.). Upper Saddle River, NJ: Prentice Hall.

Hoffmaster, B. (2004). 'Real' ethics for 'real' boys: Context and narrative. *The American Journal of Bioethics, 4,* 40–41.

Hospers, J. (1972). *Human conduct: Problems of ethics.* New York: Harcourt Brace Jovanovich.

Husted, J. H., & Husted, G. L. (1993). Personal and impersonal values in bioethical decision making. *Journal of Home Health Care Practice, 4*(4), 49–64.

Husted, G. L., & Husted, J. H. (2004). Nursing ethics. In J. Daly, S. Speedy, D. Jackson, & V. Lambert (Eds.), *Professional nursing: Concepts, issues, and challenges* (pp. 174–191). New York: Springer Publishing Company.

McKeon, R. (Ed.). (1941). *The basic works of Aristotle.* New York: Random House.

Mill, J. S. (1843). *A system of logic.* London: Oxford Press.

Polanyi, M. (1948). *The study of man.* Chicago: The University of Chicago Press.

Wurzbach, M. E. (1999). Acute care nurses' experiences of moral certainty. *Advanced Nursing, 30,* 287–293.

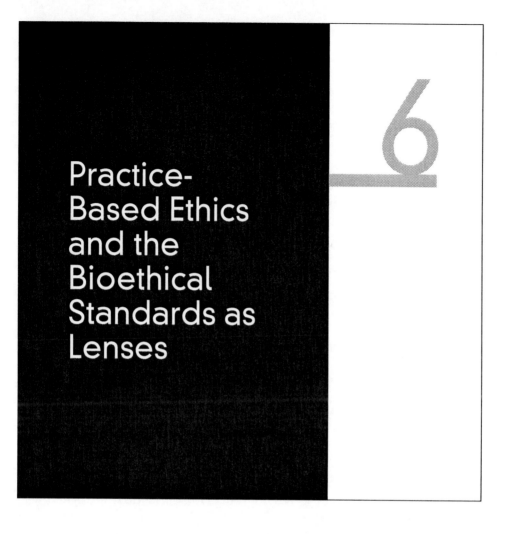

Practice-Based Ethics and the Bioethical Standards as Lenses

6

In the objective relationship between the mind of a person and the reality known by the person, there are three kinds of "things."

- There are "things" in the world outside of the mind that exist whether any mind is aware of them or not.
- There are "things" in the mind that do not exist outside of the mind, but there is still something in the world outside the mind that serves as a foundation to that which is in the mind.
- There are "things" in the mind that have no counterpart in the world outside of the mind.

The first kind of "thing" really exists in the world. This includes such things as this chair, that tree, the gust of wind blowing that newspaper, those hills in the distance, and so on. Whether or not anyone is seeing them or touching them, these things actually exist in the world outside of consciousness.

The second kind of "thing" does not exist out in reality. But something exists out in reality that serves as the basis of this thing existing in the mind. For instance, furniture exists in the mind. Outside of the mind there is no such thing as furniture. But for its own use, the mind observes these four chairs, this table, that sofa, this bookcase and groups them all together according to what they have in common, under the concept "furniture." The chairs, table, sofa, and bookcase all exist in the real world apart from the mind. But, in addition to the chairs, table, and sofa, there is no eighth thing—furniture—existing out in the real world.

The third kind of "thing" exists only in the mind. This includes such things as leprechauns, the tooth fairy, square circles, unicorns, and so on. These things exist in the mind in the sense that they can be imagined. But there are no leprechauns, tooth fairies, square circles, or unicorns in the real world outside of the mind.

Furniture does not exist in reality apart from the mind as do chairs, trees, wind gusts, and hills. But, unlike leprechauns, tooth fairies, square circles, and unicorns, furniture does not exist in the mind without a reference to reality. The existence of furniture in the mind has a foundation in the chairs, tables, sofas, bookcases, and so forth that exist in the real world.

The bioethical standards are not a kind of thing in the world. They are not independently existing realities. Their existence depends on independently existing things. They have a certain kinship to various qualities or properties of things in the world; as colors and shapes are properties of entities, the standards are properties (virtues) of ethical agents.

> The bioethical standards are not a kind of thing in the world. They are not independently existing realities. Their existence depends on independently existing things.

- There is no such thing as autonomy out in the world; there are only autonomous agents. Agents have this in common: They are all unique.
- There is no such thing as freedom out in the world; there are agents who possess or lack freedom.
- There is no such thing as objectivity out in the world apart from knowers who know what is objective.
- There is no such thing as self-assertion out in the world; apart from agents who exercise self-governance.
- There is no such thing as beneficence out in the world; there are only agents who do good and fail to do good.
- There is no such thing as fidelity out in the world; there are only agents who uphold or fail to uphold the terms of their agreements.

The bioethical standards are "things" that exist in the mind and have a foundation in reality. People possess these properties in common, but one by one. Individuals are autonomous. They act freely. They have a need for objectivity, self-assertion, and beneficence. They make agreements, and they are faithful to these agreements. It is these properties of people that keep a biomedical professional's awareness of the bioethical standards tied to reality out in the world—the reality of her patients.

For a biomedical professional to function on an ethical level, there must be something tying her awareness to the people of whom she is aware. This something is the bioethical standards.

Everyone is autonomous. Everyone is free. The standards pertain to everyone — to humans as human.

But, for a biomedical professional to function on an ethical level, there must be something tying her awareness to more than "people." There must be something tying her awareness to her individual patients.

Practice-Based

Through a process of analysis and induction, symphonology, the study of agreements was born. It had nursing practice as its model. It is a practice-based ethical theory in that it was modeled from nursing. It is applicable to practice in any health care setting or with any patient population. It enables the health care professional to make decisions that are contextually justifiable.

If nursing practice is not, in and of itself, unethical; if, in principle, it violates no one's rights and breaks no agreement implied by rights; if it is humanly desirable (that is, its reason-for-being is to benefit human individuals), then it provides excellent criteria for an ethical system. For these are the criteria of an excellent ethical system. No rights violations are built into the nature of nursing practice. The purpose of this practice is to increase the power of patients to take independent actions. It is humanly desirable. It serves human virtues. At its best, it can provide matchless criteria for an ethical system. Symphonology, a practice-based ethical system, is one who's fundamental definitions of *human purpose, benefit, desire, right, good, justifiable,* and so on are the same definitions that guide competent nursing practice. For practice, and for a practice-based ethical system, four things happen simultaneously: the patient becomes a partner in his care, he is recognized as an ethical equal, the nurse becomes his agent, and the context becomes the standard of judgment.

> Through a process of analysis and induction, symphonology, the study of agreements was born. It had nursing practice as its model.

A practice-based system of ethical decision making is a context-based system. It is one that inspires objectively justifiable actions. And, insofar as a system is context-based, it is if the context is fundamental rather than merely superficial, practice-based. Happiness is a long-term value for a practice-based ethics; immediate but lasting success is the goal of ethical action. A bioethic can be context-based on two levels:

> For practice, and for a practice-based ethical system, four things happen simultaneously: the patient becomes a partner in his care, he is recognized as an ethical equal, the nurse becomes his agent, and the context becomes the standard of judgment.

- Insofar as it is a response to the needs that brought the patient into the health care setting.
- Insofar as it is an integral part of professional practice, modeled on professional practice.

Awareness of the ethical situation is the foundation of a relevant practice-based ethic. Unless the causal processes forming the context of the situation

6.1

**Intelligible causal
sequences.**

Unbroken Chain

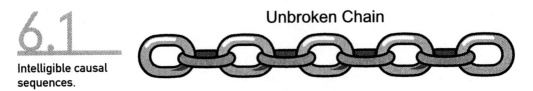

are perceived, no relevant ethical action is possible. Nursing provides the ideal milieu for the perception of these processes.

Through a practice-based ethic, a nurse can attain a very high degree of competence or excellence. A practice-based ethic, like nursing practice itself, is based on agreement. In each case, agreement produces competence.

The aim of clinical practice is to heal, nurture, and strengthen a patient's:

- Ability to control his immediate time and effort.
- Ability to pursue benefits and avoid harms.
- Ability to deal with his circumstances.
- Ability to live his life span successfully.
- Commitment to himself and his life.

These virtues are acquired for the time when he is part of the health care setting and when he leaves.

The aim of a practice-based ethic is the same. These virtues are healed, nurtured, and strengthened inside the health care setting. The aim is to produce intelligible causal sequences (Figure 6.1). The promise of a practice-based ethic is that the intelligible causal sequences that are established in the health care setting can be continued by a patient after discharge and by a nurse throughout her lifetime.

Intelligible means that sequences are open to understanding and capable of being fitted into both the context of immediate awareness and a system of abstract knowledge. *Causal* means that sequences are initiated and controlled by the actions of an agent or directed to an agent's purposes by her time and effort; volitional efforts purposefully link past events and future events. *Sequences* are a series of future events intelligibly and causally linked to a series of past events.

> *Intelligible: You know and he knows what is going on. Causal: You cause and/or he causes what occurs. Sequences: Whatever occurs is intelligible and causally connected.*

The Milieu

The Milieu is the health care arena taken as a learning device. Everything is there to be observed and understood—the nurse as agent, the patient, the values, the actions and direction of the actions, their progress or regress, the foreseeable consequences. All are there to be observed by a nurse and continued or changed.

For many centuries, the heroes and heroines of medicine and nursing, known and unknown, held an ideal in mind and slowly brought it into, at least, partial being. They produced over time the modern health care setting. It is the Milieu. The Milieu is an environment that can be understood best when:

- Events can be predicted.
- Functioning, to a large extent, can be controlled.
- Intelligible causal sequences can be established.

The Milieu can provide guidance and be replicated.

The intelligibility translates into predictability. Causality overcomes the absence of connection. Directed sequences displace unpredictable episodic occurrences. More and more it reveals how it can become possible to control an intelligible progression—in practice and in ethical interaction.

The agent–patient context is, for a nurse, an exemplar to enable her to maintain that which is ideal in the health care arena. It is an ever-present illustration of intelligible causal sequences.

In the evolution of nursing, the next development can be, and ought to be, the establishment of intelligible causal sequences in the activities of a nurse returning her patient to a condition of autonomous optimism and stability—the psychic force of his virtues that are a natural part of his independent uniqueness.

"When a nurse, as an ethical agent, learns how to identify the various parts of an ethical context and their interrelations, she has developed a significant practical skill. When she is able to understand the individual human values that make each context what it is, she has developed a . . . [valuable] skill and competency" (Husted & Husted, 2004, p. 646).

If a machine was invented that could accomplish this and effectively act on this understanding, its value should be immediately recognizable, and it would be worth a very high price. There is, although they are rare, such a machine, but she is not a machine.

The Analytic Process

The bioethical standards as ethical lenses are:

- Human nature.
- A blueprint of the nature of human nature.
- A description of what it is for a patient to experience himself as human.
- Objects of awareness through which each person is able to come to an understanding of the internal state of others.
- Critical indicators of ethical states and of everything of which ethical states are a precondition (e.g., ethical decision/agreement/interaction/justice).
- Basic motivators of ethical agreement and interaction.
- Instruments to evaluate one's ethical decision-making process.
- Principles of human action.

Every bioethical dilemma is, to a greater or lesser extent, unique. There are good reasons for this. Every patient's circumstances are unique. Even more so, every patient is unique. Uniqueness is not threatened by dilemmas but patients are. The ways they are threatened and the ways out of their dilemmas are shaped by uniqueness, thus, the importance of uniqueness.

A health care professional's first task, in order that she might understand her patient's dilemma, is to understand her patient. The direct and relevant way to do this is to study her patient's fundamental virtues—his character structures as described in the bioethical standards. This journey begins with the least complex character structure—self-assertion. Self-assertion, more than any other character structure, is revealed to a health care professional very near to the perceptual level. She can observe it. It requires a minimum of analysis to detect the presence or absence and the nature of her patient's self-assertion. What uncaused actions does he initiate? What predictable changes can be brought about by these actions?

From there, analysis proceeds through the character structures (or virtues) as they become more complex, more abstract—further from the perceptual level and more in need of analysis. Finally, analysis arrives at the virtue that includes or fails to include (thus failing to be a virtue), all the others—the patient's self-created autonomy.

In using the standards as lenses onto the character of another, one proceeds most quickly and efficiently through these steps:

- Self-assertion: The simplest, most basic expression of a patient's individual nature.
- Beneficence: The extent to which his time and effort is self-consciously devoted to the pursuit of benefit and/or the avoidance of harm.

What benefits does he consider worthy of attention? What possible harms occupy his concern? Why, and to what extent, does he consider, rightly or wrongly, changes beneficial or harmful? Why, and to what extent, is he in rhythm with the purposes of the health care setting?

- Objectivity: The degree to which he is in cognitive contact with himself, his thought-processes and motives, plus the clarity and absence of distortion in his cognitive contact with his circumstances.

Do his evaluations and actions reveal that he is in an objective cognitive contact with his context? Are his motives and efforts well or inefficiently directed?

- Freedom: The degree to which he is still engaged with the long-term plans he had before losing his agency.

Self-assertion: The simplest, most basic expression of a patient's individual nature.

It is his ability to perceive and stay in the context of his life before his disability (to the extent that these plans are still feasible), or whether he has abandoned the entirety of his life and shrunk his consciousness down to an exclusive concern with the here and now.

Is he still allied with the life he was living before the onset of disability, or has he joined with his disability and adopted a new life style? Has he redefined his life unnecessarily?

> ▓ Fidelity: The degree to which he is concerned for the needs of his life, health, and well-being; the extent to which he is faithful to who he is; if he is still the autonomous person he was.

Does he know himself as well now, after the onset of his disability, as he did before he became disabled? Do his actions and his lifestyle still reflect who he is, or do they reflect the power of external forces working through him? Does he still have an interest in the values he held before the onset of his disability?

> ▓ Autonomy: The extent to which he has retained his independent uniqueness by keeping his virtues interwoven and in rhythm.

Autonomy is remarkably complex. But it is the goal one ought to keep in mind when moving through the process of analysis from self-assertion to fidelity. Even if a health care professional never gets beyond the point where she can foresee how her patient will, generally, exercise his time and effort in action, his self assertion, her understanding of her patient will already be above average.

Nurture

That which is personally advantageous for a nurse is to nurture—as she was motivated to do when she made the agreement with herself that she would become a nurse. Odds are, when she made this agreement with herself, it was a decision to be an excellent nurse and to nurse virtuously (effectively).

The development of her virtues, if she makes this her goal, is, at the same time, the realization of her rational self-interest. If her agreement with herself was to be a nurse and to nurse virtuously (i.e., excellently), then she ought to do this primarily for her own sake and her own benefit. In this way, the motivations of her actions will provide the maximum benefit for herself and for her patient. These will be two effects of the same motivation.

Quite obviously, given the nature of the biomedical professions, every professional action is, fundamentally, an interaction. Her excellence and success, therefore, depend not only on herself but also on her patient. The power of her interaction is, to some extent, dependent on the power of her patient's response. In order to maximize the efficiency of her virtues, she must be capable of strengthening her patient's virtues. The excellence of interaction depends upon the virtues of those who interact.

> If her agreement with herself was to be a nurse and to nurse virtuously (i.e., excellently), then she ought to do this primarily for her own sake and her own benefit.

Her action, in strengthening her patient's virtues, at the same time enables her patient to realize his rational self-interest, which was his motive for coming into the health care system.

For her to interact optimally, her patient must be capable of responding. In order to perfect her professional virtues, her power to act well and successfully, she must be capable of increasing the strength of his ability and willingness to act well and successfully. This can be achieved through attention to her patient's character. It can be achieved most efficiently through attention to his individual virtues—through attention to the bioethical standards.

So, as she is analyzing him through his virtues, she can, at the same time nurture and strengthen his virtues and her own.

A Different Door

> Myself when young did eagerly frequent
> Doctor and Saint, and heard great argument
> About it and about, but evermore,
> Came out by the same door wherein I went. (Rubáiyát of Omar Khayyám)

The experience that Khayyám describes is quite common for students of ethics. They never get across the room. They "[come] out by the same door wherein [they] went." They hear "great argument" concerning the nobility of this or the glory of that, and when the first joy of learning has past, they realize that they have learned nothing related to their lives or intentions. If they do not become aware of this, they are worse off.

Sometimes, there is an ethical dilemma of which one may be unaware. If you have ever been a patient, you can understand this because as a patient you know that the health care professional is not aware of all the things with which you are dealing. But, as you gain an understanding of your patient, and you act from this understanding, you may very well resolve a dilemma without even being aware of the fact that a dilemma existed. This is much better than not being aware of it, not acting on it, and failing what you might have done for your patient—failing to do for him what he would have done for himself—and failing to do for him what you would have done for yourself.

In either case, whether a dilemma arises, it is desirable that you understand as much as you can about the patient under your care. We cannot know the mind of another person directly. Here again, the bioethical standards come in. They come in as lenses onto the psychology of your patient. Using the bioethical standards as lenses enables you to see and understand other people. They enable you to see your patient as an autonomous person.

The uses of the bioethical standards are manifold. Insofar as they are used as lenses onto the character of an ethical agent, they reveal:

- Interactions between the character structures.
- Weaknesses and strengths of an agent's character.
- Reliability of an agent's actions.
- Objects of implicit awareness through which each agent is able to communicate without understanding the internal thoughts of others.

- Virtues, or that which makes possible the virtue, of an ethical agent.
- The resources that make possible the enjoyment of life.
- The objectivity of one's awareness that enable one to enter an ethical relationship.
- The limitations on what can be agreed to in the agreement.

Understanding

Understanding the nature of another person can be compared with understanding something like a piece of hard cherry candy. How does a child first come to understand the nature of a piece of cherry candy? First, he sees an opaque redness. Then he can smell the cherry aroma of the piece of candy. He can feel its firm roundness; tap it on the table and hear its hardness. He can then taste its cherry sweetness. And now he knows the nature of a piece of cherry candy. You can understand a piece of cherry candy on a sensory level: You smell it and you taste it.

One cannot understand a person on a sensory level, not by looking at him or even by listening to him. But one can understand him, in the same way one can understand that piece of cherry candy. One can come to understand him by discovering the characteristics that make him what or who he is. The characteristics that make a person who he is cannot be grasped on a sensory level. But they can be grasped through the bioethical standards acting as lenses.

Your patient is a unique individual and, to be understood, must be understood as a unique individual. All too often, a health professional looks on her patient globally as a homogeneous and undifferentiated living organism—more or less like herself. She understands herself inadequately and only with great difficulty. Therefore, in the short time she has, she finds it nearly impossible to understand her patient. But the person that is her patient can be understood as a living, thinking organism characterized by a high degree of autonomy, that is, uniqueness.

If you see your patient as an alien mass, not surprisingly, you will not understand him. If you discover him as structured by the virtues characterized in the bioethical standards and you are open to the character structures that make him who he is, you will find it remarkable how efficiently you can understand your patient.

As she engages in the nurturing process, a nurse must examine the principles that structure and motivate a patient. This is an essential, defining part of a nurturing process. In order to do this, one who would nurture must gain an understanding of the principles involved. The most effective way to come to understand these principles is to study them in those whom one is nurturing. One nurtures these principles in one's patient. This is the art of one's profession.

Here the bioethical standards serve as lenses. They come in as principles explaining your patient's motivations. Ethical interactions with a patient are interactions with a patient's motivations. They also come in as lenses onto the general psychology of a patient. Using the bioethical standards as lenses enables you to see and understand other people. They enable you to see your patient as an individual person.

Dilemma 6.1

Bonnie is a 17-year-old teenager who has had 2 years of extensive treatment of a particularly difficult form of leukemia. She has had a bone marrow transplant, chemotherapy, and virtually all options for treatment. Through all of her treatments, improvements, and relapses Bonnie has kept in touch with two very close friends. At her last admission to a regional cancer treatment center the family was told there were no further options and Bonnie would not live more than, at most, a few weeks or months.

She is now at home, very weak, needing almost constant care. She still shows a lively interest in what is occurring, she seems to find humor in little things, and she constantly wants to listen to her favorite music cassettes. Her mother is in charge of all treatments and has issued orders to everyone that Bonnie must not be told her prognosis. These orders are reiterated to each home care nurse. She has even gone so far as to restrict visits from Bonnie's father, from whom she is divorced, and Bonnie's close girlfriends, fearing they will "let it slip" that Bonnie is terminal. She refuses to leave Bonnie's room when anyone else is visiting and usually tries to direct the conversation making comments such as, "When you get better . . ." Bonnie knows she is dying; she frequently asks Carrie, her hospice nurse, "How much time do I have left?" "Why won't anyone let me talk about my dying" and more insistently "I am not afraid to die, but I need to talk to my friends about this." You have spoken to her mother about Bonnie's concerns, but she refuses to listen to any discussion about telling Bonnie the truth. What should you do? (Turkoski, 2003)

The Standard of Self-Assertion Acts as a Lens

The character structure that serves as the bioethical standard of self-assertion is an agent's power to initiate his own actions. It is the power of an agent, thereafter, to control his time and effort.

> The character structure that serves as the bioethical standard of self-assertion is an agent's power to initiate his own actions.

If you would know your patient, you must look at how he reacts to the things that demand his time and effort and, if possible, why he reacts in this way. He is a private individual, which means, in effect, he owns the being he is. His time and effort—his living—is his own. His relationship to his living is intimate. His actions and motivations—his control of his time and effort—imply who he is. Gain an understanding of how he uses his time and to what he puts his effort, and you will know him quite well. Sometimes a patient will act against who he is. At this first stage of your ethical awareness, you will be able to recognize this.

This is the first level of knowledge one can have of another. Analysis through self-assertion gives the least complex understanding of a patient, but it is far better than no understanding at all. In some cases, it will be the only knowledge of a patient a nurse can gain. Without that knowledge, she might have no knowledge on which to base decisions and actions. This is the best basis upon which further understanding is built.

> He is a private individual, which means, in effect, he owns the being he is.

The Standard of Beneficence Acts as a Lens

The character structure that serves as the bioethical standard of beneficence is an agent's power to relate himself appropriately to the sources of pleasure and pain. It is the power to act to acquire the benefits one desires and the needs one's life requires.

If you would move to a higher level of understanding, look at the way your patient relates himself to pleasure and pain. Discover how he defines benefits and how he acts to gain benefits and to avoid harm. When you have gained this level of awareness, you will have no trouble interacting with your patient without any likelihood that you might violate his rights. You will have a workable idea as to what he would and would not give "voluntary consent." And, even when for some

> The character structure that serves as the bioethical standard of beneficence is an agent's power to relate himself appropriately to the sources of pleasure and pain.

reason he cannot give consent, you will have a basis on which to judge where his consent would and would not be "objectively gained."

His actions suggest his attitude toward potential benefits and potential harms. When you explicitly understand what his actions suggest, you will have a bit of ethical understanding wonderfully helpful to fill your ethical role successfully.

The Standard of Objectivity Acts as a Lens

The character structure that serves as the bioethical standard of objectivity is an agent's power to achieve and sustain his awareness of his thought processes and his circumstances, which is to say, his context.

If you would know your patient, look at how clearly he is aware of himself and how he engages with the reality of his situation. It is important to know him in this way because he is dependent upon that reality for his life, health, and well-being. If you understand his reactions, you understand the way he relates himself to the world. If this is possible, it is the way you need to understand him.

> The character structure that serves as the bioethical standard of objectivity is an agent's power to achieve and sustain his awareness of his thought processes and his circumstances, which is to say, his context.

A patient's behavior reveals much about his awareness of objective reality and, more important, his attitude toward it. You gain an objective understanding of him when you make this as explicit as the situation allows. Objectivity is a value to everyone. It is especially a value to a nurse, even more than to a patient. But a nurse's objectivity is the best asset a patient has.

The Standard of Freedom Acts as a Lens

The character structure that serves as the bioethical standard of freedom is the power of an agent to take self-directed, independent, sustained long-term actions guided toward the agent's own values and by his own motivations.

If you would move to a still higher level of understanding of your patient, you must look at his freedom (what he can do and what he cannot do), his desires, and the purposes he has set for himself.

> The character structure that serves as the bioethical standard of freedom is the power of an agent to take self-directed, independent, sustained long-term actions guided toward the agent's own values and by his own motivations.

When you recognize how your patient focuses his attention, what he focuses it on, and why and how he takes long-term actions, this gives you—and your patient—a very great advantage.

The ways he uses his freedom—his evaluation of his present situation and the long-term actions he plans to take—reveal a great deal about him. If you become aware of this, you will have a far deeper understanding of him. You will interact with him better if you know who he is. And it helps to know who he is—if you want to understand what he wants to do.

The Standard of Fidelity Acts as a Lens

The character structure that serves as the bioethical standard of fidelity is the power of an agent to adhere to the terms of a decision or agreement. It is an individual's commitment to an obligation he has accepted as part of his role.

> The character structure that serves as the bioethical standard of fidelity is the power of an agent to adhere to the terms of a decision or agreement.

If you would know your patient, look at the attitude he has toward himself. His attitude toward himself shapes who he is.

You ought to do what is best for your patient. This is difficult unless your patient wants to do what is best for himself. In order to reach this level of awareness of your patient, you must understand his attitude toward himself. You must know something about what he values. You must know the way he relates himself to his choices. It helps if you know how strongly he values himself—his fidelity to himself. If his fidelity to himself is weak, you may be able to strengthen it.

> You ought to do what is best for your patient. This is difficult unless your patient wants to do what is best for himself.

To do for himself everything he can do, he must be faithful to himself. To do for him everything you can do, you must be faithful to your agreement with him. If you are faithful to your agreement with him, you are being faithful to yourself as a health care professional. At the same time, nothing you can do will better strengthen his feeling of self-worth and his desire to exercise fidelity than your obvious expectation of his fidelity to himself. Your fidelity to him achieves this better than anything you can do.

Dilemma 6.2

Kim, a 19-year-old, is brain-dead as the result of severe head trauma she suffered in a Jet Ski accident. Her mother indicates that Kim had always said, "I'd donate my organs to help someone else live." Her father, who remains extremely distraught, refuses to even talk about the issue. Both look to you for support. What would you do? (Haddad, 2002, para. 1).

The Standard of Autonomy Acts as a Lens

The character structure that serves as the bioethical standard of autonomy is the rational animality, the uniqueness, independence, individual identity, and ethical sovereignty over himself as an agent of an agent.

All of these lead to and create the unique person who is your patient. If you are to know another person and if you are to interact effectively with him, you must understand his uniqueness—the final product of the bioethical standards. You must know how this person is different—how he is who he is. You begin with the knowledge that he is an individual, reasoning organism. From this, you try to discover as much about him as you can through the other bioethical standards.

> The character structure that serves as the bioethical standard of autonomy is the rational animality, the uniqueness, independence, individual identity, and ethical sovereignty over himself as an agent of an agent.

Dilemma 6.3

During the performance of a laparotomy for the removal of an ovarian cancer, Dr. Richmond discovers the presence of precancerous gonads in Amelia, his 17-year-old patient. This is a condition (testicular feminization) that occurs once in every 50,000 females. Most women who have the condition are not gratified to discover it. Dr. Richmond believes he has a duty to reveal this detail of her condition to Amelia because "she has a right to know it." (Adapted from Minogue & Taraszyewski, 1988)

Lenses In Focus

Ingrid makes an ethical analysis of each of her patients. She proceeds in this way:

She attempts to determine areas of her patient's life where he will desire control of his time and effort while he is in the health care setting. She begins with her patient. She does not begin with an empty abstraction, such as the idea of self-assertion. She begins with evidence gleaned from her patient's actions and purposes.

6.2

Lenses in and out of focus.

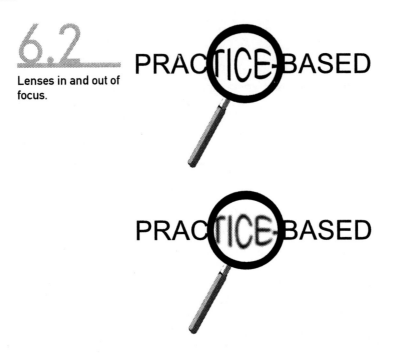

She stays on the alert for areas where she can do her patient some good. She stays alert for areas where she might do him some harm, or prevent some harm from coming to him.

She engages in a close analysis of the context. She does this in order to determine if, and where, she might harm her patient by stumbling over the standard of objectivity. She seeks to discover where her patient will benefit by receiving some item of information. Her patient is the center of her ethical attention.

She seeks to learn the areas of her patient's desire for freedom. She does this also by learning about her patient. She does not reflect on the concept of freedom in her mind. She engages in ethical interaction with a person. She does not engage in ethical interaction with a concept.

One can get in touch with reality by talking to it through concepts. One cannot get in touch with reality by talking to concepts.

She nurtures his life, health, and well-being. She does this by nurturing his commitment to himself.

All of these lead her to the uniqueness of her patient. She comes to this by learning about her patient. She does not do this by examining her concept of uniqueness. She knows that her ethical interactions will be with a unique patient. It will not be with the idea of uniqueness that she carries around in her mind.

Lenses Out of Focus

On the contrary, for Dora, a nurse who works with Ingrid, her center of attention is on her vague understanding of her guiding standards and not her patient (Figure 6.2). She regards standards as deontological rules and rules as her standards. In ethical matters, she gives her attention to these rules rather than to the well-being of her patient.

Dora's process of ethical discovery is not governed by the nature of her patient's situation. She feels a responsibility to the rules themselves. Only the rules, as she understands them, possess ethical relevance for her. Used in this way, her standards as rules make it impossible for her to stay in tune with the context.

Ingrid's use of standards assumes that the efficiency of a nurse's ethical actions is measured by the benefit the nurse's actions yield. Since she assumes this, the center of her ethical concern cannot be abstract, ethical rules. The center of her context must be the nature and the needs of her patient. But the center of Dora's ethical context is a rule. Dora assumes that the benefit of a nurse's ethical actions is measured by the mechanical conformity of her mechanical actions to an externally related standard. The center of her ethical awareness is rigid, abstract, ethical rules. Ingrid does not attempt to benefit a standard. Dora does.

A nurse who works for a telephone-based service receives a call from a young man who reports that he is going to commit suicide and discloses his plan for the time, place, and method. The nurse determines the threat is serious and calls 911 in the caller's area. The emergency response team arrives in time to save the young man. After the caller recovers, he contacts the advice service, furious with the nurse for 'infringing' on his right to commit suicide. (Malloy, 1998)

The caller shares Dora's ethical perspective.

The bioethical standards are means to ends beyond themselves. They are not ends in themselves. There is no way, in the standards themselves, to show that the standards have any value.

Fidelity is of no value to fidelity. Freedom cannot be benefited by having its freedom respected. Obviously, these ideas are utterly senseless. But, they are ideas that, in one way or other, inspire many actions in the health care setting.

> The bioethical standards are means to ends beyond themselves. They are not ends in themselves. There is no way, in the standards themselves, to show that the standards have any value.

Bob is an elderly, feeble, senile man who has entered the hospital for diagnostic studies. On her shift, Dora cares for Bob, and Ingrid cares for him on hers. Bob wants to get up and ambulate. In the context of his condition, it is foreseeable that he might fall and injure himself. Ingrid quiets him, but does not allow him to ambulate. Dora, terrified by the term "paternalism," does allow Bob to ambulate. Bob falls and fractures his hip.

Dora claims that the reason she allowed Bob to ambulate was out of respect for his right to self-determination. In Bob's context, Dora's claim does not justify her action. She placed the well-being of self-determination above the well-being of her patient. More often than not, the benefit to a patient in not being restrained outweighs the possible harm (Janelli, 2006). But this is context dependent. And no abstraction, including self-determination, forms a context.

It is only the circumstances and the knowledge and awareness of reasoning, desiring, and acting agents that form that context.

Ingrid claims that the reason she did not allow Bob to ambulate was through a fear that he would fall and injure himself. Unless what she did took place in a very peculiar biomedical context, Ingrid's claim justifies her action. Ingrid placed the well-being of her patient above the well-being of self-determination.

It is often difficult to know where and how a standard ought to be applied. Rational, ethical action on the part of a nurse without reference to the nature of her patient is impossible. On the other hand, the bioethical standards, outside of the context, do not and cannot outline the context. The context must determine the application of the bioethical standards. They are very broad abstractions, and some way must be found to bring them down into a patient's context.

Dilemma 6.4

Rodney is one of Lynetta's patients in the intensive care unit. He is dying from cirrhosis of the liver. Rodney asks Lynetta for a small drink of water. The order left by the physician placed Rodney on NPO because of the actively bleeding ulcers in his stomach and intestine.

Despite all of his medical problems, Rodney is alert and thirsty. He knows the probable consequences of a sip of water and, yet, continues to want it. Rodney's physician is called in the hope that he will change the order. He will not. He says that he wants to be conservative and is afraid that the water would trigger more bleeding. Despite this, Rodney still continues to plead for a drink of water. What should Lynetta do?

Musings

We have established that:

- Nursing as an intelligible activity relies on the nurse–patient agreement.
- The existence and nature of the nurse–patient agreement implies the appropriateness of the character structures as bioethical standards.
- The bioethical standards guide us in the most effective way of keeping the nurse–patient agreement.
- The more intelligible a nurse's practice, the more effective and rewarding.
- The bioethical standards reflect those aspects of human nature that make the nurse–patient agreement possible and desirable.
- Self-assertion clearly expresses the self-governance of individuals.
- Objectivity is a biological device whose purpose is the well-being of individuals.

■ The freedom described in the bioethical standard of freedom is the ability to pursue one's life and guide one's actions through objective awareness. This is a freedom only possessed by individual people.

■ Fidelity is a virtue that can be practiced only by individuals, one by one.

Every person is unique. So is every bullfrog and every waterfall. And the weather every winter is unique. The uniqueness described in the bioethical standard of autonomy is not the uniqueness of bullfrogs, waterfalls, or winters. It is the uniqueness of individual persons.

Wherever nursing has a logical foundation, it is an activity essentially involving individual nurses and their individual patients. Every other nursing activity (e.g., education, administration, research) is an outgrowth of this.

Study Guide

1. What is necessary for a theory to be called practice-based?
2. As you are aware, a lens, for example, in eyeglasses, is to make things clearer, more accessible to one's view. Take each of the bioethical standards as lenses and apply them to your knowledge of yourself. It will be a great learning experience.
3. Now do the above with someone you know very well. What have you learned?
4. What does looking at the standards as lenses add to your knowledge of the patients?

References

Haddad, A. (2002). Ethics in Action: Honoring a daughter's wish to donate her organs. *RNWeb, 65*. Retrieved June 18, 2004, from www.reweb.com

Janelli, L. M. (2006). Physical restraint use: A nursing perspective. *Medsurg Nursing, 15*, 163–168.

Khayyám, O. (1983). *Rubáiyát of Omar Khayyám*. New York: St. Martin's Press. (Original work published 11th century)

Malloy, C. (1998). Managed care and ethical implications in telephone-based health services. *Advanced Practice Nursing Quarterly, 4*(2), 30–33.

Minogue, B. P., & Taraszyewski, R. (1988). The whole truth and nothing but the truth. *Hastings Center Report, 18*(5), 34–36.

Turkoski, B. B. (2003). A mother's orders about truth telling. *Home Healthcare Nurse, 21*(2), 81–83.

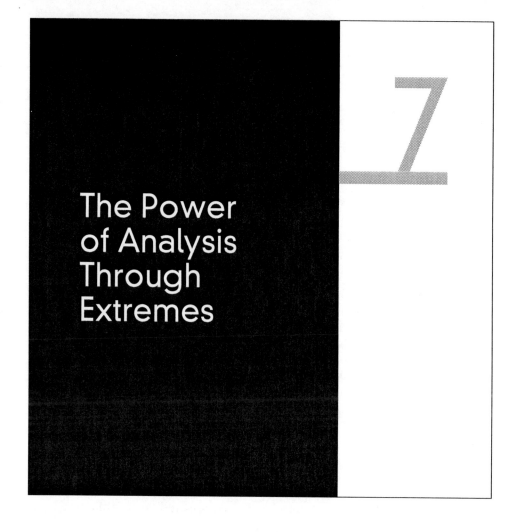

The Power
of Analysis
Through
Extremes

7

Preface to Chapter 7

The Crocodile Paradox

One balmy day on a south sea island paradise, a woman was washing her laundry in the sea. Her baby was lying on the sand a few yards away. A crocodile lurked in the nearby bushes. All of a sudden, while the woman was distracted by a spot of bear fat on a lace scarf, the crocodile rushed over and snatched her baby.

The woman pleaded, "Please don't eat my baby." Crocodiles, as any crocodologist will tell you, are remarkably straightforward, reliable, and sincere. To tell the truth, their attention tends to be narrow and their awareness dominated by instinct and tradition. Nonetheless, they have a charming sense of humor.

The crocodile decided to amuse himself by offering the child's mother this mocking bargain: "If you can tell me what I am going to do, I will give your baby back to you. But if you cannot, I will eat your baby."

This was rather unkind because the crocodile was determined to eat the baby. If the woman said that the crocodile would not eat the baby, she would not be telling him what he was going to do and so he would eat the baby. If she replied that he was going to eat the baby, this would be what he was going to do only if, in fact, he did eat the baby.

What a dreadful impasse! Hum. We will have to think about this.

> Ethical blunders are committed and harmful things are done in the health care setting as a result of a health care professional choosing the wrong person with whom to interact. The patient himself is the wrong person when the actions he proposes to take are ethically unjustifiable.

Ethical blunders are committed and harmful things are done in the health care setting as a result of a health care professional choosing the wrong person with whom to interact. The patient himself is the wrong person when the actions he proposes to take are ethically unjustifiable.

Extremes analysis will establish the nature of the case through the standards. Awareness of this nature will be awareness of what is to be done, for whom it is to be done, and why it is to be done. Awareness of the right person for whom one ought to take an action is a precondition of awareness of what action ought to be taken and why. Analysis by the appropriate standards can then guide the awareness of how it is to be done.

The right beneficiary has been found if:

- His autonomy is such that a rational, controlled, and nonaggressive agreement can be formed;
- It is justifiable for the actions that are to be taken to be guided by his freedom;
- The contextual demands of objective awareness are justifiably understood from his vantage point;
- His self-assertion rightly determines the expenditure of his time and effort, and ought to have input into decision making and choice;
- Benefit and harm are well defined by him and appropriate to the context; and
- His vision of fidelity (i.e., of the agreement) is appropriate.

The wrong beneficiary has been found when:

- His autonomy is such that a rational, limited, and nonaggressive agreement cannot be formed;
- The way he proposes to use his freedom in the context is such that it would not be possible to justify his decisions and actions;
- He cannot exercise objective awareness in guiding his actions;
- His irrational control of his time and effort would frustrate effective ethical decision making and choice;
- His understanding of benefit and harm is nonobjective or aggressive; and
- His vision of fidelity lacks respect for the rights of others.

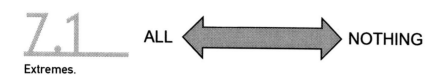

7.1

ALL ⟷ NOTHING

Extremes.

Analysis Through Extremes

When you have eliminated all that is impossible, whatever is left, however improbable, must be the case. (Sherlock Holmes [Doyle], 1930)

Extremes is a method of analysis through which a health care professional can clarify a bioethical context by identifying the relationships—the rights and responsibilities—of the people involved in that context. It involves carrying a situation to ridiculous extremes in a thought experiment in order that issues become clear (Figure 7.1). While some dilemmas do not lend themselves to extremes analysis, it is a very powerful instrument for analyzing those that do.

> Extremes is a method of analysis through which a health care professional can clarify a bioethical context by identifying the relationships—the rights and responsibilities—of the people involved in that context.

The value of analysis through extremes arises from the fact that it is usually easier to determine what is the wrong thing to do than it is to determine what is the right thing to do. Determining the wrong thing to do greatly assists one in determining the right thing to do.

The discovery of that which is definitely wrong—that which is ethically "impossible"—is a powerful tool when what is definitely right is not self-evident and not easy to discover.

> The value of analysis through extremes arises from the fact that it is usually easier to determine what is the wrong thing to do than it is to determine what is the right thing to do.

What is right and what is wrong is right or wrong in relation to the standards. To ascertain that a certain approach would be the wrong application of a standard helps one to discover the right application. Even where the right application of a standard is vague and unclear, the wrong application will probably be more evident. And its wrongness—its ethical invalidity—will clarify the right approach and the right application.

For an objective and contextual awareness, under ideal circumstances, the right thing or things would be visible, and the wrong thing or things would also be visible. This clear vision can be achieved by focusing on the extremes of each standard taken as a right (e.g., the right to freedom, the right to objectivity, etc.). Through this, one can determine whether the ethical nature of the health care setting would be better expressed in giving absolute and complete support for each standard as a right to a certain beneficiary, or whether it is best that this beneficiary should enjoy no right to the exercise of the virtue since the way in which he would exercise it would involve unethical actions and establish unethical conditions. This will establish the nature of the case overall and the most appropriate action to be taken.

The questions to be asked are: Which extreme—absolute support for a beneficiary or no support for a beneficiary—will most perfectly:

- Maintain the rationality and objectivity of the agreement;
- Satisfy appropriate commitments and expectations; and
- Avoid the violation of a right.

Extremes analysis proceeds by determining what the final results would be of one person or another having absolute control over the exercise of each standard. This is in contrast to that person having no control over the exercise of a standard. Through this analysis, it can be seen which alternative is more just and desirable. When this is determined, the ethical status of each beneficiary, and the actions that are and are not appropriate to the context will become evident.

Case Study Analysis Through Extremes

In analyzing these cases, we will focus on the context by determining whether the beneficiary's (normally the patient) complete control of the standard or the

Case Study #1

Maggie, a nurse in the cardiac stepdown unit of a distant hospital, enters the room of 23-year-old Peter, just as Peter's girlfriend is storming out. Peter's girlfriend is obviously angry. When Maggie approaches Peter's bedside, she sees that Peter's sutures have torn and he is hemorrhaging. Maggie explains the situation to Peter and tells him that she is going to take the steps necessary to stop his hemorrhaging. He tells her that he does not want her to stop his hemorrhaging. He has broken up with his sweetheart and he has nothing left to live for. He wants to die.

absolute control of that standard by another would be relatively more rational, more objectively desirable, and more justifiable. The following is an absurd dilemma in every way but one: It perfectly illustrates the nature of an agreement that a rational nurse would not make, and how such a dilemma ought to be resolved. This is the same type of analysis one would make in preventing suicide for a patient with a mental health diagnosis.

This puts Maggie in a dilemma. She has an agreement with Peter that she will act as his agent—to take those actions that he cannot. On the other hand, Peter has made a very unusual request of her. Should she take whatever steps are necessary to save Peter's life or, as the agent of her patient, should she simply accede to his wishes?

In other words, is Maggie (and by extrapolation every nurse) only "the agent of a patient, doing for a patient what he would do for himself if he were able." If this were the case much of a nurse's education would be wasted. A nurse is a person—a rational animal. She has an active sense of balance and proportion. She is more than her definition. If a person were capable of being nothing more than the agent of a patient she would not be capable of being a nurse. A nurse should substitute her judgment for her patients only in the most extreme cases. This is a most extreme case.

As we analyze this case, this is what is revealed:

In this case, should absolute consideration for Peter's autonomy be the guiding standard of interaction or should no consideration be given to Peter's autonomy? Peter is a unique, rational animal. His uniqueness is formed from his rational animality. The course of action Peter proposes turns a whimsical, emotional state, which obviously he feels very intensely, against his rational animality. This course of action turns Peter against his own nature. If his uniqueness is such that the emotions engendered by a romantic disappointment would inspire him to turn against his life, this is contrary to the essential nature of rational animality. It is irrational. He ought not to be supported in this, since no professional agreement could possibly demand irrationality on the part of the professional. No one, including the nurse herself, ought to assume that her professional agreement should replace her human understanding with duties. A nurse must expect to encounter and accept unusual religious practices or personal outlooks to which people have dedicated themselves, but never a spontaneous whimsy like Peter's.

> She has an active sense of balance and proportion. She is more than her definition.

In this case, is it more appropriate that Peter should exercise absolute freedom or no freedom whatsoever? The decision he has made would negate his freedom—an unhindered future—through his death. Since Peter has abandoned his freedom, it is appropriate that the health care professional give no consideration to his plans to destroy himself. This is the best possible and most logical course of action the health care professional can take.

Should Peter's perspective be regarded as absolutely objective and definitive and be given all consideration, or as entirely nonobjective and be given no consideration? When objectivity is reduced to the level of emotional stimulus and response, objectivity is abandoned. Peter, himself, has abandoned his objective awareness.

Should Peter's right to exercise self-assertion be absolute, or should no consideration be given to Peter's power to control his time and effort? When Peter abandoned objectivity, he abandoned his power to control his time and effort.

> When objectivity is reduced to the level of emotional stimulus and response, objectivity is abandoned.

Should perfect consideration be given to the benefits Peter plans to pursue or should no consideration be given to this? Peter sees his greatest benefit in abandoning all the benefits of his future life. In the context of his life, the harm he has suffered is nearly insignificant. He already has abandoned beneficence toward himself.

Should Peter's present state of fidelity to himself determine his nurse's action or have no influence on her course of action? Fidelity to an event (his suicide) has displaced fidelity to himself—the self that could live a long and satisfying life.

The bioethical standards are many things. Because of each thing they are, they cannot be dispensable.

It may be that Peter's future life would be so marred by the loss of his sweetheart that his life would, objectively, be not worth living. But for the health care professionals attending him, it is impossible to see that this would be so. In Peter's present emotional state, it is impossible for him to see that this would be so. Therefore, while it might be a mistake to interfere with him, it is far more probable that the benefits the health care setting provides are better brought about by ignoring his wishes and restraining him—even forcibly if necessary—in order to get the hemorrhaging stopped.

Maggie has a responsibility to do for Peter what Peter would do for himself if he were able, but in his present emotional state he is unable to do anything for himself. She has a professional agreement with Peter. But no rational person would make an agreement with another to care for his life and health and, at the same time, let him die on what can only be understood as an emotional whim. Health care professionals are expected to be rational beings—the more rational the better. A person who is rational, whether health care professional or patient, cannot logically be expected to make an irrational agreement or keep an agreement by taking an irrational action.

> But no rational person would make an agreement with another to care for his life and health and, at the same time, let him die on what can only be understood as an emotional whim.

In many circumstances when a patient wishes to die, his wish is rational, condoned, and ought to be condoned. Peter's case does not fall into this category.

Now that Peter is in a better emotional state and well on the road to recovery, we can return to our sojourn on the desert island.

Resolution of the Crocodile Paradox

When the crocodile made his good natured but horrifying offer, this is what happened:

The mother replied, "When you offered me this agreement, the implication was that you would listen to my reply. You said, 'If you can tell me what I am going to do, I will give your baby back to you.' I cannot tell you anything unless you listen to what I say. You will not hear what I say unless you listen to what I say. So, what you are going to do is listen to what I say and then you will give me back my baby, because I told you what you are going to do." Immediately the crocodile lost his air of urbane gentility, and with a surly lack of grace, returned the woman's child. He had failed to consider the implications of what he said. That which is implied in a context is often the most important part of the context.

> That which is implied in a context is often the most important part of the context.

Nothing can establish the validity of a proper resolution nearly as well as drawing out the absurd implications of its contrary. The implication to be drawn from Peter's dilemma is quite obvious. Implications seldom are obvious, but quite often extremes analysis allows one to confidently draw out the relevant implication. For instance, the implication of Maggie letting Peter die would be that bioethical interaction, in its most serious moments, can be determined by a hysterical, emotional tantrum.

This, along with the implications of the self-righteous idea that bioethical interaction must be determined by cultural traditions in certain cases requires that the professional–patient agreement shall have not ethical authority.

Case Study #2

Elizabeth is from a large and well-to-do family. She is 24 years old and living on the streets. Her family has paid to have her admitted to several, private, psychiatric facilities for treatment of her schizophrenia. Elizabeth always signs herself out. Since she is judged not to be dangerous, she cannot be held against her will.

Elizabeth's symptoms can be well controlled with psychotropic medication. However, she does not take the drugs and says she does not like the way she feels when she is on her medication. She writes beautiful poetry and says she finds "my own reality" much more interesting than the boring and tedious life she experiences when on the medication. She prefers the friends she makes on the street to the dullness of "so-called normal people."

Her sister arranges to have her poetry published and sends the meager proceeds to her. She is occasionally picked up for vagrancy and brought in for treatment. Her parents are always contacted. Elizabeth does not maintain contact with them otherwise. Eloise, a social worker, has been assigned to her case. What should be done? (Davis, Aroskar, Liaschenko, & Drought, 1997)

In this case, should absolute consideration for Elizabeth's autonomy be the guiding standard of interaction or should no consideration be given to Elizabeth's autonomy? Elizabeth is a rational animal, but her conventional reason has gone on vacation. She is living in "a world of her own." Nonetheless, the way she is living violates no one's rights. As far as we know, she is asking no one to make a commitment to her and she has no expectations of anyone.

A series of interdependent questions suggest themselves in this case: How can the greatest potential harm be avoided and how can the greatest potential good be produced? Is it more desirable for Elizabeth to be happy in her world, than unhappy in ours? Should Elizabeth sacrifice her happiness for the sake of reason or demand of reason that it serves her happiness?

Elizabeth can avoid the greatest potential harm—the loss of her happiness—by continuing her present lifestyle. Happiness is, and unhappiness is not, desirable. If it is necessary, at present, in order for Elizabeth to be happy to remain in her world, then this is her best decision, even in a strange way her most rational decision.

> Is it more desirable for Elizabeth to be happy in her world, than unhappy in ours?

In this case, is it more appropriate that Elizabeth should exercise absolute freedom or no freedom whatsoever? The ultimate goal of psychiatric care should be to bring Elizabeth to a state where she is able to control and preserve her existence and to flourish. (In this, the goal of psychiatry is no different than the goal of medical science.) At present, her activities do not threaten her survival. They allow her the only form of flourishing she can enjoy. In Elizabeth's strange and uncommon case, she has a right to absolute freedom.

Should Elizabeth's perspective be regarded as absolutely objective and definitive and be given all consideration or as entirely nonobjective and be given no consideration? In this unusual case, there is a, at least apparent, conflict between objectivity and reason. In several cases cited in this book, the resolution suggests that the power to reason ought not be sacrificed for the sake of objective awareness.

This is particularly true when the revelation of a new objective fact would be so emotionally devastating that it would be impossible for the hearer to exercise reason. When awareness of an objective fact, in the immediate moment, makes it impossible to reason about one's course of action in the future, objectivity loses all value.

> *The alternative here for Elizabeth is not a subjective awareness unrelated to objective reality, but objective awareness tied to a smaller context—a context with which a patient is psychologically and cognitively able to deal.*

As an ethical tool, objectivity and reason do not refer to a person's ability to do crossword puzzles or balance a checkbook. Reason and, therefore, objectivity are tools to achieve flourishing and happiness. In Elizabeth's case, happiness would not be achieved by adopting a more conventional lifestyle. So, in a very real sense, it would be irrational for her to change her lifestyle. If any way could be found to enable her to be happy in a different reality, then this might be acted upon. But, at present, there is no such way.

Should Elizabeth's power to control her time and effort be absolute or should no consideration be given to her power of self-assertion? The arena of Elizabeth's life and her agency is maximized in her present lifestyle and the friends she makes on the street.

Elizabeth's life is more purposeful and much more interesting than the boring and tedious life that she experiences when on medication. It is a great temptation to try to control the lives of others or, somewhat more beneficently, to try too hard to help others control their own lives. Sometimes the best thing to do is to do nothing.

Should perfect consideration be given to Elizabeth's plans to pursue her own sense of beneficence or should no consideration be given to this? Elizabeth's desire is to continue the lifestyle she is living now. And no way can be discovered that would enable her to experience her life in this way under different circumstances (e.g., living at home on medication).

Should Elizabeth's present state of fidelity to herself determine her course of action or have no influence on her course of action? Elizabeth, in her own reality, is experiencing life in an emotional state that many people might envy. Considering that Elizabeth's family is well-to-do, they might exercise fidelity to her by adding something onto the meager proceeds that Elizabeth's poetry brings to her.

Gentle coercion to induce Elizabeth to adopt a more self-controlled lifestyle, of course, is justified. Placing Elizabeth in a state of slavery to appearances is not.

The implication of compelling Elizabeth to conform would be that a humdrum and conventional lifestyle is an ethical standard. A standard so important that, in enforcing it, every individual standard can be violated.

> Gentle coercion to induce Elizabeth to adopt a more self-controlled lifestyle, of course, is justified.

Case Study #3

Jerry is an AIDS patient. He has a rare lymphoma with several large tumors in his abdomen. Jerry is responding to treatment and will probably be able to return to his home. He has asked his physician and his nurse to keep his confidence. He does not want his wife or his homosexual partner to know that he has AIDS. The physician encourages him to tell his wife and lover, but Jerry refuses. He says that he is very careful about using a condom, and he does not want to upset his present lifestyle with his wife and lover.

Should absolute consideration or no consideration be given to Jerry's unique desires?

Jerry's disease has robbed him of many potential benefits he would have enjoyed without it. He is now imperiled at every turn. Whatever happens may strip him of one of the few benefits he has left. If Jerry were to lose the relationship he has with his wife and/or his lover, the quality of his life would be greatly diminished. In addition to everything he now faces, either loss would be a type of "little death." But suffering the little death of a destroyed relationship is insignificant in comparison to the real death that Jerry's wife and/or lover would suffer if he were to infect them.

Jerry's physician has no right to allow these two people to be placed in jeopardy based on Jerry's promise to practice safe sex. Jerry's nurse also has an ethical obligation to speak out if this is necessary.

Should absolute consideration or no consideration be given to Jerry's freedom? The uniqueness of a person's position does not give him the freedom to threaten another person's right to life. Even more so, it does not give a biomedical professional a right to cooperate with him in this by maintaining a life-threatening confidentiality.

> But suffering the little death of a destroyed relationship is insignificant in comparison to the real death that Jerry's wife and/or lover would suffer if he were to infect them.

Should absolute consideration or no consideration be given to Jerry's outlook on the situation? One cannot develop as an ethical agent and one cannot flourish as a human being without taking certain actions and developing certain attitudes. One does not maintain an ethically developed attitude toward one's own life if one does not inform another person that his or her life is about to be placed in danger. By informing Jerry's wife and lover, the physician would honor his own life and, at the same time, fulfill his human and professional obligation to them.

Should absolute consideration or no consideration be given to Jerry's self-assertion? The range in which one has a right to exercise one's time and effort has rigid ethical boundaries. It stops far short of any action that would endanger the life of another person. The fact that one might be careful while exercising this action is not relevant.

Should absolute consideration or no consideration be given to Jerry's benefit seeking? Jerry's physician has an opportunity to extend a significant degree of beneficence toward Jerry. This opportunity is very much outweighed by the harm Jerry's physician has the opportunity to do to the others. It is the function not only of epidemiologists but of all health care professionals to prevent or stop the spread of disease. There is no obvious reason why AIDS is an exception.

Is absolute consideration or no consideration due the health care professional agreement? What consideration ought to be given to the rights' agreement? The biomedical professional–patient agreement is not an agreement that can include a clause allowing them to conspire together to violate the rights of others.

If Jerry can exercise absolute freedom, he need not even take precautions. If he has no freedom, then, while he will be inconvenienced, no one's life will be placed in jeopardy. His view of the situation cannot be regarded as objective. Sexual passion is not noted for producing objective judgments. Only by breaking a confidence with Jerry can his wife and lover be endowed with an objective awareness to which they have a right. One's control of time, effort, and sexual passion seldom go well together. No one whose life is endangered can really be thought of as exercising self-assertion. Life must be given precedence over sexual passion. The benefit to Jerry is relatively trivial. The detriment to his wife and lover could be fatal. A health care professional has no right to exercise fidelity to a patient when this would violate the rights of a third party. Out of respect for his own life, the physician should exercise a greater fidelity to potential victims.

> A health care professional has no right to exercise fidelity to a patient when this would violate the rights of a third party.

The implication of maintaining Jerry's confidence is that a health care professional ought to keep his professional agreement, even if this means violating the rights' agreement. But if violating the rights' agreement is justifiable, then there is no ethical reason to keep the professional agreement. The rights' agreement is the foundation of the health care professional/patient agreement. It is a fact that legally, he would be liable if he knowingly infected his partner. Use of a condom is not an excuse for not informing one's partner. Here, the law and ethics are in harmony (Thomas, n.d.).

Case Study #4

Alfred came into the hospital 4 days ago for a coronary bypass. The surgery went well, and Alfred seems on the way to recovery. A few hours ago, his family was in to visit him. The room was filled with quiet conversation, and the family seemed to share a sense of intimacy.

It is now time for Alfred's first heparin injection. Lois, his nurse, has just come into his room to give him his shot. For no apparent reason, Alfred refuses the medication. Lois knows that Alfred's failure to take the medicine puts his life in jeopardy. She explains to him the reason for the drug and stresses its importance. On the one hand, Lois's reasoning tells her that Alfred should take the heparin. There is every reason why he should take it, and no apparent reason for him not to take it. On the other hand, Alfred is adamant. He absolutely refuses the shot of heparin. He also refuses to discuss the reasons why he will not let Lois give him the injection. There is no apparent reason why Alfred's freedom does not give him the right to make this decision. There seems to be an irresolvable conflict between Lois's reason and Alfred's freedom.

If you think about the ethical dilemmas that Alfred's case involves, three things are obvious:

1. Justifiable ethical decisions depend, not on the facts of the ethical context, but on those facts that are known. Justifiable ethical decisions cannot depend on facts that are not known. No decision of any sort can be made on the basis of facts that are not known or on the basis of a person's refusal to recognize or reveal them.
2. An ethical agent may often feel guilt over the results of a decision that was made on inadequate knowledge. The guilt the agent assumes may very well be worse than the unfortunate result of the decision. If the agent made the decision on an objective reading of all the knowledge that was available, the decision would be perfectly justifiable regardless of its results. Alfred ought to be fully informed concerning the foreseeable consequences of his decision.
3. An ethical agent's reasoned beliefs are sufficient to justify ethical actions. There is nothing whatsoever that an ethical agent can act upon except his reasoned beliefs. There is no need for an ethical agent to do better than he can do.

The health care professional might invite Alfred to come along on an analysis through extremes, while someone is on the phone locating Alfred's family. Lois might dialogue with Alfred as follows:

You have every right to decide what is going to happen to you, but if you refuse the heparin, you may suffer a stroke or a heart attack. You may very well kill yourself or become paralyzed.

Do you want to make these decisions entirely alone without any expert input (autonomy)? If you give your attention to yourself and the circumstances here in this room, you will probably enjoy a long life (freedom).

Do you want knowledgeable guidance? Do you want to look through the eyes of people who can see the consequences of different decisions? Do you want to control everything that goes on in this room or do you want to make it an informed cooperation? If you keep your thinking narrowed down to your present mood, you may change your mind when it is too late (objectivity).

Do you want to make your decision without any knowledge of its consequences or what these consequences would mean to you [self-assertion]? Six feet under, there is nothing to which you can react. You will never again react to family or friends. You will never decide on where you want to visit or where you want to go on vacation. You will never again drink a cool beer on a warm day or spend an evening reminiscing with your wife in a quiet restaurant [beneficence]. [The best thing a health care professional can find out about a patient is those things in life he most enjoys. These are always useful as spurs.]

There are a lot of decisions you do not have to make right now. You do not have to decide where you want to go in the next several weeks or what you want to do. But I think you are going to want to be around to make those decisions.

Alfred, you will be dead a long time. How about taking a few years to complete a good life [fidelity]? Okay? [The offer of an agreement.] Let's get at it. [The assumption of an acceptance. This is an example of "gentle coercion".]

> The best thing a health care professional can find out about a patient is those things in life he most enjoys. These are always useful as spurs.

If he still does not want to take his heparin, he may, in self-defense, reveal the reasons why not. Then you will have much more to work on with him. But hopefully, in this way you can show him—without telling him—the unique person he is; the way he is reacting to his present condition makes him the wrong person—making the wrong decision for himself.

To act otherwise would imply that force is a valid form of ethical interaction, or that his experience of comfort and control in the present moment is more important than his experience of comfort and control throughout the rest of his life.

Discovery Versus Choice

> That which will be discovered will be the lesser of two harms, or the lesser of two benefits, or the existence of a harm opposed to a benefit.

The outlines of a context can be discovered by analysis through the standards. Analysis of potential benefits and harms—the most fulfilling exercise of the standards as virtues is revealed through their foreseeable consequences. That which will be discovered will be the lesser of two harms, or the lesser of two benefits, or the existence of a harm opposed to a benefit.

The ethically appropriate beneficiary can be discovered in the structure of the context by analysis through extremes. Not only this, but there is always the possibility that another dilemma, perhaps more important than the first, may be discovered through extremes analysis. Extremes analysis will reveal what is certainly the wrong person, thing, time, way, extent, and reason.

> Extremes analysis will reveal what is certainly the wrong person, thing, time, way, extent, and reason.

When it is perfect, an agreement will be with the right person. When agreement is not with the right person, it is radically imperfect. That which would ordinarily be the right thing to do will be the wrong thing to do, and every category will be failed.

The Perfect Bioethical Agreement

One who is the right person when no right is violated becomes the wrong person when a right is violated. The right person, when interactions are in sync with the nature of the health care setting and the nurse's role, becomes the wrong person when interaction is out of sync. The right person under the terms of a rational agreement, when the agreement becomes irrational, becomes the wrong person.

> One who is the right person when no right is violated becomes the wrong person when a right is violated.

When there is no possibility of an innocent person's rights being violated, when the agreement between a patient and the health care system is consistent with the nature and purpose of the health care system, and when the agreement is free of irrational terms, the bioethical agreement is perfect.

The fact that extremes analysis has revealed one person to be the right beneficiary of ethical interaction does not imply that he is to be the exclusive beneficiary of ethical actions. Others must be considered, albeit, in an indirect way and to a lesser extent.

If one went from extremes analysis to an exclusive concern for the rights of one beneficiary, one would have discovered the context, only to abandon it. The purpose of extremes analysis is to establish the right beneficiary and what is right for that beneficiary. It does not, and cannot, give one a license to ignore balance and proportion in relation to everyone else involved in the situation.

For instance, your patient wants to talk to you about the condition of his wife, but you see that the patient in the next bed, who is not your patient but is unattended, is in intense pain. You check and discover that he has not been given his pain medication. You arrange for him to get his pain medication. Then you go to your patient to discuss his distressful situation. A health care professional's agreement with a patient does not include the proviso that she will not assist someone who is in severe pain before consoling the patient with whom she has an agreement. This is an example of giving up a smaller good to gain a greater good.

> The fact that extremes analysis has revealed one person to be the right beneficiary of ethical interaction does not imply that he is to be the exclusive beneficiary of ethical actions. Others must be considered, albeit, in an indirect way and to a lesser extent.

> The purpose of extremes analysis is to establish the right beneficiary and what is right for that beneficiary.

You are about to give your patient his aspirin as ordered. He believes that this will help him to sleep. A visitor in the patient's room has a heart attack. You give the aspirin to the visitor. You would do this even if it meant that your patient would have to toss and turn all night. But then, after the person who had the heart attack has been treated, you would, of course, obtain aspirin for your patient. This is an example of giving up a smaller good to prevent a greater harm.

You go into a drugstore to buy medicine for your husband who will die without it. The pharmacist informs you that he will sell the drug to you, but only at a wildly inflated price—a price that you cannot pay. A dilemma arises: Under these circumstances, would you be justified in stealing the medicine from the druggist? Should the druggist or your husband be the beneficiary of your ethical action?

It would be understandable if you were to place a greater value on the life of your husband than on the property rights of the druggist. Many people would be inclined to forgive you if you were to steal the medicine. Then, later on, you could reimburse the druggist the normal cost of the medicine. The druggist has an implicit agreement with his customers that he will charge a standard price for his medicine. He proposes to break this agreement. You hold him to it. This is an example of doing a smaller harm to prevent a greater harm.

You have promised your kids that you will take them to an amusement park. Your neighbor is rushed to the hospital. She must have a delicate operation and she wants you to go with her to help her understand what is happening during the process. Obviously, it would be more rational of you to make your neighbor the beneficiary of your action. But, because of this, you would certainly not conclude that you should never again take your children to an amusement park. This is an example of doing a smaller harm to attain a greater good.

Guidelines

Freedom and objectivity for various reasons are the most powerful standards for extremes analysis. Most instances of analysis through freedom will reveal how freedom is to be exercised and if its exercise will produce irrational consequences or involve a violation of rights. Most instances of objectivity will reveal what justifiable decisions and choices will be achieved and whether they would presuppose an irrational agreement.

> Freedom and objectivity for various reasons are the most powerful standards for extremes analysis.

It is very rare that it happens when one analyzes through the extremes of two or three standards, that the others are going to show something different. After two or three, the others will follow suit unless the first, second, or third, or one of the next three were analyzed inappropriately.

Most instances of self-assertion will reveal what would motivate self-assertion—and whether this will result in excess or deficit—whether the agent's control of his time and effort is commensurate with the terms of the agreement.

Most instances of analysis through beneficence will reveal how the idea of beneficence squares with the nature of the health care system or whether it presupposes an irrational agreement—an agreement inappropriate to the health care system.

Most instances of analysis through fidelity will reveal what fidelity requires—whether, for instance, it might require a violation of rights.

The greatest value of autonomy is in confirming analysis through the other standards. There is a venerable philosophical axiom—*Operatio sequiteur esse*—that describes the fact that the characteristic actions of an existent arise from the nature of the existent. So it is with the nature—the autonomy—of a person. The knowledge of who he is follows on and requires the awareness of what he does and why.

Another effective way to discover the autonomy—the individual nature—of a person is through his passions. The patient's emotional reaction to circumstances may be the most reliable indicator of the condition of his autonomy. Therefore, a flawed autonomy will be demonstrated by emotional reactions toward the wrong thing, or the wrong person, for the wrong reason, at the wrong time, in the wrong way, and to the wrong extent. This will reveal a lack of justifiable cause and effect actions and reactions (Aristotle as cited in McKeon, 1941).

Autonomy is the interwoven character structure that produce a person's actions and that he experiences as himself. The fact that he is likeable and attractive or upsetting and unattractive is in the eyes of the beholder. It forms no part—nothing—of his autonomy.

Only an autonomy that produces irrational or coercive decisions and actions is a flawed autonomy.

Study Guide

1. What can be learned from the crocodile and the importance of the implicit to ethical decision making?
2. What are the main purposes of analysis through extremes? How is it used?
3. Extremes analysis is a useful tool. It is *not* meant to be used as definitive, only as a guide, a very helpful guide. Could you use this in your personal life? How?
4. Give an example of where extremes analysis might be most useful in your practice.

References

Davis, A. J., Aroskar, M. A., Liaschenko, J., & Drought, T. S. (1997). *Ethical dilemmas & nursing practice* (4th ed.). Stamford, CT: Appleton & Lange.

Doyle, A. C. (1930). *The complete works of Sherlock Holmes, Vol. I: The sign of fours*. New York: Doubleday.

McKeon, R. (Ed.). (1941). *The basic works of Aristotle*. New York: Random House.

Thomas, J. C. (n.d.). *Please don't say anything: Partner notification and the patient-physician relationship*. Retrieved October 25, 2006, from http://www.ama-assn.org/ama/pub/category/print/11504.html

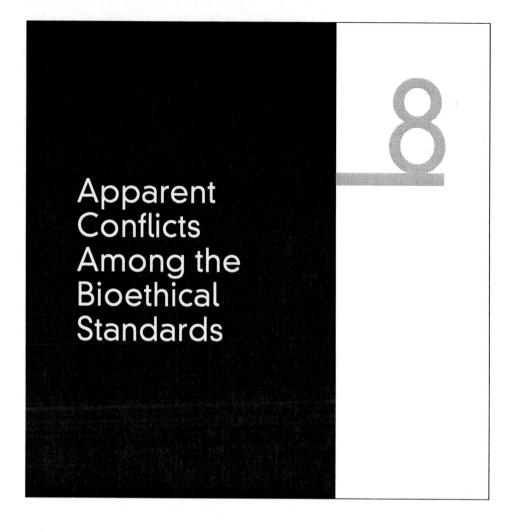

8

Apparent Conflicts Among the Bioethical Standards

Actions that are ethically appropriate in relation to a certain patient at one time, may not be ethically appropriate in relation to the same patient at a different time. Actions that are ethically appropriate to one patient at a certain time may not be appropriate in relation to a different patient at the same time or if the actions are taken in a different way. The bioethical standards signify virtues which, working together, constitute the character of a rational being—specifically, insofar as he is an ethical agent. It is these virtues that place the agent in a context, that make the context what it is in relation to the agent (or patient), and that shape the agent's motivations and actions.

Each virtue shapes its own peculiar sort of motivation and the interacting of the virtues produce the nature and the nuances of an ethical agent's motivation in any specific circumstance.

Fidelity as a virtue determines the strength or weakness of an agent's motivation. Fidelity is, so to speak, the virtue of an agent's decisions and agreements.

> Fidelity as a virtue determines the strength or weakness of an agent's motivation.

Beneficence is the intensity of his motivation to pursue benefits and/or defend himself against harm. Beneficence reveals the strength of his self-interest and the appropriateness of his motivations. Beneficence is the virtue of his practical reason.

Self-assertion motivates one to search out possibilities of advantageous changes in one's immediate circumstances. Self-assertion is shown in his activity and self-control, or their absence. It is the virtue of an agent's volition.

Objectivity is the virtue of maintaining an uncluttered awareness of one's circumstances and one's place in his circumstances. The evidence of this is given in the competency of his action—whether he is motivated through understanding. This is the virtue of his awareness.

Freedom denotes an agent's interest in and concern for the value of his life and the values of his entire lifetime. Freedom is the virtue of his rational self-interest. It is shown in the degree to which he is appropriately oriented to his future and the reality of his lived world.

Autonomy is his character. It is the interweaving of all of these.

Nurses can, and ought to, use the bioethical standards as instruments of ethical analysis. A patient's virtues or vices will imply his motivations. His motivations will suggest his present intentions. And these will suggest his probable values or decisions, and his actions. Two problems can arise for a nurse in her use of the standards as instruments of analysis in her discovery of the character of her patient and in the tenor of their relationship:

1. She can be uncertain as to her application of a bioethical standard.
2. She can feel a lesser or greater confidence in her application of a particular standard than is justified.

These problems arise because it is possible for conflicts to arise in the nurse's understanding of the appropriate application of the standards. We will now turn to those conflicts.

Here is a conflict among several standards. Whatever resolution is possible, it seems it must come from outside the standards. But then it would come from outside the nurse/patient agreement since that agreement can only be understood in terms of the bioethical standards, which are the motivators of that agreement.

In different ways the nurse and patient:

▨ Want to clarify and retain the knowledge of who they are (their self-awareness)—a competent professional and one able to retain his competence.

▨ Look forward to their life span with confidence and anticipation—retain enthusiasm for her profession and knowledge that he will be able to continue to meet his responsibilities.

Dilemma 8.1

Fred is an 85-year-old man who suffers from senile dementia. He is depressed and aggressive. For some time, he has undergone antidepressant treatment, which has made it easier for him and his caregivers. However, he suddenly refuses to accept the treatment after he has heard that it is given to insane people. He says he is not insane and so he now refuses to accept the medication. There seems to be no way to convince him to take the medication. His wife, who visits him each day, is desperate. She urges the physician who visits the nursing home to give her husband the antidepressant, by force if needed. She wants him to have the medication for his own sake and for hers. She doubts that her husband fully understands the consequences of his rejection of the medicine. The physician consults the nurse who is responsible for him, who agrees to use force. The antidepressant is given to the man by injection, while several people hold him down. (Tannsjo, 1999, p. 329)

- Know that their ambitions and decisions are objectively justified—she will not have to defend her ambitions and desires against objective facts and the objective facts do not threaten his ability to meet his obligations.
- Retain the capability of controlling one's time and effort—her abilities make her a skilled and reliable professional and make him capable of functioning independently.
- Continue one's pursuit of benefit and successful avoidance of harm—continuing to enjoy the benefits of success and avoiding the drawback of failure, and continuing one's state of capability and avoiding a state of incapacity.
- Maintain fidelity to one's knowledge one's motivations and one's values—maintaining fidelity to oneself and one's profession through fidelity to one's patients and maintaining fidelity to the value of life.

But a nurse is the agent of her patient, doing for her patient what he would do for himself if he were able. This always takes place within a context. The nurse–patient agreement establishes the fact of this relationship. The context establishes the nature and purposes of the relationship and actions that can and ought to be taken. No other actions are ethically justifiable. And nothing can come from outside of this relationship. There are two possible approaches to a resolution. Both involve the standards in one way or another.

> The context establishes the nature and purposes of the relationship and actions that can and ought to be taken. No other actions are ethically justifiable.

Autonomy and Freedom

A person's freedom is his ability to take independent actions toward relatively long-term goals. His right to freedom is his right to make independent and long-term choices and decisions and to act on these choices and decisions.

Dilemma 8.2

A health care professional is determined that a patient shall exercise his right to make decisions regarding his treatment. The patient wants the health care professional to make the decisions.

It can be argued that:

- The patient is exercising his freedom by delegating responsibility to the professional.
- The nature of this patient's autonomy is such that this is the best way he can exercise his freedom.
- A patient's relationship to a health care professional always, to some extent, involves this delegation of responsibility.

Also, it can be argued that:

- The patient is not exercising his right to freedom in refusing to exercise it.
- The patient is not expressing his autonomy, but abandoning it.
- In matters concerning the course of his life, it is ethically desirable that a patient delegate as little responsibility as possible.

In the life of a nurse, a large number of apparent conflicts arise between autonomy and freedom. They sometimes arise out of a failure to differentiate between the two.

The standard of freedom involves a patient's right to take uncoerced actions, actions motivated by his own independent purposes and judgment. A biomedical professional's refusal to accept a patient's decisions and choices is a violation of the bioethical standard of freedom. The professional's efforts to coerce actions from her patient are another form of the same violation.

> The standard of freedom involves a patient's right to take uncoerced actions, actions motivated by his own independent purposes and judgment.

A person's autonomy is his independent uniqueness. His right to autonomy is his right to be what he is. Every form of intolerance or coercion is directed against someone's autonomy.

The difference between autonomy and freedom is shown by a consideration of the way each standard is violated.

Autonomy and Objectivity

Patients sometimes experience a psychological disequilibrium, which interferes with their being able to participate readily in health care decision making. They may retain the ability to think logically in other areas, but in this area their thinking is distorted (Howe, 1993). Health care professionals need the ability to help these people see the consequences of ill-considered decisions. This is an ethical ability.

A nurse has an ethical obligation to recognize the fear of a patient who is more fearful than most. This is one way a professional recognizes the autonomy of her patient. Each patient has a right to be who he is, and some patients are more fearful than others.

Dilemma 8.3

Rachel is a nurse whose patient, Ken, is dying. She and Ken are old friends. Rachel knows that Ken is probably unaware of the seriousness of his condition, and she knows that Ken is terrified of dying. She also knows that Ken has many business and personal affairs that he would want to get in order if he knew of his condition. Rachel is, as the saying goes, caught on the horns of a dilemma. If she reveals his condition and incites terror in him, she will be ignoring Ken's present personality structure. This would be a violation of his autonomy. If she does not tell him and enables him to get his affairs in order, she will be violating the standard of objectivity.

Since they are old friends, Ken might expect Rachel to tell him that he is dying. At the same time, his behavior might have given her no opportunity to do this. But Rachel's behavior might lead him to believe that he is not dying, which is not true. If she knew that her behavior might mislead him and she could have prevented this, then, in respecting his autonomy, she violated the standard of objectivity. On the other hand, in respecting the need for objectivity, she may violate his autonomy.

Note that, whatever Rachel does, she must find some way to apply what she does know to what she does not know. Rachel is in a double bind. Neither autonomy nor objectivity will enable her to work her way out of this dilemma.

Autonomy and Self-Assertion

An individual person's right to self-assertion is an outgrowth of autonomy, an outgrowth of his right to be who he is. One thing that every person is, regardless of other differences or similarities, is an independent individual. Every person is self-assertive by nature. One cannot deny (violate) the self-assertion of another without, at the same time, denying (violating) his autonomy. Nor, of course, can one violate the autonomy of another without violating his self-assertion. On the other hand, if a nurse rigorously accepts a patient's autonomy, she cannot violate his self-assertion.

> Strictly speaking, every right is a right to take an action. However, there is a sense in which it can be said that one has a right to be autonomous. One has a right to be whatever one is, for example, a male, a lover of classical music, a hiker, a scholar. To be what one is is not an action. One does not take an action in the immediate moment to be these things. They are, simply, what one is—a result of one's development. "The right to one's autonomy" is not just a figure of speech. It is a right in as strong a sense as the right to take a nonaggressive action. It denotes the ethical propriety of accepting the uniqueness and the differences of any person with whom one interacts. It is this uniqueness and these differences that produce a person's actions. It would be absurd to make the self-contradictory claim that a person has a right to take particular nonaggressive actions but no right to possess the character structures that are the source of these actions.

Autonomy is individual and independent uniqueness. A person's right to autonomy is that moral property whereby he has the right to be dealt with according to his uniqueness. A person's right to self-assertion is his right to self-ownership—his right to control his time and effort, which includes his right to be free of undesired and undesirable interactions or relationships.

Dilemma 8.4

Rick works as a copyeditor. He is a 27-year-old homosexual with a long history of kidney disease. Three years ago, he tested positive for HIV, but he has been symptom-free and his T-cell count has been above 400. Ten months ago, he suffered kidney failure, but since then he has been doing well on dialysis. He now wants to receive a kidney transplant from his 49-year-old mother, Mrs. Raymond. He has been very insistent that she donate a kidney for him, and she now agrees to the procedure. She knows that he is HIV positive. The psychiatrist, who evaluated both Rick and his mother, reports that both are extremely guarded in their communication and that their relationship seems complex and troubled. The case comes to the Ethics Committee. Should the mother's consent be accepted as a free and autonomous choice? (Rhodes, 1992, pp. 75–76)

Like any conflict that arises between autonomy and self-assertion, it is not a real but merely an apparent conflict. The conflict arises only because one or both terms (autonomy and/or self-assertion) are ill-defined.

Like any conflict that arises between autonomy and self-assertion, it is not a real but merely an apparent conflict. The conflict arises only because one or both terms (autonomy and/or self-assertion) are ill-defined.

> Mohan and his wife are asleep when their house catches on fire. Mohan manages to get out of the

house. He is taken to the hospital in an ambulance. For a long time, Mohan cannot get information on what has happened to his wife. Finally, he is told that she is dead. He begins to cry. He asks Kathleen, his nurse, to see that he is left alone.

Mohan's physician is contacted by the coroner about arrangements for the disposition of the body of Mohan's wife. Mohan and his wife are Hindu and no one knows what should be done. The physician instructs Kathleen to ask Mohan what he wants done. Kathleen tells the physician that Mohan is grieving and wants to be left alone for the time being. The physician angrily orders Kathleen to go and get the information he asked for. Now Kathleen faces an apparent conflict between the need to violate an aspect of Mohan's autonomy (the fact that he is a Hindu) and his self-assertion (the fact that he wants to be left alone).

If Kathleen breaks in on Mohan's mourning, this will be a violation of his self-assertion. The only way it could be otherwise would be if Mohan does not enjoy self-ownership, but is owned by his physician or perhaps by his religion. That he is owned by his religion suggests that the autonomy that ought to be respected is not the uniqueness of Mohan but only one aspect of his uniqueness—his religion. It suggests that Mohan can be dealt with, not according to his uniqueness but according to the uniqueness of his religion.

The idea that Mohan's self-assertion might be the property of his physician is even more absurd. There is no way to make the idea that Mohan is owned by someone or something other than Mohan himself ethically intelligible. On the other hand, Kathleen would also violate Mohan's right to self-assertion. She would do this because his physician decided that the practices of Mohan's religion are more important to Mohan right now than his experience of the loss of his wife. This is not her decision to make. In asking to be left alone, Mohan made a decision from his autonomy concerning his self-assertion. If he has a right to autonomy and self-assertion, then, of necessity, he had a right to make that decision.

It might be argued that it is not Mohan, but his physician who decides what interactions Mohan finds desirable or undesirable. There is no reason to believe that Mohan would order his priorities in this way or turn his self-ownership over to his physician in this context. The conflict between Mohan's autonomy and his self-assertion is merely apparent. Both have been violated. There has been no conflict between them. No, even apparent, conflict between autonomy and self-assertion is possible. At least two other relevant series of events are possible here:

1. Kathleen does not disturb Mohan. The coroner takes the body of Mohan's wife and handles it through the usual procedures. In this case, apparently, Mohan maintains his self-assertion, but his right, and his wife's right, to autonomy may be violated.

Surely there must be a conflict here. But if we look at this series of events as it is, this is what we find. It is neither Kathleen nor the physician who violated Mohan's rights. If, in fact, anyone violated Mohan's rights, it was the coroner. Furthermore, note that no conflict between self-assertion and autonomy arises because the coroner does not become involved with Mohan's immediate control of his time and effort. Depending on other factors—the context of his knowledge and the intentions that motivate his actions—the coroner may be guilty of violating Mohan's autonomy or that of Mohan's wife (of course he is not).

2. It is possible that Mohan may require nursing and/or medical interventions. In this event, Kathleen must use careful contextual judgment. She must balance the importance of honoring Mohan's rights against the importance of the nursing or medical interventions.

If all Mohan needs to have is his morning care, it would be absurd for Kathleen to break in on his self-assertion. If he needs a vital medication, it would be absurd not to.

One does not have rights desire by desire, but in the context of one's life and over the whole span of one's life. What is and what is not a right is implied by the reigning agreement and is shaped by one's nature—and the context.

Whatever Kathleen does, she cannot escape a need for keen ethical judgment. No ethical agent can ever escape a need for ethical judgment.

Autonomy and Beneficence

> Perhaps no ethical dilemmas that a nurse faces are more common than those that arise through apparent conflicts between the requirements of beneficence and the recognition of autonomy.

Perhaps no ethical dilemmas that a nurse faces are more common than those that arise through apparent conflicts between the requirements of beneficence and the recognition of autonomy. For the biomedical professions as a whole, the most difficult and the most severe dilemmas arise through apparent conflicts between these two standards. These dilemmas do not arise in the context of the situation. They arise, whenever they do, in the context of the understanding or, more precisely, misunderstanding of the health care professional or her patient.

Dilemma 8.5

The classic case of a conflict between autonomy and beneficence is the case of a comatose Jehovah's Witness who needs a blood transfusion. His autonomy demands that, since he cannot explicitly communicate contrary wishes, it can be assumed that he would not want the transfusion. The standard of beneficence, on the other hand, demands that the professional act to bring about good. To allow a patient to die when he could have been saved is a very great failure to bring about good. Still, to give a patient a transfusion and save him, under these circumstances, might violate the standard of autonomy.

Autonomy and Fidelity

The primary responsibility for fulfilling the agreement between nurse and patient naturally lies with the nurse. It cannot be otherwise. The patient is a patient—one who is, to a greater or lesser extent, passive—unable to initiate action. Agency, the ability to initiate action, resides in the nurse. A patient is one who is affected by the action of an agent.

> The primary responsibility for fulfilling the agreement between nurse and patient naturally lies with the nurse.

Dilemma 8.6

Henry has a low tolerance to pain. He is very high strung and fearful. He makes such demands on his nurse Irene's time and energy that she cannot adequately attend to her other patients. Does Irene's recognition of Henry's autonomous nature demand of her that she ignore her responsibility to her other patients? Or does fidelity to her agreement with her other patients override her obligation to recognize Henry's autonomy?

The ethical situation that Irene faces is a dilemma that cannot be resolved by reference either to autonomy or to fidelity. The resolution demands a careful consideration of the definition of a nurse's profession (Husted & Husted, 1996).

Freedom and Objectivity

An apparent conflict between the standards of freedom and objectivity can arise whenever two or more people are interacting.

Dilemma 8.7

Bobby is 4 years old. He has a problem with bed wetting. Bobby has asked Marilyn, his nurse, not to tell his parents, and she has agreed. Bobby's parents are, perhaps, overly concerned with his bed wetting. When his parents come to visit, they ask Marilyn whether Bobby has been wetting the bed. If Marilyn tells them the truth, this will be perfectly in line with the usual understanding of the demands of the standard of objectivity. It may also interfere with the spontaneous and positive interactions between Bobby and his parents. It will interfere with the actions Bobby wants to take. Instead of being open and accepting, Bobby's parents may be harsh and forbidding.

In order to facilitate Bobby's freedom of action, Marilyn would have to practice deception. She would have to lie to Bobby's parents. One bioethical standard requires Marilyn to facilitate her patient's freedom of action. Another places a moral obligation upon her to deal with Bobby's parents on the basis of objectivity. The two together pose a dilemma for Marilyn. The dilemma apparently cannot be solved by reference to either standard alone.

Freedom and Self-Assertion

If any person enjoyed total and complete self-assertion, a question as to his right to take free action could not arise. But patients are in a situation where they cannot expect to enjoy complete self-assertion. If a patient had total and complete self-assertion, he would have no occasion to interact with another person. If he had no occasion to interact with another person, there would be no one to interfere with his freedom of action.

Responsibility with respect to a patient's right to self-assertion also involves a responsibility to respect his freedom. Self-assertion (a person's right and power to control his or her time and effort and freedom) and a person's right and power to choose and pursue long-term actions guided by objective awareness are, obviously, intimately connected. But one does not necessarily depend upon the other.

> Responsibility with respect to a patient's right to self-assertion also involves a responsibility to respect his freedom.

Linda stops a former patient passing in the street to ask how he is. This is a way of interfering with her former patient's action, but it is an entirely blameless way. It is not a violation of his self-assertion. This form of interfering with a person's action is of no ethical importance. Interruptions of a patient's freedom of action through an invasion of his self-assertion can occur in two ways:

1. Linda interrupts a patient's action even though the goal of this action is one upon which the patient places a high degree of importance and Linda knows this.
2. Linda does not interfere with any important action her patient wishes to take. However, she subjects him to a constant series of minor interruptions. She violates his right to take actions simply by the repetition of minor obstructions to his self-assertion and Linda knows this.

> Occasions can arise when not interfering with a patient's action would mean a loss of his power of self-assertion.

Occasions can arise when not interfering with a patient's action would mean a loss of his power of self-assertion. For instance, if a nurse fails to interfere with a patient's actions when these actions might, foreseeably, injure the patient. There are also occasions when invading a patient's self-assertion will result in preserving his power of self-assertion. This occurs, for instance, every time a nurse awakens a patient (invades his self-assertion) in order to give him his medication (and thus ensure his future power of self-assertion).

A dilemma involving the standards of freedom and self-assertion could oc-cur in this way:

Dilemma 8.8

A caller phones the nurse's station and speaks to Lotte, Ray's nurse. The caller tells Lotte that he is Ray's lawyer. He tells her that he was to come in today for Ray to sign his new will, but he is unable to get there today. He asks Lotte if he might come in the next day to see Ray. Lotte knows that there is a strong possibility that Ray might not live that long.

If she tells the caller of Ray's condition, she may violate the standard of self-assertion. She has no way of being certain that the caller is Ray's lawyer. There is a definite possibility that the caller is a speculator who could use a prior knowledge of Ray's impending death to profit by undermining the value of Ray's corporation. If she does not tell the caller of Ray's impending death, there is a possibility that this will interfere with Ray's freedom to take actions that are vitally important to him. It will require a particularly keen attention to the context to resolve this dilemma.

Freedom and Beneficence

An apparent conflict between freedom and benefi-cence is a conflict in which a patient's desire to avoid acting stands in opposition to his well-being.

> An apparent conflict between freedom and beneficence is a conflict in which a patient's desire to avoid acting stands in opposition to his well-being.

Dilemma 8.9

Margaret is 87 years old. She is very feeble and is kept restrained in a wheelchair. She complains to her nurse, Sandra, that she wants to be "untied" so that she can walk around. Sandra knows that there is a very good chance that if Margaret were to walk around, she might fall. If she fell, she could severely, painfully, and permanently injure herself. This would cause her to lose the safe freedom of action she already enjoys. Untying Margaret would violate both beneficence and freedom. Assume, however, that the only freedom Margaret could enjoy, since she cannot sit for any length of time, would be to walk around. A small change in the context changes a fairly clear-cut situation into an ethical dilemma. A minor change in the context will often have major ethical repercussions.

Freedom and Fidelity

Dilemma 8.10

Charlie, a heart attack patient, is having a heated argument with a business associate. He regards the favorable resolution of this argument as being of extreme importance to his career. Ingrid, Charlie's nurse, wants to call a halt to this argument, but Charlie wants to continue it. Ingrid believes, rightly, that this argument places Charlie's health and, possibly, even his life in jeopardy. It is Charlie's life to do with as he wills. If Charlie has a right to live, then he has a right to take chances. Life requires one to take chances.

At the same time, Ingrid has had Charlie's health care placed in her hands. Her knowledge of the requirements of effective medical care is much greater than Charlie's. She has a responsibility to protect Charlie's life and health.

If Charlie exercises his right to take free action, Ingrid cannot exercise fidelity to her agreement. In order to exercise fidelity to the nurse–patient agreement, she must interfere with Charlie's freedom of action.

Nurses, generally, tend to argue in favor of Ingrid's right to interfere with Charlie. At the same time, they tend to argue against Sandra's right to interfere with Margaret.

But, in relation to the bioethical standards of freedom and fidelity, there are no fundamental differences between the two cases. From this perspective, these cases are identical. The difference is in the context. Each case places a patient's right to take certain actions in opposition to a nurse's responsibility to protect his well-being. Once again, the dilemma must be resolved by means of the contextual application of the standards. Nurses tend to argue rightly. Margaret is 87 years old. At this age, whatever pleasure and comfort she might gain is worth some risk, which can be minimized. Charlie is not 87 years old. If he is 47, he is risking, perhaps, 40 years. This risk cannot be minimized.

Objectivity and Self-Assertion

If a nurse is to defend her right to self-assertion—her own right to self-ownership—she must take certain positive actions. She must actively maintain her right not to disclose any fact if this disclosure would threaten her right of self-ownership and place her in an unfavorable condition. If a nurse is to defend a patient's right to self-assertion, she must have the same attitude toward her patient. She must maintain her right not to disclose any fact when she is aware that this disclosure would threaten her patient's right of self-assertion.

Two nurses, Sybil and Janet, work together and maintain a friendly relationship with one another. This relationship includes going out to dinner together occasionally.

Sybil and Janet are both aware that, at some future time, together they may be in competition for the position of head nurse. This awareness has never before influenced their relationship. One evening, Sybil tells Janet that a mutual friend has said that Janet is a recovering alcoholic. She asks Janet if this is true.

In fact, Janet is a recovering alcoholic. She can affirm that she is a recovering alcoholic or she can deny it. Or she can refuse to discuss the topic. If Janet does not deny this fact or if she refuses to discuss the topic, then Sybil will have every reason to believe that the information she has received is accurate.

It is quite possible that Sybil could use this information to prevent Janet's being considered for the position of head nurse. Then again, Sybil might never use the information in this way. It is very possible that Sybil is simply "making small talk" and is not at all thinking of violating Janet's right to self-ownership.

Janet faces a dilemma. If she tells the truth, and friends are justified in expecting the truth from each other, she surrenders her right to self-assertion. If she decides to maintain her self-assertion, she will have to lie to Sybil.

Let us look at a different situation:

Dilemma 8.11

Karen has entered the hospital and had an abortion. Her husband, Steve, a salesman, has been out of town. He locates Karen's nurse and asks her why Karen is in the hospital.

This presents a dilemma. Karen's nurse knows nothing about the circumstances surrounding the relationship between Karen and Steve. If she tells Steve that Karen has had an abortion, she may be violating Karen's right to control her time and effort. If she does not tell him, she is violating the standard of objectivity—and probably for no reason. If she refuses to tell him anything, her refusal might cause Steve great anxiety. It might also sow the seeds of distrust in his mind.

It would be very desirable if a nurse had a way to deal with such dilemmas before they arose. But sometimes, the nature of the context cannot be determined before the dilemma.

Objectivity and Beneficence

Apparent conflicts between objectivity and beneficence produce a great number of ethical dilemmas.

Apparent conflicts between objectivity and beneficence produce a great number of ethical dilemmas.

Dilemma 8.12

Hugh is dying. Lucy, his nurse, believes that his death is imminent. She remembers that Denise, his wife, had expressed a desire to be with her husband when he dies. Hugh and Denise had agreed to be with each other at the end so that the person who died first would not die alone. Lucy calls Denise to tell her of her husband's condition. It is a rather long time before Denise arrives at the hospital. Denise is blind and she must find someone willing to drive her to the hospital. By the time she arrives, Hugh has died.

Before Lucy takes her into her husband's room, Denise expresses how glad she is to have arrived before his death. She spends several minutes in the room with her husband. She does not know that he was already dead when she arrived. If Lucy tells Denise that her husband died before she arrived, she honors the conventional standard of objectivity but fails the test of beneficence. If Lucy tells her that she was with her husband while he was still alive, Lucy violates the standard of objectivity but meets the test of beneficence. This poses a dilemma.

Objectivity and Fidelity

By the nature of things, conflicts between the standards of objectivity and fidelity cannot arise. Fidelity to the nurse/patient agreement entails objectivity in two ways:

1. The terms of the agreement must be objectively understood.
2. Actions that satisfy the standard of fidelity must be understood objectively.

But, in some unusual cases, a seeming conflict can arise:

Dilemma 8.13

Ike is Joan's patient. Ike's prognosis is poor. For reasons known only to himself, Ike does not want his wife, Helen, to be told of his prognosis. There are a number of legal and practical arrangements that must be made, and Helen needs to know the facts of Ike's condition.

If Joan reveals Ike's prognosis to Helen, she violates the agreement she has with Ike and she has lied to Ike. But doesn't Joan have an ethical obligation to Helen? If she does not tell Helen the truth, it will mean an avoidable future hardship for Helen. Joan is not certain that Ike understands this.

Joan faces a dilemma that cannot be resolved either by reference to objectivity or by reference to fidelity.

Self-Assertion and Beneficence

Taken to the extreme, either self-assertion or beneficence would make the exercise of the other impossible.

If any person had the isolation of perfect self-assertion, it would not be possible for another person to act benevolently toward him, nor would it be necessary. If a person enjoyed perfect self-assertion—if he enjoyed perfect control over his time and effort—this would entail that he would succeed in achieving the objects of all his actions. In this case, no one could act benevolently toward him. No one could bring any value into his life that he could not achieve in his own time and by his own effort.

If any person had the means to unlimited beneficence no one would be foolish enough to interfere with his self-assertion.

Let us look at a more common dilemma:

Dilemma 8.14

Doris brings Shawn, her 5-year-old son, into a clinic to be treated for injuries sustained through a fall. Alice, the nurse who treats Shawn, recognizes that his injuries are much more consistent with battering than with a fall. Beneficence seems to demand that Alice report her belief that Shawn is a battered child. She cannot do this, however, without creating an invasion of Doris' self-assertion. Whatever she does, she ought to do it only with full awareness.

Self-Assertion and Fidelity

A nurse has a moral obligation to remain faithful to her agreement with her patient. However, her obligation to exercise fidelity does not end with her obligation to her patient. As an ethical agent and as a nurse, she also has an obligation to exercise fidelity toward her colleagues and toward her employing institution.

She also has an obligation to exercise fidelity toward a patient's family members when, otherwise, their rights would be violated.

> nurse has a moral obliga-
> n to remain faithful to her
> greement with her patient.

Apparent conflicts between the standards of self-assertion and fidelity are rare, but here is one possibility:

Beneficence and Fidelity

There are no conflicts between beneficence and fidelity.

A hypothetical conflict would take something like this form: John is going to have his leg amputated. Suddenly, he changes his mind. He asks not to be anesthetized. Marilyn, his nurse, is determined that he shall receive the benefits for which he entered the hospital. The operation is performed.

Dilemma 8.15

Dan is in a nursing home suffering from Huntington's chorea. He will remain there until his death because he is no longer able to care for himself. He and his ex-wife have been divorced for the last 4 years. She comes in occasionally to visit him with their two children, Lauren (age 6) and Brian (age 9). Dan has made it quite clear to the physician and nurses that he does not want his ex-wife or children to be told his diagnosis. But if the children do not know of his condition, they will not be able to make an informed decision about having children of their own. Does Dan have a right to have his request honored?

Such an event, of course, could never occur. For this reason, no actual conflict between beneficence and fidelity has been shown.

For Marilyn to maintain fidelity to her agreement by coercing John into going through with the operation would involve an absolutely unjustifiable breach of his freedom. The agreement cannot be met in this manner. A dilemma that is resolved by coercion is not really resolved. A dilemma that is created by coercion is resolved by pointing out the coercion.

Musings

The bioethical standards can ease a nurse into the bioethical context. They can make it easier for her to resolve ethical dilemmas. But conflicts in the interpretation of the bioethical standards can arise (Figure 8.1). When this occurs, they cannot be resolved in the context they have created. A wider context must be formed.

8.1

Only apparent.

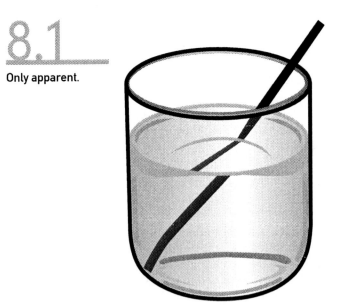

Study Guide

1. Think about your own life and how you have been conflicted in what you want to do versus what your rational nature guides you to do. Exercise your ability to critically think about this and to see where your thinking has gone astray.
2. Take a patient who is doing something very destructive to his health—a patient with COPD who is smoking, a diabetic patient who refuses to stay on any kind of diet, and so forth. Most always these patients, as with all patients, will say that they want to be well and yet their behavior says otherwise. How might you help this patient to be motivated to regain his health?
3. Could the use of gentle coercion be of some help in the above situation?

References

Howe, E. G. (1993). The vagaries of patients' and families' discussing advance directives. *Journal of Clinical Ethics, 4,* 3–7.

Husted, G. L., & Husted, J. H. (1996). Ethical dilemmas: Time and fidelity. *American Journal of Nursing, 96*(11), 23.

Rhodes, R. (1992). Cases from Mount Sinai School of Medicine, CUNY. *American Philosophical Association Newsletter on Philosophy and Medicine, 91,* 75–76.

Tannsjo, T. (1999). Informal coercion in the physical care of patients suffering from senile dementia or mental retardation. *Nursing Ethics, 6,* 327–336.

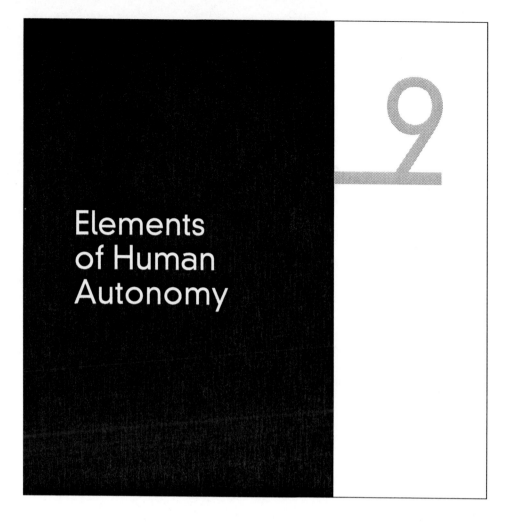

Elements of Human Autonomy

In our backyard, there lives a free-spirited bird named Ickarow. One day, some time ago, the way he tells it, Ickarow noticed that when he flies from tree to tree, the air presses against his body, slowing the rate of speed he could otherwise attain. Ickarow, oblivious to the need for analysis, has decided to fly up above the air so that he will be able to fly faster, more easily, and efficiently.

"Poor misguided Ickarow," we say. But is not a professional who hopes to arrive at an objectively justifiable ethical decision without a prior exercise of observation and analysis fully as misguided as Ickarow hoping to fly in a vacuum? She has lost her context as fully as Ickarow. She will never understand the ethics of her profession, no more than Ickarow understands the mechanics of flying.

Analyzing Autonomy

Ethical decision making must be preceded by ethical judgment. It cannot be any better than the judgment on which it is based. Before an ethical agent can know what to do, he or she must understand the independent uniqueness of who is involved, the nature of the circumstances in which it is being done, and why it is being done. This knowledge is gained only through judgment. A perfected judgment is enriched by the elements of individual autonomy. The validity and value of every later judgment must be formed in the light of the first judgment—the assessment of autonomy.

The autonomy of an individual is the unique nature of that individual. The elements of autonomy are the elements of human nature. They are the principles that give every individual person a human nature. They are properties or characteristics possessed by a human person simply because he or she is a human person. They form the nature of the person.

The elements of autonomy will serve the following tasks for a health care professional:

- They can facilitate her acquaintance with the nature of her patient. If necessary, they will enable her to make a rigorous analysis of her patient's nature and see into his values and motivations.

If a professional's objectives are to be met successfully, the road to success is understanding the patient's unique character. The measure of her ethical competence is how well her actions reflect that understanding.

The best way to achieve that understanding is to understand what he has created out of his human nature (his virtues). While, at the same time, never forgetting the human nature out of which he created these virtues.

> The measure of her ethical competence is how well her actions reflect that understanding.

- They enable a nurse to clarify the precise nature of the dilemma she faces.

The ethical aspects of the patient's situation profoundly evolve from the way it affects him, the way he evaluates it, and in his reaction to it. Many of a nurse's ethical dilemmas arise when these evaluations and reactions are inappropriate to the situation. These evaluations and reactions arise from the way the elements of autonomy are lived by this patient. These elements are given to him. But within the limits of what they make possible, how he lives them is very revealing.

- There are certain circumstances in which, for various reasons, the elements of autonomy serve better to resolve dilemmas than do the bioethical standards.

Generally, these will be when a nurse must do more than simply interact with a patient—when she must, in effect, also act for a patient.

The elements of autonomy are especially effective in the analysis of five types of dilemma:

1. When a nurse cannot speak to her patient, but must speak for her patient (e.g., when she speaks for an embryo or an infant; when her patient speaks

a foreign language or comes from a significantly different culture; when her patient is comatose or otherwise incapable of communicating).

2. When a nurse is acquainted with her patient's unique and individual nature well enough that she can actively engage the elements of his autonomy—his objectivity just as his way of reasoning, his idiosyncratic ways of dealing with topics on which he cannot or will not deal objectively, his benefit seeking as revealing his motivating desires, and so on—into her analysis. This is very rare.

3. When a nurse joins a patient in deliberating about his future purposes and actions.

4. When a marriage partner, significant other, or a parent wants to confer with a nurse regarding decisions for a patient.

5. When her patient is a psychiatric patient. The elements of autonomy are the ethical bridge to a psychiatric patient.

One becomes autonomous when he takes his innate elements and develops them as virtues or vices.

No one can be human and be completely unfamiliar with that which makes him autonomous. Everyone is familiar with the elements of human autonomy, at least on an implicit level. It is quite advantageous for a nurse to become familiar with them explicitly.

Dilemma 9.1

Vladimir, a concert pianist, has sustained an injury that may affect his ability to play the piano. There are two operations that could be performed. One operation has a 90% chance of restoring gross movements of the hand and eliminating pain. Another experimental operation has about a 10% success rate in restoring fine motor coordination. However, if this operation were to fail, Vladimir would lose much of the gross movement of his hand. Vladimir must make a decision. The decision regards the possibility of achieving a value or the loss of a value. The value of being able to play the piano must be considered in the context of other activities that Vladimir values. The decision that Vladimir must make is an ethical decision. The action he will take, based on this decision, is an ethical action.

Vladimir must take into consideration these two essential facts: The success rate for one operation is 90%; for the other, it is 10%. When making his decision, Vladimir must consider the value he places on his ability to play the piano. He must also consider the disadvantages of losing gross motor coordination. The situation can guide Vladimir's action through the desires that enable him to understand himself and his life. By means of these desires, Vladimir can reason the relative desirability of both operations. We can assist him in this process.

In order to interact effectively with Vladimir, we will have to join him in this process. We will have to get into his ethical context—the context of his vital purposes.

Desire and the Ethical Context

Imagine a world in which desire is not a part of human nature. This world is a tropical island floating among the clouds. On this island, all the necessities of survival—fruit trees, cool water, and so on—are readily at hand. There is no motivation through discontent, no awareness that human life can be more than the basic necessities. The faculty of human desire has withered away or the inhabitants of the world never possessed this faculty.

In this world, there are no specific human realities. There are no human purposes, no human choices, and no human actions. In this world, every action is conducted on an animal level. Therefore, nothing is either good or evil. Nothing is either right or wrong.

In such a world, ethics, as a study, would be inconceivable. In this world where there is no human desire, there are no vital and fundamental goals. If there are no vital and fundamental goals, there is no need for a system of standards to motivate, determine, or justify these goals. Without human desire, human life would be unimportant. If desire were not an element of human nature, there would be no ethical realities of any sort. Ethical realities exist in the world only because desire is an element of human nature.

> Ethical realities exist in the world only because desire is an element of human nature.

Desire as "The Essence of Man"

The following is not based on a rigid exposition of Spinoza's thought. Spinoza is speaking "of the face of the entire universe" and this, "under the aspect of eternity." We are speaking of the health care arena—tomorrow and the next few days. We are in a totally different context. However, we believe that this approach is ultimately justifiable in Spinozist terms. In the meantime, we offer this as: "Variations on a Theme by Spinoza."

The great ethicist, Benedict Spinoza (1632–1688), said of desire that it is the essence of man. By "desire," we will mean all of the physiological and psychological processes that constitute the life of an individual person. Desire is defined as: . . . that, which being given, [the person] itself is necessarily [given], and, being taken away, [the person] is necessarily taken [away]; or, in other words, that without which [the person] can neither be nor be conceived, and which in its turn cannot be nor be conceived without [the person]. (Spinoza, 1685/1949, p. 89)

The term *desire*, insofar as it signifies an element of individual autonomy, has a specific meaning. It does not refer to any single desire for any single value. It does not even refer to the whole collection of a person's desires. It refers to the defining fact of human existence. It is the nature or "essence" of every individual person (Husted, 1988).

This makes desire much more than simply a psychological reality. It makes every process sustaining the life of a person, an aspect of desire. From this perspective, every fact about an individual human being, and about all human beings, could, in principle, be explained in terms of desire.

This definition perfectly defines desire in a professional context. This point is so important, and so potentially valuable to a nurse in understanding her profession, that we will examine this definition of desire on a simpler level than we have presented it, and in detail:

> This makes desire much more than simply a psychological reality. It makes every process of a person, as a living thing, an aspect of desire.

- There is a minor difference in the chemical composition of males and females, but basically every person has the same chemical composition.
- Everyone's physiology is basically the same.
- Everyone has the same world to think about.
- Everyone's life depends on the same basic conditions.
- All people are limited, in the same ways, in the actions that they can take.
- Everyone has the same rights to life and action.

Despite all this, each and every person is different—is autonomous—in a vitally important way. There is one human attribute in which every individual person is different from every other. This attribute is human desire—as a psychological reality.

We define desire as including, "all of the physiological and psychological processes that constitute the life of an individual person." This gives the concept of desire an organic grounding. Without this organic grounding, human desire may easily seem to be either arbitrary—whimsical, transient, and, therefore, unimportant, or a passion—a behavior entirely determined from influences outside of the agent. This would make it of no greater ethical value than any other externally determined passion, for instance, tripping on a stone. But desire is an expression of the essential being of a human agent.

Given an organic, vis-à-vis, a purely psychological grounding, it follows that, for example, a tree in the actions of its roots and leaves exhibits a form of desire. In humans, the same kind of organic actions occur. A human is unaware of these actions and the accompanying circumstances of his organism. These vital and fundamental actions we can refer to as a form (albeit a primitive form) of desire. Desire, of course, includes those conditions and actions of the organism of which a human is conscious and the conscious ideas that motivate her to take purposeful action. All of these constitute the desire of the ethical agent.

Desire and the Nurse's Orientation to Nursing

A professional ethic, at all odds, should be appropriate to the profession whose members it is set to guide. Every profession arises out of human purposes and desires. Nursing and the biomedical sciences arose out of the desire to regain

Dilemma 9.2

Mr. Judd, age 64, comes into the hospital to have a tumor (later discovered to be benign) removed from his jaw. During the surgery, he suffers a cerebral vascular accident (CVA). Three weeks after the CVA, the physician asks the family about withdrawing food and fluids, and allowing Mr. Judd to die naturally. Mr. Judd has no living will or durable power of attorney for health care. His wife and children turn to Amanda, Mr. Judd's primary care nurse, for advice. On assessment, Amanda finds that Mr. Judd responds occasionally to simple commands, such as, "Squeeze my hands," "Turn your head," "Blink your eyes," and so on. Based on these observations, Amanda tries to talk to the physician. The physician insists that food and fluids be withdrawn. He believes that Mr. Judd will never get any better. Are there any further steps that Amanda ought to take?

health and well-being, as well as to alleviate pain. Therefore, a nursing ethic ought to be appropriate to this desire. Without human desire regarded as important, what would be the need for nurses: What important human purpose could nurses and nursing serve?

> Nursing and the biomedical sciences arose out of the desire to regain health and well-being, as well as to alleviate pain. Therefore, a nursing ethic ought to be appropriate to this desire.

A nursing ethic needs a logical basis for empathy with the desire to regain health and well-being. Without this basis, a nursing ethic becomes pointless. There will be no necessary and permanent connection between dilemmas and ethical analysis. Dilemmas will be subject to being resolved by convention and convenience.

An explicit empathy with human desire, as such, is the only logical basis for empathy with an individual's desire. If a nurse does not have empathy with human desire as such, she will not have empathy with a patient's desire for health and well-being. On what basis could a nursing ethic, for instance, approve of the desire for health and well-being, while not approving the desire for autonomy, freedom, and, ultimately, happiness? No health professional who lacks empathy with desire as a human reality has a stable empathy for any individual patient or any individual person. Caring is empathy for another person's desires, or it is quite cold and impersonal.

No bioethical standard is desired by a patient for its own sake. The reason for this is very simple. No bioethical standard exists in isolation from the purposes to which agents direct it.

> No bioethical standard is desired by a patient for its own sake.

Wen is in the hospital. His nurse, Evelyn, is quite aware of Wen's uniqueness. Evelyn's recognition of Wen's uniqueness, however, is utterly valueless to Wen. In itself, uniqueness is without any ethical importance. Uniqueness becomes autonomy—an ethical standard and concern—insofar as a person expresses this uniqueness by acting on his personal desires.

If Evelyn recognizes that Wen is an accountant, a wood-carver, a husband, the father of two children, and that he lives beside a river, her recognition of Wen and his circumstances is of no great ethical advantage. How could it be? The census taker who talks to Wen in his workshop recognizes this much.

Another nurse, Jennifer, begins with the awareness that Wen is motivated by desire. She recognizes that Wen desires to earn a living, perfect his skill at carving horses, retain the love of his wife, happiness for his children, and to return to his home beside the river. Jennifer empathizes with Wen's desires. This fosters understanding between Jennifer and Wen. It provides the basis for an ethical interaction between them.

A nurse will seldom, and perhaps never, encounter an ethical dilemma that she can resolve with a ballistic accuracy. Ethical dilemmas involving unique and "inconvenient" desires lend themselves, less than any other, to a clear-cut resolution.

Dilemma 9.3

Nine-year-old Wally was badly burned in a fire at his home. Iris, his nurse, comes to take him for debriding. Wally begins to cry and tells Iris he does not want to go. His face trembles, and he screams, "I'll go when my Mommy comes." Wally's mother was killed in the fire. Without any further discussion, Iris agrees not to take him.

The short-term benefit that Wally received by not undergoing the pain of debriding might not, all things being equal, compensate for the long-term detriment. But then, Iris must consider the possible effect on Wally if he is told under these circumstances that his mother is dead. Iris has, in a sense, done Wally some good. She may have done him greater harm. It is not possible to calculate the amount of good or harm that Iris has done Wally. The harm Iris did was permanent. Perhaps the good was also permanent.

Everyone desires to give and receive that which is good. Everyone desires to avoid that which is harmful. But in every concrete situation, it is not always easy to recognize what is good and what is harmful. Perhaps it is the last skill that a nurse masters.

Desire and Ethical Decision Making

In a solitary context, what any person ought to do, among other things, is determined by what he wants to do and what he can do. What action he wants to take depends on why he is acting—the nature of his purposes. There are other principles of ethical action to be considered. But ethical decision making begins in desire and is appropriately shaped by concern for every element of autonomy.

> In a solitary context, what any person ought to do, among other things, is determined by what he wants to do and what he can do.

In an interpersonal context, there would never be any reason for ethical decision making if it were not for desire. Agents form an agreement and begin to interact. They need a way to define the purposes of their interaction. They need a way to keep their desires in harmony. The desire that originally motivated them provides that way.

Self-Preservation of Desire

It is desire that brings a nurse into the nurse–patient agreement—her desire to be a nurse. The patient's desires are, so to speak, forced upon him. It is these desires that determine the decision a professional ought to make and the actions she ought to take. The desires that illness or injury force upon a patient make nursing what it is.

> *In one way or another, whatever a person does and whatever a person is are determined first by desire. Spinoza, tells us that, "Desire is the essence of a man, that is to say, [desire is] the effort by which a man strives to persevere in his being" (1685/1949, p. 201).*

At one end of our existence, this desire motivates us to fill our basic needs. On the other end, it inspires the highest creations of the human mind.

But desire can be thought of as more than this. It can be thought of as the energy of life. All the processes that preserve and enhance the life of the organism arise from desire. Life desires itself. From metabolism to reason, two forms of the energy of life, these processes serve to preserve and/or enhance the life of the organism. Reason does this fully as much as any other vital process. Reason, itself, can be thought of as a form of desire. It is a process that produces understanding. The achievement of understanding satisfies the desire for understanding. Understanding serves human agency and human life.

A person lost in a forest might feel a desire to create shelter for himself. He might examine all the resources about him and figure a way to build a shelter. If he cuts his arm, the laceration will likely heal itself. In several ways these processes—to feel, to examine, to build, and to heal—are very different. But they are alike in one very significant way: each is a way nature has programmed the living organism to preserve its existence as a living organism. In a widened sense of *desire*, each process can be thought of as a form of desire.

In the case of a patient, there is the most intimate connection between these different forms of desire. A patient's rational decision to enter the health care setting is motivated by his desire to regain his health. His desire to end the pain he suffers and to regain his health arises from and is an extension of unconscious bodily processes. These physiological processes are those that the body sets in motion in the healing process.

We can view the whole process—the healing processes by which the body regenerates itself, the conscious feeling of desire, and the reasoning process that produces the decision—as three expressions or steps of one natural drive. In one way or another, this whole process can be seen as the working of desire.

We can also view this process mechanistically. We can look at it as three different processes, one following on another and each moving in a different direction. If we do analyze the processes in this way, we view them like billiard balls striking one another on a billiard table. Then we have carved the patient into three parts—a body, an emotional capacity, and a mind.

To do this would be in conflict with biomedical thinking. Biomedicine has begun to think of the patient as a unitary being—one who is to be understood holistically. It would also be in conflict with the patient's thinking. The patient is not a mind bringing a body into the health care setting. Nor is a patient a body bringing a mind into the health care setting.

If we look at humans holistically, we see their lives, as they live them, as conscious and embodied desire. In humans, reason is the instrument by which this desire preserves itself. Desire begins the process. Reason is the way that desire keeps it (keeps itself) going.

The biomedical arts are ways in which people preserve their lives. Medicine is the child of desire and reason.

Reason and Desire

Desire is, like fire, a useful servant but a fearful master. (Author unknown)

Every person is inspired by a desire to pursue the good as he sees it. The good is the object of desire. The good is, as Thomas Aquinas observed, a form of the true. The true is the object of reason.

That which can be good, however, is good only if it is true, only if it actually exists or can be brought into existence. The pursuit of the good ought to be guided by the knowledge that it does exist, either actually or potentially. It ought to be known that that which is pursued is truly good. This must be discovered by reason.

Ethical action is the pursuit of vital and fundamental goals. The goals of the health care professions are vital and fundamental values. For the health care professions, as for all ethical action, it is reason that makes the pursuit of these values possible.

> That which can be good, however, is good only if it is true, only if it actually exists or can be brought into existence.

Socrates said of reason that it is man's means to pursue the good. Aristotle said of reason that it is man's means to happiness. For the American logician and philosopher of science Charles Sanders Peirce, reason is important because it is man's means of refining his beliefs. For novelist–philosopher Ayn Rand, reason has ethical importance because it is man's means of survival.

Where there is good or the possibility of good in the world, where happiness is possible, where belief needs to be refined, and where survival is a problem that must be faced, there is an ethical universe. This universe calls for practical reason and ethical action.

In an ethical universe, desire is a human's source of action. Reasoning power allows a person to discover intelligible relations in his or her experience of the world. Reason allows the individual to adapt his or her actions in the pursuit of that which he or she experiences as good. In this sense, reason is the comrade-in-arms of all ethical action. Reason is the choreographer of intelligible causal sequences.

A human is, in the classic definition, a rational animal. Imagine what your condition would be if you entirely lacked reason. Your relationship to your reason is so intimate that your condition cannot be easily imagined if you were deprived of reason. Without the use of your reason, you would have no more autonomy, freedom, or self-ownership than an earthworm. Animals, when they are not driven by basic needs, do little more than sleep.

> Reason is the choreographer of intelligible causal sequences.

It is through reason that nurses are able to consider the rationale for their actions, the scope and extent of their participation in decision making, and the manner in which decisions are to be made and to be implemented (Milstead, 1999). A nurse who totally lacked reason would not be able to understand or to act on the bioethical standards. She would, in fact, not be able to act on or to understand anything at all. To the extent that she does lack reason, or is unable to exercise it, she is unable to act or to understand. Even minor lapses of reason—such as occur when under stress and unless she has made awareness of the character structures second nature—may make it temporarily impossible for her to be guided by the bioethical standards.

Each of the bioethical standards arises as a form of desire and is activated in response to desire or is based upon some form of desire. In an ethical sense, each is also a virtue, a form of reason or knowledge. Each virtue is reasoning desire.

Dilemma 9.4

Donna is a nurse in the neonatal intensive care unit. Maureen, her patient, has given birth to a very premature infant. The infant does not weigh quite 2 pounds and cannot breathe spontaneously on his own. The amniocentesis reveals that the infant has Down's syndrome. A sonogram shows that the baby suffers from a severe heart defect. Maureen asks Donna for information and advice. Her baby has only about a 5% chance of living. If the baby does live, he will have severe mental and physical handicaps. The neonatologist wants to treat the baby aggressively. Maureen asks Donna if she should allow this treatment.

Considering the limited potentiality of this baby's life, the demands of beneficence are not easy to determine here. But they must be determined. Beneficence has to be a part of life for life to flourish. At the same time it is, at least, open to question whether beneficence always demands preserving life. Life needs beneficence very much in the same way it needs justice. When a nurse diligently fulfills her part of the nurse–patient agreement, she acts beneficently. She also acts as she has agreed to act. Therefore she acts with justice.

Reason as the Basis of the Bioethical Standards

All of a patient's choices, values, and actions begin in desire. A nurse ought to easily understand this. All of her choices, values, and actions begin in desire. Those choices and actions that do not begin in her autonomous desire are not hers. Not surprisingly, she experiences them as alien. She experiences them as something outside of herself. The patient's experience of his desire is precisely the same. A patient, being in a state of enforced passivity, experiences most of his choices and actions as alien and not his own. He experiences them as being forced upon him. A nurse has a significant advantage in understanding her patient if she understands this part of his experience. Her task—for his benefit and hers—is to make them the product of his virtues.

Everyone's choices, values, and actions begin in desire. These, however, should not be allowed to continue in desire alone.

A professional's ethical thinking begins as a meditation on desire. But, very early on, it should be turned over to reason. This is true because of the nature of ethics—the structure of the world we live in, the nature of desire, and the irreplaceable necessity of reason. Ethical action is action toward vital and fundamental goals. Any action taken toward vital and fundamental goals must be sustained by reason. Otherwise, there would be no way for a nurse to be aware—and no way for a patient to be aware—that they are vital and fundamental goals and ought to be pursued as vital and fundamental goals.

Dilemma 9.5

Little Sandy is in the hospital to have his tonsils removed. Sandy is screaming and crying. He does not want to have the operation. The surgeon brings in the consent form for Sandy's mother to sign. Sometime later, Sandy's nurse gives him the preoperative medications.

This seems to be an easy case with which to deal. It seems this way only because we take so much for granted. Sandy's tonsils are infected. It would be reasonable for them to be taken out. On the other hand, Sandy is already an autonomous individual. Autonomous individuals have rights.

At first glance, this situation seems to present no particular problems. Sandy must be operated on. All the same, ask yourself these questions:

1. Does Sandy's mother have an ethical right to sign the consent form?
2. Does Sandy's nurse have an ethical right to give him the preoperative medications?
3. Does the surgeon have an ethical right to operate on Sandy?
   Now, assuming that Sandy has no rights protecting him against this procedure (and, in every culture, we take it for granted that he has not), consider these questions:

4. When and how will Sandy acquire the rights that would protect him against this procedure?
5. Do Sandy's mother, the surgeon, and the nurse have rights that would protect them against undergoing this procedure involuntarily?
6. If so, when and how did Sandy's mother, the surgeon, and the nurse acquire these rights?
7. When and how will Sandy acquire the rights that his mother, the surgeon, and the nurse possess?
8. Will Sandy ever acquire the right to decide for his child? If so, when, why, and how?

We must assume that, at some time in his life, Sandy will acquire the right to decide for his child. If he does not, then neither did his mother ever acquire the right to decide for him. It seems as though reason is on the side of Sandy's tormenters. In reason, Sandy ought to have the operation. In reason, there is no reason for Sandy not to have the operation. There is no reason except Sandy's desire not to have it.

At the same time, it is a fact that Sandy is an autonomous ethical agent. If Sandy's autonomy will not protect him, nothing ever will.

The most rational course of action to be taken is for Sandy to have his tonsils removed. Can the reason why the others possess the rights they do be because reason is on their side? Does Sandy lack rights in this circumstance because reason is against him? Sandy's case shows the fragile interweaving of reason, autonomy, and individual rights.

It seems, then, that a conflict between reason and autonomy is built into the nature of rights. On the one hand, people possess rights "by virtue of their rationality." On the other hand, they can interact with others only if others give their "voluntary consent" to the interaction. This voluntary consent, in addition, must be "objectively gained." People possess rights by virtue of their capacity to reason. But they can interact with others only according to the autonomy of those others.

> On the one hand, people possess rights "by virtue of their rationality." On the other hand, they can interact with others only if others give their "voluntary consent" to the interaction.

Conflicts can arise, even among benevolent people, over the question of rights. Most of these conflicts involve:

- One person's belief that reason demands or justifies an action.
- Another person's belief that this action would violate his autonomy—his right to be what and who he is.

Everyone has a right not to be aggressed against, coerced, or defrauded. This is the implicit agreement. It is the basis of ethical interaction. In addition to the universal rights agreement, a special implicit agreement is formed between nurse and patient. Special conflicts can arise here. Conflicts sometimes arise as to what constitutes aggression, coercion, or fraud. Although one person's reason tells him the other's rights have not been violated, the other's reason will tell him they have. Here autonomy must prevail. Some middle ground must be found between the reasoning of one person and the autonomy of another.

Dilemma 9.6

Roger is an elderly man who was brought into the hospital because of dehydration as a result of the flu. While Roger is in the hospital, his physician realizes that Roger's pacemaker needs to be replaced. The physician and nurse go in to talk to Roger about the scheduling of the operation. After the physician leaves, Roger tells his nurse that he has no intention of having the operation. The last time he had a pacemaker put in, he suffered a stroke that left him confined to a wheelchair.

Even at his advanced age, Roger has autonomous purposes for his life. When he analyzes the benefit of having the pacemaker replaced (another year of life) against the drawbacks (the possibility of having another stroke and becoming completely dependent on others, or the possibility of not surviving the operation). he decides that his most reasonable course of action is not to have his pacemaker replaced.

On the other hand, when his pacemaker runs down, Roger may die immediately. This certainly seems to place reason on the side of Roger's physician. The physician feels, not without probable justification, that reason is on her side. The operation to replace the pacemaker would probably be a success and would give Roger another year of independent living. Whatever rights Roger has in this situation, he does not have by virtue of any reasoning he has done. What Roger has to gain is objectively much greater than what he has to lose. It is almost beyond doubt that the course of action suggested by the physician is the course of action Roger should take. The physician believes that Roger is old and senile. She has Roger declared incompetent, and the operation is performed.

This situation places the rights that Roger has by virtue of his autonomy into conflict with the rights the physician has by virtue of her reasoning. Ask yourself these questions:

1. Was the physician justified in the course of action she took?
2. Do a health care professional's education, training, and experience give her extraordinary rights?
3. What is the ethical role of a nurse in this situation?
4. The judge who declared Roger incompetent may have been legally justified. Was he ethically justified?

One final question:

5. Is there any significant difference between Roger's situation and Sandy's?

If reason is allowed to override autonomy in conflicts among rights, this will solve a large number of problems. At the same time, it will create an infinite number of problems. From then on, if at anytime anyone feels that his or her reason justifies a course of action, he or she will have a right to violate the autonomy of another. Under these circumstances, no one will have any rights at all.

If one is to have any rights, then reason cannot be allowed to override autonomy. Suppose that the reasoning behind one person's argument is superior to the reasoning behind another's. Ignoring the fact that, in most cases, it would be difficult or impossible to prove this, there would always be a third person whose reasoning is superior to the second. Then, there would be a fourth whose reasoning was superior to the third. This could go on forever. No ethical decision could ever be made.

> Spinoza deals with the question of good and evil on its most basic level. He describes good and evil thusly: "We call a thing good which contributes to the preservation of our being, and we call a thing evil if it is an obstacle to the preservation of our being, that is to say, a thing is called by us good or evil as it increases or diminishes, helps or restrains, our power of action" (1685/1949, p. 196).

Reason and beneficence counsel a nurse to look at the issue of good and evil from her patient's point of view. Unless she does this, it is impossible for her to form and keep an agreement with her patient according to the purposes that brought him into the health care setting. This point of view and these purposes are the reasons why there is such a thing as the health care professions. A professional cannot ethically dispense with them in her ethical decision making.

We have already defined desire to include much more than the well-known psychological state. A nurse understands her patient best if, by desire, she understands all the processes that contribute to her patient's survival and the enhancement of his life. The psychological state of desire is the best known process of this type, but every process that contributes to the survival of the organism belongs to the same family.

By including every such process under the concept of desire, a nurse can have a well-balanced understanding of her patient. The patient's psychological state is only a small part of the context. Only this understanding of his desire enables the professional to interact with her patient in his entire context. This understanding of desire, as an element of autonomy, is the understanding of a person. For a nurse to know her patient as a living reality is far more important than it is for her to know any isolated psychological state.

The Different Aspects of Life

To gain understanding of the role of ethics in a patient's life, we must define *life* inclusively, in the same way we define desire. As a bioethical element, life includes the entire context of a living person. As we shall see, any narrower definition would not be adequate for an effective bioethics. Under life, we must understand every process and action, including reason and desire, by which an organism maintains its survival and enhances its state of being.

We have a very limited understanding of life if we look at it only as a natural curiosity. We have an adequate understanding of life only if we understand it

To gain understanding of the role of ethics in a patient's life, we must define *life* inclusively, in the same way we define desire. As a bioethical element, life includes the entire context of a living person.

from the perspective of the subject who is living it. In order to do this, it is desirable to understand life from our own perspective.

For bioethics, an adequate understanding of life will include such things as:

- The body's physiological processes.
- The integration of these processes.
- Basic needs common to all animals—food, water, air—which are directly and immediately tied to the animal's survival.
- Basic needs common to all human beings: shelter, clothing, companionship, freedom from pain, and so forth.
- The life of consciousness: perceptual experience, conceptual thought, emotion, and so forth.
- The higher-order needs and values of human beings: purpose, creativity, hope, self-ownership, and so forth—values that are directly and immediately tied to a human level of existence.
- The value of various activities: walking, flying an airplane, cooking, working, and so forth—conditions of physical self-expression.
- The meaning of "aesthetic" values: Music, reading, painting, hobbies, discussion, and so forth—those conditions under which a person examines and/or experiences his life at its best.
- That with which a person is engaged and to which he is committed—the meaning, to a person, of the products of his acts of choice.
- Memories of the past.
- Anticipations of the future.

A nurse can define life from the perspective of an outsider. There are, however, a number of reasons why she ought to define life from the perspective of the living subject.

1. Medical science defines it from this perspective. If medical science thought of life simply as physiological survival, there would be no such thing as psychiatry, physical therapy, plastic surgery, and so forth.
2. If a nurse defines her patient's life solely in terms of its basic physiological processes, she will never be able to deal with ethical questions concerning risk, euthanasia, abortion, cloning, and so forth. If she defines life in terms of its basic physiological processes, then she will never truly experience her patient. She will be very much in the position of a novelist who, when she looks out at the characters in her novel, never really sees beyond herself.
3. If life, as an ethical concept, were defined in terms of physiological processes, then life as an ethical concept would pertain to all organic matter.

All organic matter is characterized by physiological processes. All organic matter has basic needs that must be met if it is to survive. If a nurse broadened her understanding of life as an ethical concept, to denote all physiological processes, she would have to broaden her understanding to include all living matter in her ethical concern. If she concerned herself with the freedom, self-assertion, and so on of all organic matter, she, herself, could not survive. Nurses, in common with everyone else, need to consume organic matter in order to remain alive. It would be strange indeed if a bioethical standard logically demanded the self-destruction of the health care professional who recognized it.

A nurse's ethical concern is not with organic matter, it is with a patient. It must be with a patient in his entirety. This is the only kind of patients there are—patients in their entirety.

> A nurse's ethical concern is not with organic matter, it is with a patient. It must be with a patient in his entirety. This is the only kind of patients there are—patients in their entirety.

Her ethical commitment to her patient does not arise from the fact that he is organic matter. It arises from, and is formed by the fact that his life is all the things it is. A patient's life is his autonomy. In addition to his physical needs and processes, his life is his desire, his reason, his purposes, and his power of agency.

4. If, on the other hand, a nurse defines her patient's life entirely in abstract terms, she will never be able to deal with her patient on an ethical level. People involved in ethical interaction are individual and concrete. Only an understanding of life as one element of an individual patient's autonomy will serve to guide ethical action. People are too different and life is too many things for the individual to be understood in entirely abstract terms.

It is not possible for a nurse to deal with her patient's life entirely on an abstract level. If it were possible, then she would hardly have to deal with her patient at all. Only if a nurse defines the life of her patient as she defines her own life will she look at her patient as an ethical agent looks at another person in an effective ethical interaction.

> Only if a nurse defines the life of her patient as she defines her own life will she look at her patient as an ethical agent looks at another person in an effective ethical interaction.

In every case, the benefits that accrue to the patient logically imply the benefits that accrue to the professional. Their interaction ought to enhance both of their lives. This is the place for a concern for life to begin.

A nurse's agreement is not with organic matter. Nor is the life that is at the center of her agreement a disconnected abstraction. Her agreement is with the virtues of an individual human being.

Life as the Basis of the Bioethical Standards

A health care ethic that is not appropriate to patients—and to health professionals—is riddled with problems. The chief problem is that it is not an intelligible field of study. Not every ethical system is automatically intelligible. Ethics is, or ought to be, derived from a study of individual people as living, rational beings. There is no intelligible ethic of redheads or of diabetics. There is no intelligible ethic of poets or of long-distance runners. An intelligible ethic relevant only to males or only to females is impossible. Such an ethic would be a mistake or a prejudice masquerading as an ethical system.

> Ethics is, or ought to be, derived from a study of individual people as living, rational beings.

A rational, solitary ethic is one whose motivations can be justified by the benefit it brings to the person who follows it. A rational, interpersonal ethic is one whose motivations can be justified by reference to the benefits and harmony it brings to the interaction of the people who are guided by it. Human survival, on every level, is contingent upon rational belief. Rules and conventions are not substitutes for rational belief. They weaken the conditions of human survival.

Life as the Preconditioned of All Action and Values

Nothing can be sought or desired by anyone unless that person is alive. Life is the precondition of all values. As Spinoza (1685/1949) describes it: "No one can desire to be happy, to act well, and to live well, who does not at the same time, desire to be, to act, and to live, that is to say, actually to exist (p. 206)."

In the field of ethics, one faces two options:

▓ One can choose a ritualistic ethic. This is an ethic based upon and arising out of rules, customs, and conventions.

This action is not interaction. It is not constant. It is episodic. When the occasion for ethical action arises, nurse–patient interaction ends. A nurse essentially abandons her practice in order to interact with a duty, an emotion, a number, or a social pretense.

▓ One can choose a symphonological ethic. For a health care professional, a symphonological ethic is an ethic based on her patient's purposes, and the nature of her professional practice as codified in the nurse–patient agreement.

Nursing is far more intelligible under a symphonological ethic. If a nurse follows rules and conventions, her ethical actions are objectively purposeless. They are imposed from outside. The final value of her ethical system is "what a professional is supposed to do." This is not the same thing as the life, health, and well-being of her patient. To pursue the well-being of a patient is to act purposefully. This is the highest potential of the profession. It is the highest potential of a nursing ethic. A nursing ethic ought to be all about what nursing practice and human life are all about.

Life as the Final Value

Life is the entire state of a living being. As an element of human autonomy, it is the state of the person that one experiences as one's self in one's world.

The fact that something is valued by one person provides no motive to any other person to value it, unless the second person values the first person intensely. Before one can value anything else, one must value one's self. Things are valued by a person because the person is valued by herself and her valuing is respected by herself.

In the health care setting, if judgment and choice are to be determined by reference to the rights and values of a patient, then the question of the central term of the nurse–patient agreement is not problematic. The central term is the patient's life.

Consider this:

▪ Life is the precondition of all of a patient's other values.
▪ Life is the precondition of a patient's rights. To respect a patient's right to autonomy, freedom, and so forth, and not to be concerned for his life and well-being is, very much, to miss the point. At the same time, to be concerned with a patient's life and well-being, and not to respect his right to autonomy, freedom, and so forth, is to have lost one's ethical direction.
▪ Life is the purpose of a patient in entering the health care environment. A patient's concern for his life, in all those aspects of his life that are of a nurse's professional concern, must be shared by his nurse, or there is no easily understood reason for her being his nurse. Life is the central term of the agreement that a nurse makes with her patient.
▪ A patient's motivation in entering the health care environment is the fact that his capacities and potentialities are radically circumscribed. When a patient regains his capacities and potentialities, his life is very much expanded.
▪ A patient, except in the most extreme circumstances, can have no rational desire before his desire to live. However, in extreme circumstances, a desire for death is not an irrational desire. It arises from a recognition of the nature of life.

> However, in extreme circumstances, a desire for death is not an irrational desire.

Ronnie is an 8-year-old child who is dying. He comes in every week for a transfusion. One day, he says to Leah, his nurse, "I don't want this anymore." Leah explains what will happen if he does not get the transfusion. Ronnie says that he knows and he still does not want the transfusion. Leah gets the parents, physician, and other consultants together and tells Ronnie's story. Ronnie takes control of his life with Leah's help. (Woods, 1999, p. 428)

The Role of Purpose

It is possible to make ethical decisions with an individual person, either oneself or one's beneficiary, serving as the reference point of ethical analysis. A person does this when he or she makes human purposes the center of his or her ethical system.

There are few consistent followers of either a ritualistic or a purposive ethical system. Most people haphazardly form the ethical system they adopt. They form it out of a combination of what they have been taught by Aunt Maude or

Uncle Jeffrey and their observations of effective, or merely pretentious, ethical actions in real life.

Ethics, as a formal study, arose from the necessity of making decisions in the face of adversity.

A person can observe what succeeds and what fails early in life from the experiences of the everydayness of family living, the give and take of playing with play-mates, and the demands of school work. A person can observe this but not everyone does.

> Ethics, as a formal study, arose from the necessity of making decisions in the face of adversity.

Amy, a nurse on a cardiac step-down unit, is a case in point. Her ethical system is much more influenced by the ethical instruction force-fed to her by her Aunt Maude and Uncle Jeffrey than it is by her experience of successful and failing human interactions.

Her actions are much more ritualistic than purposeful. Her actions have more in common with singing a song or reciting a poem than with cooking a meal or mowing the lawn. The goal of singing a song or reciting a poem is simply the activity itself and nothing beyond it. The goal of cooking a meal is the finished meal. The goal of mowing a lawn is having an attractive lawn. Amy's ethical actions have no purpose beyond the actions themselves. Her ethical actions, like singing and reciting, are their own reason for being. In the context of a person's everyday life, there is certainly nothing wrong with singing a song or reciting a poem. These can be enjoyable activities. But purposeless activity is very inappropriate to a bioethical context.

Body and Mind

The Aristotelian, life-centered ethic has been under attack ever since the time of Rene Descartes (1596–1650), and especially since the systematic deontology of the philosopher Immanuel Kant (1724–1804). Since Kant, formalism and rit-ualism have been elevated into a worldview.

Descartes began his philosophy by arguing to establish the existence of the mind. Following that, he extended his analysis to establish a proof of the existence of bodies. He regarded minds and bodies as different in nature and different in kind.

A ritualistic ethic is one that concurs. In addition, it implicitly or explicitly holds that:

- Ethical principles are what they are apart from the desires, choices, and purposes of ethical agents.
- The reason for being of an ethical principle is to direct an ethical agent in the control of evil impulses.
- The desires, choices, and purposes of ethical agents are either ethically irrelevant or ethically undesirable.
- Agreement and interaction are unnecessary to interpersonal ethical ac-tions.

A purposive ethic (an ethic in the Aristotelian tradition) is one that holds, along with Aristotle and Aristotelians, that a human person is a unitary being—that there is no moral opposition between a person's consciousness and the physical body. In each case the view on how a human person is constituted complements the view of what is right and wrong for a human person. Modern biomedicine is much more Aristotelian than Cartesian. Human nature at its best potential is much more Aristotelian than Cartesian.

The Anatomy of Purpose

When circumstances, resources, knowledge, and ability make one's purpose foreseeably possible to achieve, then purpose and action are justifiable. When it is foreseeably impossible, then purpose and action are not justifiable.

To pursue a purpose that includes a number of other valuable purposes is more justifiable than it would be otherwise. If one purpose excludes a number of other valuable purposes, it is for that reason less justifiable than it would have been or completely unjustifiable.

Desires are formulated into purposes. There are three types of purpose that determine the ethical aspects of a situation:

- **A purpose set by an individual agent's desire and decision.** Desire motivates an agent's action toward every goal. Desire is the dynamic principle that is the basis of every human purpose.
- **A purpose set by the recognition of rights.** By recognizing the rights of others, one sets uncoerced cooperation as the principle of purposive interaction.
- **A purpose projected and acted upon among individuals through explicit agreements, promises, and so forth.** This purpose must always be motivated by desire and, ethically, must recognize the rights of everyone involved.

For a decision and action to be justified:

- Its goal must be a predetermined purpose.
- There must be a reason to believe that it will tend to accomplish this purpose.
- It must not be prohibited by the nature of the nurse's professional role.
- It must not violate the rights of the patient.
- It must not interfere with the understanding that brings them together.

Purpose as the Basis of the Bioethical Standards

Purpose is the mental set of a desiring being. It also describes action directed toward vital concerns, needs, and values. Finally, purpose signifies the needs and values that an agent's actions are directed toward. Purpose is the central element of a practice-based ethic. In any action that a person takes, success or failure depends upon whether the person accomplishes his or her purpose. In an ethical context, whether an aspect of the context is good or evil depends upon whether it assists or hinders the purposeful actions that are called for in the context. The intentional quality of the action is determined by the purpose—the object of the action. An ethical action is defined in terms of its purpose.

The practical quality of an action is determined by its appropriateness to the achievement of its purpose. Purpose intends some envisioned progress. Progress is achieved through a conscious process. This process follows the context in which progress is most complete or most probable. For nursing, this conscious process consists in the standards of the profession. These standards lead a nurse to exercise intelligent cognitive discrimination and insight into the contextual relationships that make progress possible.

A person's actions always include the mental set—the intention that inspires the action. Intentions always include the object of the action—the goal for which the action is intended.

If a person's purpose is to gain happiness, then those actions that will bring about conditions that produce happiness are right and good. Those actions that bring about conditions that undermine happiness are wrong and harmful. The alternative is the agreement or the disagreement between context, actions, and their purpose.

For purposes of returning a patient to a state of agency, those actions that bring about the physical and psychological conditions of agency in a patient are right and good. Those actions that undercut the physical or psychological conditions of his agency are wrong and harmful.

> If a person's purpose is to gain happiness, then those actions that will bring about conditions that produce happiness are right and good.

Steven is in the hospital with peripheral vascular disease. His nurse, Joy, is educating him about how he must care for himself when he leaves the hospital. In order to do this, Joy:

- Tries to find out all she can about Steven so she can advise him according to his specific situation.
- Gives him all the information he needs so that he can enjoy the maximum freedom of action.
- Tells him whatever he needs to know in order to enable him to gain and retain his power of agency. She tells him nothing that he does not need to know or that might hinder his gaining and retaining his power of purposeful action.
- Allows Stephen the isolation he needs in order to make autonomous decisions.
- Does whatever she can in order to promote Stephen's welfare. She does nothing that might hinder Stephen's welfare, nothing that might hinder his power to take autonomous actions.

The Facets of Purpose

The standard of any action, including ethical actions, is the purpose that the agent means to accomplish by the action.

Question: "Why did the chicken cross the road?"

Answer: "To get to the other side."

If a chicken, or a person, wants to walk across the road, then getting to the other side is the standard of success. If a person wants to learn to use a computer, then his or her standard of success is the ability to use a computer. If a student wants to learn to fly, then the standard of success is being able to take off, stay up, and come down. If a nurse wants to recognize the self-assertion of her patient, then that patient acting on his self-assertion, is the standard of the nurse's success.

Every event that fulfills an agent's purpose is an event that signals the success of an ethical agent. The reason for being of ethical decision making is to guide the action of an ethical agent to realize such events.

The world presents various alternatives to an ethical agent. An agent chooses from among alternatives according to his or her desires. When an agent chooses from among alternatives, this act of choice forms a purposeful frame of mind. A purpose is the object of a desire that a person brings to the forefront and retains in his or her attention.

A choice is an objective relationship between a state of desire and a possibility that a person perceives in the world. A choice is a mental action that closes off alternative mental actions of choice. All action is purposeful behavior.

> A choice is an objective relationship between a state of desire and a possibility that a person perceives in the world.

Any purposeful ethic involves choice. An ethical system not based on purpose and choice is ritualistic and formalistic. It is like reading poetry to oneself. A ritualistic or formalistic ethic cannot motivate actions appropriate to nursing. It cannot guide a nurse's actions appropriately. It cannot enable her to objectively justify the actions she takes. It can no more be a professional ethic than tea leaf reading can be a technology.

A nurse armed with a formalistic ethic would not know what questions to ask of a context. Nor would she know what would constitute the answer to a contextual ethical question. A process of ethical justification has to do with these questions and answers. Such a process is simply an explanation of the questions a person has asked and the answers upon which she has acted.

Reason and Purpose as the Foundation for Ethical Decision Making

Purpose as an element of autonomy, in and of itself, is of primary importance in resolving an ethical dilemma. Each of the other elements of autonomy is important only as it relates to purpose.

Dilemma 9.7

Jody Smith, a retired nurse with three adult children and numerous adult grand-children, lives in a small rural area on a limited income. Two months ago, she fell and broke her left hip. After surgery for an artificial hip replacement, she was transferred to a rehabilitation center where she had a left-side cerebrovascular accident (CVA). Upon her readmittance to the acute care facilities, she received aggressive therapy for the CVA. Completely paralyzed on her left side, Mrs. Smith has decided that she no longer desires aggressive therapy and frequently asks the staff why she cannot die in peace. "The rehabilitation is so painful and I'll never walk again. What's the use?" Both the physicians and her family are much more optimistic. The orthopedic surgeon is convinced that Mrs. Smith will walk again, and the neurologist believes that Mrs. Smith will make a full recovery and be able to return home and care for herself. Both physicians have excluded Mrs. Smith from their conversations, assuring her children that she will be "as good as new." They ignore Mrs. Smith's request to discontinue anticoagulants and rehabilitative therapy. She refuses to cooperate with the physical and occupational therapists. She will not take her medications, and refuses to perform simple tasks, relying instead on staff members to meet her activities of daily living. What should be done? (Guido, 1998)

The Role of Agency

The Nature of Ethical Action

Imagine, if you will, that you are taking a stroll over a very large lawn by a wood side. As you walk, you pass one by one, a rock, a tree, and then a horse. Finally, you pass a young woman and a young man.

From the viewpoint of the rock, nothing is either good or evil. Whatever happens, it is a matter of perfect indifference. But in order to experience the ethical aspects of what you see during your stroll, imagine that one thing, if only this one thing, is good in relation to the rock. There is a very weak sense in which the (only) good for the rock is to retain its structural integrity, to retain its "rockhood." Obviously, the rock is not conscious of a desire to re-main in existence. That is not important. What is important is this: There is nothing morally outrageous in the fact that the rock exists and remains in existence.

Now you pass a tree. This is a very different kind of thing. The rock is inert and inanimate; the tree is alive. To stay alive, the tree must sink its roots into the earth to draw stability and sustenance from the ground. So you encounter a sort of progression, a change in the way of being. Even so, there is nothing here in the living and acting of the tree that is morally undesirable. Life is not, in itself, an ethical disaster.

Now you come to the horse. The horse is also alive. It is alive in an even stronger sense than the tree. The horse is conscious of its environment. It moves about from place to place in a manner that follows from its nature. The horse eats grass from the ground and apples from the tree. Yet, even in this behavior of the horse, there is no basis for a rational moral indignation. The existence of the horse is not a moral calamity.

So it is also with the man and woman. Here again one comes to a different kind of being—the man and woman are not only conscious, they are conscious on an abstract and conceptual level. Yet, there is nothing any more intrinsically immoral in the existence of reason in the man and woman than there is in the animality of the horse. There is nothing more morally undesirable in the animality of the horse than there is in the treeness of the tree. There is nothing more morally undesirable in the treeness of the tree than there is in the rockness of the rock.

In a nursing context, an ethical system that would seek to work around the "disaster" of a patient's being human and being alive would be a tragic mistake. It would be the opposite of an intelligible, practice-based system.

Action Versus Passion

The term *action* in ethics has a very specific and technical meaning. It can be most easily understood in relation to its correlative, *passion*. Action and passion are both forms of behavior.

A passion is any behavior that an entity undergoes through a force external to itself and not as an outcome of any act of self-determination. An action is a behavior that an agent initiates. The agent determines the execution of the action, the occurrence, and the nature of the behavior. Scratching an intolerable itch or behavior exhibited under the influence of an overwhelming emotion, such as fear, are instances of passion. The falling of a leaf, the careening of a billiard ball, the behavior of a nail in the vicinity of a magnet are also examples of passion.

> A passion is any behavior that an entity undergoes through a force external to itself and not as an outcome of any act of self-determination.

Making and completing long-range plans, meeting an inconvenient ethical responsibility, engaging in a difficult, unfamiliar thought process, and testing one's self with a heavy weight are various types of action. These, of course, are things that leaves, billiard balls, and nails cannot do.

In relation to a force that precludes volitional choice and compels behavior, an (potential) agent is passive. This meaning of the term *passive* is retained in the adjective and in the noun *patient*; indeed, both terms have the same root. A patient is a person who is passive—a person who is incapable of actions according to normal capabilities.

Action, on the other hand, involves these preconditions:

- An agent's awareness of the situation in which he is to act.
- An agent's awareness of himself as a rational being, plus his specific awareness of himself in relation to the situation in which he is to act.

■ An agent's implicit awareness of his capacity for self-determined behavior. All these capabilities can be possessed by a patient. What the patient lacks, to a greater or lesser extent, is the fourth capability.

■ The capability to translate his awareness into an action intended to bring about a desired result.

These preconditions of agency belong to every agent and are not inherently problematic. However, these potential assets of an agent can become problematic under the influence of a dilemma—when an agent may forget possession of these abilities, distort his or her relationship to them, or be unable to estimate what he or she can accomplish through them.

A nurse may find the physical or mental condition of her patient's functioning as a kind of dilemma, causing him to lose his awareness of, or even his interest in, his powers of agency. The demands of effective nursing under these circumstances call upon a nurse to rekindle this awareness if possible. This requires that she recognize the difference between her patient's passive acceptance of various circumstances and his actual exercise of agency. An action actually expresses the nature and intention of the agent, whereas passive acceptance does not.

Dilemma 9.8

After her gall bladder surgery, Ruth Sparrow had a serious problem, but not with her health. The surgery was successful and she was doing well. The problem was money. Her bill was close to $20,000 and she had no savings to fall back on to pay for it. She said to the hospital: "I will give you a kidney, if you will mark my bill paid in full." They turned her down. Then she ran an ad in the paper: kidney runs good, for sale—$30,000 or best offer. While she received many crank calls some were serious and asked for her blood type. The ad was pulled by the paper since it is against federal and state laws to buy or sell a human organ or tissue. What do you think? (Bioethics Case Study, 2000).

Agency as the Basis of the Bioethical Standards

A person's agency is the power to act on autonomous desires that spring from his or her own reasoning. Agency makes a human life what it can be and will be.

Agency requires autonomous desire. Without autonomous desire, behavior is involuntary. Involuntary behavior does not arise from agency. For instance, if a person is jostled in the street and bumps into a wall, that behavior does not arise from agency. His behavior, as we have discussed, is a passion—it arises from a force outside of his agency.

> A person's agency is the power to act on autonomous desires that spring from his or her own reasoning.

Agency requires reason or autonomous thought. Behaviors that arise entirely from the emotions, as well as reflex behaviors, are not actions. Actions express the specific nature of the agent who acts. Only rational beings possess agency. Only reason in action expresses the specific nature of a rational being.

If ethical action does not properly begin with attention to agency, with actions that arise in a patient's autonomous desire and reason, then all of bioethics is misdirected. The health care setting is designed to promote the regaining of agency in the service of a patient's individual purposes. For this reason, every bioethical standard has the same purpose.

- The standard of autonomy protects those actions of a patient that express his unique character structure.
- The standard of freedom protects actions arising from the individual agency of a patient.
- The standard of objectivity supports the actions that arise from the individual agency of a patient. It does this by allowing him to act on his own knowledge and awareness.
- The standard of self-assertion protects the self-governance of a patient insofar as that self-governance is expressed in the patient's self-initiated actions.
- The standard of beneficence protects the actions of an agent and his power of agency.
- The standard of fidelity protects his objective attention to his self-interest and to the values he pursues, as well as a person's self-awareness of the interactions of several agents as they act toward interwoven purposes.

Try to imagine applying the bioethical standards to a machine and you will see the essential relationship between the standards and the patient's agency.

Agency, Rights, and the Ethical Interaction

Imagine a desert island with only one inhabitant, Debbie. With no possibility of a division of labor and none of the tools of civilization available to her, survival is a pressing problem for Debbie. Under these circumstances, what does Debbie have a right to do and what does she have no right to do? What would it be wrong for her to do?

In these highly unusual circumstances, it is obvious that Debbie has the right to do whatever she has the power to do. Her right to take action is unlimited.

> *Strictly speaking, rights exist only in situations where more than one person is involved. A right is a right against another person—a right not to be aggressed against. So when we speak of "one's rights on a desert island," we are using the term rights in an extended sense to refer to what would be equivalent to rights among a number of people.*

Debbie has the right to pursue any value that she has reason to believe will bring her benefit and the right to shun whatever would tend to her detriment.

She has as much right to pursue her values as she has to exist—and each for the same reason.

How could it be wrong for Debbie to act to sustain her life? Why would it be wrong for her to act toward the realization of her values? There is no logical reason why she should negate any aspect of her being, neither the fact that she is nor the fact of what she is.

The fact that Debbie, a thinking, valuing person, actually exists is exhaustive evidence that it is right that she should exist. The fact that she is, by nature, a being to whom the pursuit of values is appropriate is conclusive evidence that it is right that she pursue that which she values. Against the fact that she does exist, no rational evidence can be adduced to show that it would be ethically better if she did not exist. The proposition that Debbie ought to renounce her life or the pursuit of her values cannot be logically or, therefore, ethically justified. It simply does not make sense.

Debbie has the right to be what she is. Any alternative to this principle is incoherent. As a natural corollary to this principle, we must conclude that Debbie has a right to do whatever she has the power to do. Nothing she does can violate the rights of another. There is no other on the island.

Now, let us change the scenario somewhat.

One day, Michelle washes ashore. Holding strictly to the context of our problem, how has Debbie's situation changed? How is the principle that Debbie has the right to do whatever she has the power to do been modified?

Ethically, the principle is unimpaired, although two significant changes have come into Debbie's life:

1. As rational beings, Michelle and Debbie have an obligation not to violate each other's rights. Whether or not they do violate each other's rights, the obligation remains. The obligation is there, not by virtue of any arbitrary decision either might make, but by virtue of their defining characteristics, by virtue of what Debbie and Michelle have in common—their rational nature. As a corollary of this, each has an obligation to honor the agreements that she makes with the other.
2. Debbie's existential position is enormously enhanced, as is Michelle's for having found Debbie there.

If the inhabitants of the island number two or number in the millions, nothing is essentially changed. Moreover, allow yourself a little thought experiment by placing yourself in the picture. If you were Michelle or Debbie, the ethical principles governing the situation would remain exactly the same. You lack no right that others possess. You possess no right that others lack. If any ethical circumstance that might apply to a particular individual is, all things being equal, right or wrong, it can only be because it is right or wrong universally, for every ethical agent.

The Biological Function of Agency

Agency is an agent's power. It is the instrument of reason and desire. It is the servant of an agent's purposive mind-set.

The function of purpose is to move an agent from a lesser to a greater level of autonomy, freedom, objective connection to reality, self-governance, power to pursue values, and fidelity to his life. The function of agency is to move an agent from a less refined reason and a less complete knowledge to a more refined reason and a more complete knowledge. It guides reason in its vision of rational desires and in actions leading to the fulfillment of desire. It enables an agent to attain a more desirable condition of being.

Finally, agency serves to increase its own competency and strength. In taking physical actions, a person increases the strength of her body. In taking the actions necessary to increase understanding, a person increases the strength of her mind.

Dilemma 9.9

Seven years ago Beth and her husband's 2-year-old son was kidnapped. They have never found him alive or dead. Beth, age 42, is in the hospital dying of ovarian cancer. In all probability she will be sent home to die once the physician has controlled her pain. She is alert and able to get around, although she is weak. She has a living will, which states, among other things, that she does not want to be connected to any machines or to have CPR performed. The physician has written a DNR order. In order to better control her pain the physician has ordered a drug in addition to her morphine drip. You give a drug by IM injection.

Within minutes of giving the drug Beth has, what you believe to be, an anaphylactic reaction and goes into respiratory arrest. At the moment that Beth arrests, a colleague rushes into say that they have just received a call from Beth's husband. The child has been found alive and well. You know your colleague to be entirely reliable. What should you do?

Agency and Rights

In the life of every (noncriminal) individual and in the history of humanity, it becomes evident that the range and effectiveness of people's activities are greatly augmented if they do not have to devote time and effort to guarding themselves against aggression, coercion, and fraud. So, as a sort of evolutionary instrument, an implicit agreement arises among rational beings, an agreement not to aggress against, not to coerce, and not to defraud one another.

It is also the essential basis of the existence of laws. Laws arise because there is a need for them. But the need arose long before the laws. This implicit agreement arose before the laws were possible. It arose with the human ability to make agreements.

Before any laws were ever made, the necessary relations of justice existed. "To say that nothing is just or unjust except that which is commanded or forbidden by positive law is as absurd as saying that before a circle is actually drawn its radii are not equal" (De Montesquieu, 1848/1949, p. 108).

To the extent that a society is free, the laws that it recognizes as most fundamental are reflections of individual rights. These laws are an explicit statement of the implicit agreement on nonaggression. Where laws have no rational justification, where they serve no evident need, and where they have no moral basis, they are resented and notoriously difficult to enforce. Not so with laws based on the implicit agreement—perhaps not even a criminal can resent such laws.

This preexisting agreement against aggression arises from the human condition. Without it, there would be no basis for honoring any inconvenient explicit agreements. No legal system could possibly be effective. There would be no basis for agreement on a legal system. The only check on people's criminality would be the limits of their imagination and the range of their daring.

Making an agreement is not at all synonymous with having reason to believe that an agreement will be kept. Where there is no positive reason to believe that an agreement will be kept, there is no practical reason to make an agreement. Dependable explicit agreements are made possible by this implicit agreement.

We have defined rights as being: The product of an implicit agreement among rational beings, made and held by virtue of their rationality, not to obtain actions, nor the products or circumstances of action from one another, except through voluntary consent, objectively gained.

This implicit agreement gives fiber to explicit agreements and to laws. It gives moral force to every explicit agreement and every other implicit agreement. This holds true of the unspoken agreement between nurse and patient. The nurse–patient agreement is, in effect, guaranteed by the implicit agreement that constitutes rights. It is an agreement that nurse and patient have a right to expect that each will fulfill his or her role according to the purposes that motivate their interaction. It is an agreement that there will be fidelity and benevolence on each side.

The English philosopher John Stuart Mill (1806–1883) said that one person cannot advance the interests of another by compulsion. One person cannot rightly compel another person to do something because it is better for that other person to do it, because it will make the other person happier, or because, in the opinion of the first person, it would be wise for the second person to do it (1819/1988).

Rights determine the actions an agent can take. Everyone has the right to be free from the coercion of others. Everyone constantly relies on the specieswide agreement that people will not deal with each other coercively. A person can act freely in any social context as long as he or she does not coerce another. In coercing another, a person gives up the right to exercise freedom. It is well said that:

> This implicit agreement gives fiber to explicit agreements and to laws. It gives moral force to every explicit agreement and every other implicit agreement.

> [The right to] self determination is an individual's exercise of the capacity to form, revise, and pursue personal plans for life...free from outside control...In the context of health care, self determination overrides practitioner determination. (President's Commission for the Study of Ethical Problems and Medicine and Biomedical and Behavioral Research, 1982, p. 32)

She has an ethical obligation
to protect her patient from
anyone who would violate his
rights. Above all, she cannot, herself, break the rights
agreement.

A nurse, because she is the agent of her patient and through the implicit agreement she has with him, has agreed to protect the rights of her patient. She has an ethical obligation to protect her patient from anyone who would violate his rights. Above all, she cannot, herself, break the rights agreement.

Dilemma 9.10

Jason is a patient in a psychiatric hospital. He was admitted nonvoluntarily. He has been diagnosed as a paranoid schizophrenic. His physician has prescribed 5 mg Haldol and 2 mg Cogentin. Jason refuses to take the medication. He tells his nurse, Jessica, that the physician is trying to poison him. Aside from what he tells her, Jessica has no reason to believe that Jason's physician is trying to poison him. Would she be justified in giving Jason an injection of the medication against his will so that he would get the benefit of it? Would doing so violate Jason's rights?

Musings

No one can be human and be completely unfamiliar with that which makes him or her autonomous (Figure 9.1). Everyone is familiar with the elements of human autonomy, at least, on an implicit level. It is quite advantageous for a professional to become familiar with them explicitly.

To interact on a human level is to interact on a highly intimate level. People interact with each other on an intimate level when they understand each other's desires. Desire is the basis of meaning and purpose in every human life. Intimacy rests on meaning and purpose.

The interweaving of their desires is the ethical basis for the nurse–patient agreement. This agreement is seldom, and probably never, verbalized. It is an implicit agreement arising immediately between them. The ultimate basis of this agreement, therefore, is not anything the nurse or the patient says. It is what they are that determines what they ought to do.

A professional's exercise of reason is her greatest source of ethical confidence and strength. As the agent of her patient, confidence and strength are values that she offers him and herself. She owes it to herself to exercise reason in developing the virtues that her profession requires.

There is one activity more central to human life than any other. This is the discovery and pursuit of autonomous purposes. It is the activity that relates an individual's abstract aspirations and the biological functions necessary to the organism's continued survival. There is no reason why both cannot come into the health care system.

2.1

Husteds' Symphonological Bioethical Decision Making Model II.

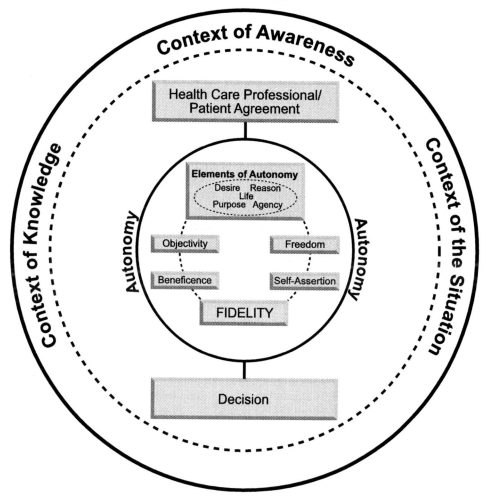

Study Guide

1. Think about your own desires and how you did or did not use reason to follow through on them. What were the consequences for you? Were there consequences to others? Could the consequences be mitigated?
2. "Desire is, like fire, a useful servant but a fearful master" (author unknown). What would this mean for the nurse or for the patient?

3. If a person does not desire to do good but does something good, what can be said about this person? What might be the consequences for a patient under this person's care?

4. If a person desires to do good but fails to use his or her rational nature (or reason), what might be the consequences for the patient under this person's care?

5. Think of a situation in which the elements of human autonomy would have helped resolve a problem regarding choices in your own life. Take this problem or dilemma through the elements to see how the decision differs or is the same as what you did. Then analyze why.

6. Does the element of life prohibit the withdrawal of food and fluids from a dying person? Would there be a context in which it would or a context in which it would not?

7. The fun parable about the chicken crossing the road highlights a number of important points regarding the role of purposes. What are some? How do they relate to your practice?

8. The action–passion distinction can create a feeling of guilt in health care professionals. Should it? What does it mean to say you cannot know what you cannot know? Can you do what you cannot do? Give concrete examples from your practice.

9. What does it mean to return the patient to a circumstance in which he or she can be his or her own agent? Why is this important? What if it is not possible?

10. Take the case of Ronnie, how would you resolve it using the elements of autonomy?

References

Bioethics Case Study. (2000). *Transplant*. Retrieved October 25, 2006, from http://www.mhhe.com/biosci/genbio/olc_linkedcontent/bioethics_cases/g-bioe-04.htm

De Montesquieu, S. (1949). *Spirit of the laws* (T. Nuggent, Trans.). New York: Random House. (Original work published 1848).

Guido, G. W. (1998). *Legal issues in nursing* (2nd ed.). Stamford, CT: Appleton & Lange.

Husted, J. H. (1988). Spinoza's conception of the attributes of substance. *The Metaphysics of Substance: The Proceedings of the American Catholic Philosophical Association, 61*, 81–131.

Mill, J. S. (1988). *On liberty*. New York: Penguin. (Original work published 1819).

Milstead, J. A. (1999). Advanced practice nurses and public policy, naturally. In J. A. Milstead (Ed.), *Health policy and politics* (pp. 1–41). Gaithersburg, MA: Aspen.

President's Commission for the Study of Ethical Problems and Medicine and Biomedical and Behavioral Research. (1982). *Making health care decisions: The ethical and legal implication of informed consent in the patient-practitioner relationship*. Vol. 1. Washington, DC: U.S. Government Printing Office.

Spinoza, B. (1949). *Ethics* (J. Gutmann, Ed.). New York: Hafner. (Original work published 1675)

Woods, M. (1999). A nursing ethic: The moral voice of experienced nurses. *Nursing Ethics, 6*, 423–433.

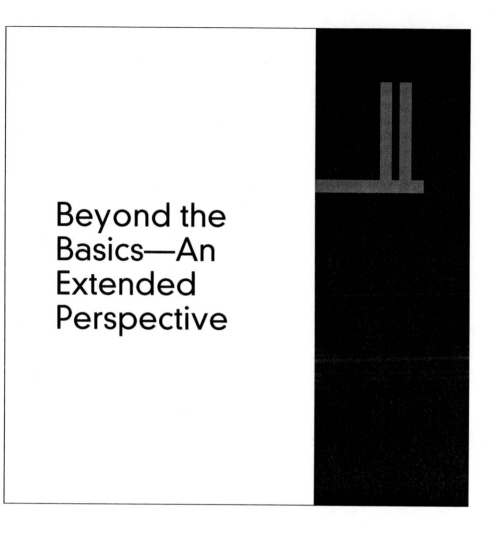

Beyond the Basics—An Extended Perspective

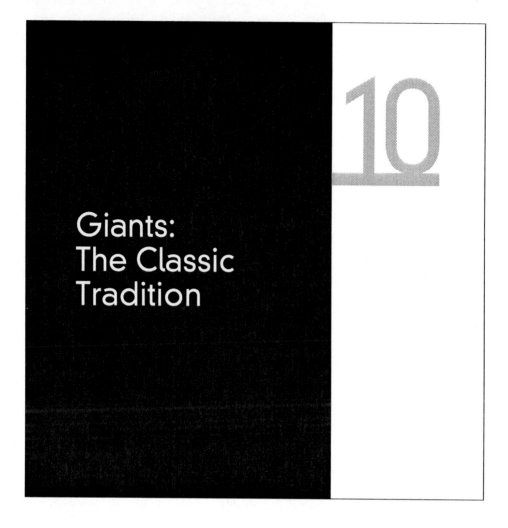

Giants:
The Classic
Tradition

The world is given to us as a book. How strange we so seldom read it.
— Eugene Aben-Moha

It all happened—or most of it—in the state of Lu in China around 550 BC. Then it happened, happened all over China. Then it happened throughout the world. And a small part of it is still with us.

Shu-Liang Heh was a soldier of legendary daring and prowess. In his old age, having nine daughters, he became very desirous of having a son. For this purpose he made an alliance with the Yen family and married their youngest daughter, Yen Chang-Tsai.

Heh and Chang-Tsai made their home near to Ni, the sacred mountain. Chang-Tsai offered prayers to the mountain to let her conceive a son. She promised the mountain she would name her son, Chung Ni in its honor.

Chang-Tsai conceived. Her pregnancy was accompanied by dreams and signs and wonders. In a dream she was told to give birth to her son in a cave on Ni. As the time of her delivery drew near, she had visions of strange animals and emissaries from other planets. When her child was born, dragons served as sentries. Lovely angelic maidens attended Chang-Tsai.

At the baby's birth, a spring of clean warm water rose on the floor of the cave to serve as a bath for mother and baby. When they had bathed, the spring dried up and disappeared. The angelic maidens blessed Chang-Tsai's son. All these events seemed to portend a remarkable future for Chung Ni.

Chung Ni

Very early on Chung Ni developed a deep interest in music and ceremony. Each of these involves structured harmony and control. He was bitterly criticized for these interests as being a waste of his time. His brilliant intelligence was obvious from his earliest years. Chung Ni (551–479 BC), who is known in the Western part of the world as Confucius, the Latinized form of Kung Fu, was going off in a different direction. He was going his own way and he would take a good part of the world with him.

Soon after his birth, monstrous animals and unearthly maidens and men ceased playing a part in Confucius life. He turned his attention to the affairs of humankind.

At that time in China, the well-being of the Chinese depended heavily on the will and character of the ruler. Confucius studied the history of the benevolent rulers of the past. He found in them attitudes and virtues that he determined ought to be possessed by all men. These he held up as the ideal—the virtues of the wise and noble rulers of the past.

In his early 20s, the fame of his learning began to spread and he gathered around him a group of students. He devoted his life to teaching. Where the teachers of the past had taught of the exploits of mythical warriors, legendary events, and methods of foretelling the future, Confucius taught of nothing but humanity, human nature, and the possibilities of human life. He was history's first thoroughgoing ethicist. It is highly probable that no philosopher has influenced the subsequent philosophy of ethics over a longer span of time than this awe-inspiring teacher. Even now he is the most revered figure in Chinese history and in the history of ethics.

In the 17th and 18th centuries, his ideas were carried to Europe by missionaries returning from China. These ideas were avidly taken up by many of the most famous thinkers of Europe. His influence on the ethical philosophy of that time in the Western world is incalculable.

Reciprocity: Confucius' Rule of Life

Several principles in Confucius' philosophy tend to produce and sustain ideally effective conditions for successful ethical action. Foremost among these guides is the principle of reciprocity. Reciprocity pertains to established patterns of interaction between ethical agents. It is established on an appropriate or acceptable balance between value given and value received. It is a recurring interchange of benefits or values. The process of reciprocity begins when a first agent accepts a benefit from a second agent and returns a benefit to the second agent. The second agent then responds in kind and this process continues as its practical value becomes obvious. These benefits need not be physical values. A benefit can be anything that a first agent experiences as something of value. For example, it can be something as simple as the smile of an infant. The infant's smile will evoke a gleeful response on the part of its mother. The end result will be a very close relationship and a lifelong trade of emotional values between the child and its mother.

The sequential acquisition of benefits and the way benefits are given and received produces trust and encourages the continuation of ethical interaction. Of all the processes characterizing human interaction, only processes characterized by reciprocity can establish and sustain:

> The process of reciprocity begins when a first agent accepts a benefit from a second agent and returns a benefit to the second agent. The second agent then responds in kind and this process continues as its practical value becomes obvious.

- An intelligible context—the participants have a clear understanding of the process.
- The events involved in the interaction being under the causal control of the reciprocating agent—each agent is active, events are not ruled by chance.
- Predictable sequential actions and responses.

These together produce intelligible causal sequences. They make ethical interactions maximally effective.

Reciprocity can best be seen in something such as one farmer helping another to herd his cattle. In return, the second farmer helps the first harvest his crop of rice. And then this practice continues. Balance and proportion are easy to see in an arrangement like this.

In the nurse–patient interaction the spirit of reciprocity can be just as strong, but the nature of reciprocity cannot be as clearly seen and cannot be balanced and proportioned easily in the same ways it can be between the two farmers.

When the reception of a benefit is not reciprocated, no trust, no intelligible context, and no commitments or expectations will be established. Reciprocity is predictable sequences of action. These sequences are controlled by the agents practicing reciprocity. They are caused by and intelligible to the agents involved.

Reciprocity produces intelligible interactions, causal power (power capable of producing an intended effect on the part of each person), and forward moving sequences. An added benefit to each is the development of his or her ethical character. This benefit enhances all the others.

> Reciprocity produces intelligible interactions, causal power (power capable of producing an intended effect on the part of each person), and forward moving sequences.

The Rectification of Names

A further principle, which humankind has not mastered and probably will not master in the next thousand or so years, would solidify the trust that reciprocity establishes and transform the world. The *rectification of names* is the principle that words should be properly applied to things, and things should be designated by their proper names. Everything ought to be understood and to function as its name implies. Everything ought to be handled as its name designates, for example, a pet ought not to be tormented; that which is called a home ought to be a place of contentment. A word ought to accurately define and identify that which it names. For instance, only that which is just—only that which sustains understanding, allows each agent the full range of his rightful actions, and allows productive sequences of action to continue—should be called justice. Otherwise, words and things will not agree, understanding will suffer, and action will be diffuse.

The Chinese regard words as names. They regard words as the names of the things that they designate. The rectification of names, then, is the correction of the way words are used to designate things—the correct use of words or language to identify that which is spoken of.

Everything ought to be understood as being what it is, for instance, celebration should be understood as having all the attributes of celebration, a father the qualities of a father, an agreement the necessary parts of an agreement. A patient ought to be understood as a patient, a nurse as a nurse, and so forth. Everyone ought to understand oneself as who he or she is. Above all, an ethical agent ought to be understood as being what an ethical agent is.

Two things are essential to ethical interaction:

- An objective understanding of each by the other.
- The objective language tools necessary to make objective understanding possible.

Confucius advised those who would nurture to, "Look closely into a man's aims; observe the means by which he pursues them and discover what brings him contentment; ask him to state his ambitions, freely and without reserve. Store away impressions. Study how to take advantage of his good points and overcome his weakness" (Confucius as quoted in Bahm, 1992, p. 34).

His advice to nurses would be to:

- Note the impressions of the patient's behaviors, which are revealed in the quality of the patient's self-assertion.
- Discover what brings the patient contentment. This reveals a patient's understanding of beneficence.
- Observe the means by which the patient pursues aims. This reveals the patient's objectivity.
- Examine his actions in pursuit of his ambitions. This reveals the quality of the exercise of the patient's freedom.
- Study his good points and his weaknesses. This reveals his fidelity to himself.
- Look into a patient's aims, which reveals a patient's autonomy.

About 2,500 years ago Confucius described nursing and nurses as symphonological. At its best, nursing still is.

"If names be not correct, language is not in accordance with the truth of things. If language be not in accordance with the truth of things, affairs cannot be carried on to success" (Confucius, *Analects*, Book 13, chap. 3).

"If names be not correct, language is not in accordance with the truth of things. If language be not in accordance with the truth of things, affairs cannot be carried on to success" (Confucius, *Analects*, Book 13, chap. 3).

This project, the attempt to reform language, was continued by Socrates in the Western world.

Socrates

Socrates is the most famous philosopher of the Western world. The adventure of his discovery has been immortalized in the *Dialogues of Plato*. The adventure began in ancient Greece about 450 BC.

The Affirmation of Life and Ethics

Inspired by the discovery that "the unexamined life is not worth living," Socrates was the first Western philosopher to systematically turn his attention to the affairs of human life. Socrates, the son of a stone mason and a midwife, saw himself as following his mother's profession with this difference: Where his mother assisted at the birth of children, he assisted at the birth of ideas. He did this through a method that he called *dialectic*. The method involved disciplined conversation. Socrates would begin by posing a question. When a member of his audience offered an answer, he would question the answer. Through this method (which has come to be known as the *maieutic method*—the method of midwifery), Socrates led his audience to draw ethical distinctions and attempt to discover the true definitions of ethical abstractions, such as wisdom, justice, virtue, and happiness. That is to say, by reflecting on concrete facts, they were led to wide ranging ethical understanding. This understanding generally proved to be both shallow and short-lived.

> Socrates led his audience to draw ethical distinctions and attempt to discover the true definitions of ethical abstractions such as wisdom, justice, virtue, and happiness

At the same time, Socrates stressed the crucial importance of context.

Context

If it is difficult to define the virtues and the vices, it is, sometimes, also difficult to know when (in what context) the same action is virtuous or vicious. If a bank robber ties up a bank teller and locks him in a room, this violates the bank teller's rights and is a vicious action. If a policeman puts the bank robber in restraints and locks him in a jail cell, this action, taken out of context, is identical to the action of the bank robber. But it is a virtuous action. The context makes the difference. The bank robber has rejected the agreements that make virtuous interaction possible. The policeman has reestablished the conditions that make virtuous interaction possible.

A girl's father tells her fiancé when he comes to visit her on a one day pass before sailing off to war that she is not at home when, in fact, she is at home and waiting for him. Her father performs a vicious act. He takes her agency as his own.

A rejected suitor, holding a large knife, awakens a father in the middle of the night to ask him whether his daughter is at home. Her father lies. He answers in the negative but, in fact, his daughter is at home. Omitting contextual factors, his actions are the same as the actions of the father in the prior vignette. But, it is a virtuous action. The difference is shaped by the context.

A man is going to hunt a rogue bear tomorrow and a visitor steals his rifle. This is a vicious action. But, if a man has become demented and has sworn to shoot his neighbor the next day, then this visitor in stealing his rifle performs a virtuous action. Even though the actions out of context are identical—stealing the rifle—the context is different. Their ethical values are completely opposed.

Socrates, the founder of ethics in the Western world, was not the first person to think about these very basic human problems. He was, however, like Confucius in the East, probably the first to think about them deeply and rigorously. He proposed a systematic examination of human experience and human life as the way to discover solutions. He discovered the role of context in ethical analysis and action and the radical necessity of doubt. Thus began, in the Western world that part of philosophy that is known as ethics. Ethics examines the ways men and women can exercise their power in order to bring about human benefit—the ways in which we can act in order to bring about the conditions of survival and flourishing.

> Ethics examines the ways men and women can exercise their power in order to bring about human benefit—the ways in which we can act in order to bring about the conditions of survival and flourishing.

Socrates was convinced that no stable virtue and no ethical action are possible without knowledge. He also believed that no ethical knowledge is possible without an understanding of the meaning of ethical terms and the contexts in which they are applied. To gain an understanding of actions as just or unjust, one must understand the essential nature of justice. To know the requirements of happiness, one must first know the defining properties of happiness. To have knowledge of virtuous action, one must first know what virtue is.

These conversations often led the people of Athens into areas where they had no desire to go. Their ethical beliefs consisted entirely of social customs and conventions. To engage them in practical reasoning, Socrates had to call their beliefs into question. To have one's beliefs called into question is a painful experience. To call one's own beliefs into question is a very unpopular activity. But no practical reasoning is possible without this activity and this experience.

As is well known, Socrates' beneficence cost him his life. He was executed by the state for teaching heresy and "corrupting the youth of Athens." Then, as now, many people would rather kill or die before engaging in practical reasoning (Vlastos, 1991).

Aristotle

It is not necessary to say much about Aristotle (384–322 BC). Aristotle was a great ethicist, although there have been greater. He was a poet. Like Confucius, he discussed the desirability of reforming language to conform to reality. He held that definitions are either true or false, and are important. However, he did not discuss this under the rubric of ethics but rather of logic and epistemology. Philosophy is ethics and more. It is also metaphysics (the study of the nature of

10.1	Examples of Virtuous Means and Their Opposed Vices		
Deficit	**Mean**		**Excess**
Cowardice	Courage		Foolhardiness
Humility	Pride		Vainglory
Indifference	Tenderness		Doting
Passivity	Firmness		Stubbornness
Mock modesty	Sincerity		Boastfulness
Apathy	Determination		Fanaticism
Indifference	Awareness		Obsession

reality) and epistemology (the study of knowledge and how it is acquired and several other topics), all of which he investigated. For many centuries, he was referred to as "the master of them that know." This nickname was well deserved. Aristotle was, among other things, a scientist, and he is the greatest philosopher of all time.

The Golden Mean

In ethics, Aristotle is best known for his doctrine of the Golden Mean (*Nicomachean Ethics*, Book II, chaps. 1109A 20–23):

Virtue is a character structure—a state or habit—appropriately suited to human action. The virtues, he tells us, are a mean between two extremes—each extreme being a vice. At the one extreme is a deficit where action is taken too weakly, where it is inadequate to the value offered by the circumstances. At the other extreme there is excess where action is taken beyond what is objectively justified. With deficit, sequences begin weakly, if they begin at all. With excess, sequences tend to self-destruct.

For instance, courage is the virtue between the deficit of cowardice (the unwillingness to take justified risks) and the excess of foolhardiness (the willingness to take risks out of proportion or unnecessary to the value to be gained) (Table 10.1).

The *virtues at the mean* serve to bring about intelligible causal sequences in action or interaction. The vices at the extremes fail. The deficit produces no causal power. The excess makes intelligibility impossible. Neither produces effective sequential interactions.

When an agent meets a circumstance with an appropriate response, her action is intelligible and it keeps her understanding relevant to the circumstances. It enables her to engage with, and control, her part of the events occurring in the circumstance. By establishing the intelligibility and a sustained understanding of events in the circumstance, maintaining power to control these events, and guiding their direction, an agent can direct sequential events to serve her purpose.

When an agent meets a circumstance with an appropriate response, her action is intelligible and it keeps her understanding relevant to the circumstances.

The application of the Golden Mean would be a virtue much more appropriate to an orator in the senate than a nurse at the sickbed. Many times senators of all ages and nations will "sin" through timidity, the failure to say things that ought to be said, and through fear of their listener's response. Or, on the other hand, drunk with their own magnificence, they will become bombastic, speaking without informing or persuading, whereas the virtuous senator will speak in terms showing good sense and good measure.

This type of advice—to stay with the Golden Mean—is not nearly so germane in the case of nurses. Nurses are seldom ineffective through timidity and are seldom bombastic.

Ideally, ethical standards will structure interactions so that they will be sequential rather than episodic. For this to be possible, circumstances and sequences must be intelligible. Agents have to know what to expect. As a basis for this, sequences must be caused and controlled by the awareness of the interacting agents. Where judgments are based on assumptions or intuition an interweaving of causally controlled effort on the part of interacting agents and understanding are not possible because of the absence of intelligibility. Interacting agents cannot establish sequential interactions, nor achieve the reciprocal benefits of sequentiality.

For the contemporary ethical systems, as we shall see, evaluation and judgments (assumptions) are based on intuitions (guesses) as opposed to evidence-based conclusions. With sequential actions, after every sequence there is at bare minimum a well founded belief that there will be a momentum of expectations and commitments continuing beyond the sequence. With the contemporary ethical systems, there is no foundation for this belief; duty, social sentiments, and emotions are unpredictable.

With the contemporary ethical systems, there is no foundation for this belief; duty, social sentiments, and emotions are unpredictable.

With the ethical action of the professional, the need for intelligible causal sequences is self-evident. The awareness of this cannot be escaped. None of the great ethicists explicitly discuss the advantages of intelligible causal sequences but all of them laid the appropriate groundwork for this.

No nurse would even question that nursing interventions have to be causal and sequential. But no one ever suggests that a nurse's ethical interventions ought to be the same and for precisely the same reasons.

When agents meet a circumstance with apathy they will not analyze the circumstance or the events that are occurring within it. Neither the circumstance nor their response to it will be intelligible. The events that occur will be caused by forces outside of the context and outside of the agent's control.

When agents engage with the circumstances and the events within the circumstances, in the manner of a fanatic, their actions and, therefore, their understanding will not be appropriate to the circumstance. In order to exercise fanaticism, they will have to falsify the nature of the circumstances to themselves and to each other. In meeting the circumstance on the level of fanaticism, their engagement with it will not be causally effective. It will not be appropriate to the nature of the circumstances or the events.

Finally, since their interaction in the circumstances will be inappropriate, it will not meet the objective demands of the circumstances as they arise. They will lack the power to control a planned and directed sequentiality. At its worst, their interaction will lack connection.

If agents meet the circumstance with a calm determination, that is, from the perspective of the Golden Mean, the circumstances will tend to be as intelligible as they can be made. Their actions and responses will be appropriate to the realities of and changes in the circumstances. There will be causal forces. They can engage with the circumstances as they come to understand the demands it makes on them. Their actions will be sequential.

An approach from the Golden Mean:

- Enables an ethical agent to act effectively and makes it possible for her to sustain activity.
- Endows the character of an ethical agent with qualities that make her actions self-controlled—neither deficient nor excessive but controlled by an objective awareness of the circumstances and of her response.
- Assures that the awareness with which an agent guides her action will not be given over to free association but will be intelligibly and causally related to the circumstances. It keeps her in the context.
- Assures that an agent's action will not be bumbling but will tend to be smooth-flowing because it will be well and naturally controlled.

A nurse instructs a patient on the health regimen for his brittle diabetic condition, such as diet, method of injection, activities, the inspection of the skin, and so forth. The patient's reciprocity is seen in his taking an active part in learning this. It is obvious that a patient's healing continues after his discharge. Reciprocity established the momentum for this. Everyday for the length of the patient's stay, the nurse can engage in meaningful conversation and emotional reinforcement of the teaching. Each exchange derives its strength from what has gone before, that is, from reciprocity—Confucius' fundamental principle, his rule of life.

Apathy for a nurse leads to burnout. For a patient, it decreases the drive to get well.

Nurturing, which is what a nurse does, is not something that an excellent or virtuous nurse does now and again in a rehearsed manner (Table 10.2). When she is not actively nurturing, she retains an inner attitude that makes her a mature, predictable, nurturing force.

> Apathy for a nurse leads to burnout. For a patient, it decreases the drive to get well.

The Categories of Effective Interaction

Aristotle has devised another elegant and highly useful analytic tool, which we will call the *ethical categories*. He combines a discussion of the Golden Mean into a discussion of the ethical categories.

The natural categories of ethical interaction are that it shall be:

10.2	The Virtue of Nurturing and Its Opposed Vice	
Deficit	**Means**	**Excess**
Distracted	Nurturing	Overbearing

- The right thing—the product of close analysis and understanding.
- At the right time—when the greatest good can be accomplished.
- For the right reason—through an appropriate motive.
- To the right extent—balanced and proportionate.
- For the right person—the person with whom one is interacting.
- In the right way—in a way that does good or at least no harm (Figure 10.1).

The ethical categories are not found in Aristotle's book The Categories, *but they are discussed in* The Nicomachean Ethics, *which we have discussed in greater length in chapter 5.*

Of Aristotle, more than any other philosopher, it can be said that he did take the world as a book and devoted his life to reading it. As a consequence, Aristotle is preeminent among philosophers.

Spinoza

An example . . . is the face of the entire universe, which although varying in infinite ways, yet remains the same. (Spinoza, *Correspondence,* Letter 64,)

The universally admired philosopher, Benedict Spinoza (1632–1697), took not the world but the entire universe—and this under the aspect of eternity—as his book. "It is the nature of reason to perceive things under a certain form of

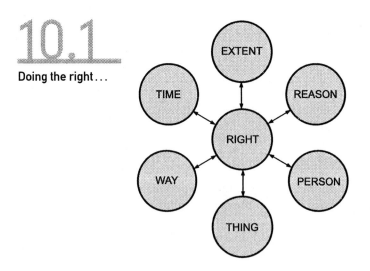

10.1

Doing the right . . .

eternity" (*Ethics*, Pt. II, Prop. 44). He read it quite well. He read the chapter on humankind so well that there has never been an ethicist the equal of Spinoza.

In Part IV of his major work *Ethics*, after a discussion of the psychology of desire, Spinoza lays out the revolutionary part of his work. He has established in his discussion of desire that it is in the individual's nature to love himself, to seek what is profitable to him, to desire everything that leads him to a greater perfection, and to endeavor to preserve his life. Then he observes that reason demands of us nothing, which is opposed to our nature (Pt. IV, Prop. 18). *Reason sanctions these desires.*

Spinoza defines *virtue* as "acting according to the laws of our own nature." It follows from this that the foundation of virtue in man is the endeavor to preserve our existence and that happiness consists in the experience of our power to preserve our existence. (Pt. IV, Prop. 18)

If one endeavors to preserve his existence, and does this through a series of rational actions, he will establish in his life a pattern of intelligible causal sequences. In Part IV, Proposition 19, Spinoza explains how this is done: "According to the laws of his own nature, each person necessarily desires that which he considers to be good and avoids that which he considers to be evil."

> Spinoza defines *virtue* as "acting according to the laws of our own nature."

By the laws of our nature, the emotion of joy reveals the desire for something we consider to be good. The emotion of sorrow reveals the aversion to something we consider harmful. These desires and aversions are not chosen by us but are internal to our nature as human beings. If they are directed by an objective awareness, and if the desire or aversion is acted on in a rational way, this will establish the intelligible sequences that characterize a life lived according to the nature of a living rational being.

Following this, Spinoza's major insights are:

Individual life is the metaphysical foundation of the existence and nature of ethics. At the birth of an ethical agent, the need and the nature of ethics comes into being (Pt. IV, Prop. 21-22). Virtue is an individual's human power that is limited only by the nature of a human being—by the effort through which an individual strives to preserve and enhance his existence.

The foundation of every virtue is the desire to exist. "No one can desire to be happy, to act well and live well, who does not at the same time desire to be, to act, and to live, that is to say, actually to exist" (Pt. IV, Prop. XXI).

Life is a process that involves changing things. An ethical agent's virtue is his power to change things—"as reason directs, from the ground of seeking our own benefit" (Pt. IV. Prop. 24). Life is the first principle of all experience and actions. "Without life no virtue can be conceived" (Pt. IV, Prop. 22).

No action one takes without understanding is a virtuous action. One is not active at all, and it is not an action. It is a passive reaction to outside influences reflecting their power rather than the power of the agent (Pt. IV, Prop. 23).

One who acts virtuously, acts according to the laws of his nature, that is, acts as directed by his reason seeking to preserve his being and to flourish. His actions reflect the power of his reason against that of outside forces acting on him (Pt. IV, Prop. 24). All this, and only this, is necessary to produce intelligible causal sequences.

> One who acts virtuously, acts according to the laws of his nature, that is, acts as directed by his reason seeking to preserve his being and to flourish.

As one acts, the efforts he makes through reason are efforts to understand. His mind regards nothing as a benefit to itself except that which contributes to its understanding (Pt. IV, Prop. 26).

Spinoza has something to say that is as relevant to a nurse as it is to a farmer or a shopkeeper or an artist or a babysitter. That is the admonition to rational self-interest.

"As reason makes no demands contrary to nature, it demands that every man should love himself, should seek...that which is really useful to him: he should desire everything which really brings man to greater perfection and should, each for himself, endeavor insofar as he can to preserve his own being. This is as necessarily true as a whole is greater than it parts" (Part IV, Prop 18).

Again, as virtue is nothing else but action in accordance with the laws of one's own nature, and as no one endeavors to preserve his own being except in accordance with the laws of his own nature, it follows that the foundation of virtue is the endeavor to preserve one's own being and that happiness consist in man's power of preserving his own being.

Far from advocating "the little pleasure of irrational selfishness," Spinoza is clearly speaking of a rational self-interest ethic. And he is entirely serious about this: "If a man knew of a certainty that he could live better at the end of the rope, than at his dinner table, he would be a fool not to rush to the gallows and hang himself" (*Correspondence*, Letter 36b).

"Men who are governed by reason, that is, who seek what is useful to them in accordance with reason desire for themselves nothing which they do not also desire for the rest of mankind, and, consequently, are just, faithful, and honorable in their conduct" (Part IV, Prop. 37).

The systems of the classic traditions are studies that can only be learned through experience, through trial and error. Trial and error is entirely inappropriate to the health care system. Before it was replaced by controlled experimental research studies, trial and error produced many of the nightmarish horrors of early medical and psychiatric practice.

The effort to rectify names cannot be completed by a nurse before she begins practice since the effort itself has not begun. The possibility of a pure reciprocity is lacking in nurse–patient interaction. One thing is possible: that a patient and nurse together can be inspired to seek their rational self-interest and no conflict between them will arise. And this is the aim of symphonology.

However, this brief history of the classic traditions serves to establish that something other than mechanical formalism or unreasoned emotions are available to guide one's ethical existence in the health care setting. The benefit of an objective standard of ethical judgment is available to nurses through a practice-based ethical system. The purposes of professional practice and ethical interaction are the same—to establish intelligible, causal, and humane sequences of interaction. The standard is not given abstractly in words but immediately, simultaneously, and objectively in events and communication.

The Difficulty of Virtue

The giants of the classical tradition recognize the difficulties of mastering the knowledge and attitudes necessary to the practice of the classical ethics.

Two of Confucius' disciples were conversing one day. One said to the other, "You are too modest, you are surely the equal of Confucius." The other disciple replied, "Our Master cannot be equaled, in the same way as one cannot go up into the heavens by climbing the steps of a stairway" (*Analects*, Book 9, chap. 25). The implication here is plain. The ethics of the classic period are difficult to the point where some aspects for some agents are impossible to achieve.

Socrates is motivated by the idea that no one can know the nature of the good and do evil. Since evil is done quite abundantly, the implication is that knowledge of the good is exceedingly difficult. The citizens of Athens found it troublesome to the point where they sentenced Socrates to death and executed him.

Aristotle mentions that the development of an ethical character necessitates the creation of a "second nature."

Spinoza ends his masterpiece with this warning: "If the way which, as I have shown, leads hither seems very difficult, it can nevertheless be found. It must indeed be difficult since it is so seldom discovered, for if salvation lay ready to hand and could be discovered without great labor, how could it be possible that it should be neglected almost by everybody? But all noble things are as difficult as they are rare" (*Ethics*, Book V). With Spinoza, ethics reached its high point and then went to pieces.

The great philosophers of the classic traditions described the final objective of their systems in different ways.

The ancients who wished to illustrate illustrious virtue throughout the kingdom, first ordered well their own States. Wishing to order well their States, they first regulated their families. Wishing to regulate their families, they first cultivated their person. Wishing to cultivate their person, they first rectified their hearts. Wishing to rectify their hearts, they first sought to be sincere in their thoughts. Wishing to be sincere in their thoughts, they first extended to the utmost their knowledge. Such extension of knowledge lay in the investigation of things. Things being investigated, knowledge became complete. Their knowledge being complete, their thoughts were sincere. Their thoughts being sincere, their hearts were then rectified. Their hearts being rectified, their persons were cultivated. Their persons being cultivated their States were rightly governed. Their states being rightly governed, the whole kingdom was made tranquil and happy. (Confucius, *The Great Learning*, chaps. 4 and 5)

For Socrates, it is the examination of life, since "the unexamined life is not worth living." The purpose of examination is knowledge. Knowledge, as opposed to enthusiasm and self delusion, is difficult and must begin in understanding.

Aristotle taught that the great value produced by ethics is happiness. Happiness is exceedingly rare and difficult to identify.

For Spinoza, the value sought and produced in the pursuit of virtue is virtue itself.

For a practice-based ethic, the final cause or objective is to nurture and strengthen the virtues of a beneficiary—the patient—and, as a result of this, to nurture and strengthen one's own virtues. No ethical concept has been more thoroughly gutted, more in need of rectification, than the concept of *virtue*.

The ethical ideal for Confucius was for everything to be in balance and serving its purpose, for everything to be knowable and known.

And reciprocity is nothing other than sustained intelligible causal sequences.

> For a practice-based ethic, the final cause or objective is to nurture and strengthen the virtues of a beneficiary—the patient—and, as a result of this, to nurture and strengthen one's own virtues.

Socrates focused on the starting point that one ought not to begin with words but with a clear awareness of what is good, of contextual factors, and with a knowledge of the true meaning of ethical concepts. The probable consequence of actions in the circumstances at hand—the context, enables one to act on the basis of understanding and foresight. As for knowledge of the nature of the virtues, Socrates believed that this was virtue itself. It is not possible to know the nature of the good and, knowing this, to do evil.

For Aristotle, the first step is that one ought always begin from and never leave what is appropriate, real, and complete. And that one, oneself, ought always be appropriate, real and complete.

Spinoza discovered that every ethical reality is fundamentally shaped by the nature of the ethical agents' life. Virtue—the excellence of an ethical agent—is found in obedience to the laws of one's nature and the nature of one's life.

All this tends to intelligible causal sequences.

Musings

The ethical systems of the greatest ethical thinkers have, implicitly, one common thrust. Whatever the approach, the trend of their thinking is to the conditions necessary to establish intelligible causal sequences in human affairs.

The giants' promise for the study of ethics is the following:

- Confucius—a better world.
- Socrates—a life worth living.
- Aristotle—happiness.
- Spinoza—virtue itself.

The ethical systems of the classical traditions are exceedingly difficult to learn and to practice. Nevertheless, nearly everyone who comes in contact with them assumes that he or she already understands and practices one or more. Everyone is more virtuous than everyone else, and easy and convenient ways have been found which make this possible.

One of the most powerful is the propensity of those who make decisions to make belief a function not of understanding but of convenience—to believe and disbelieve whatever it is convenient to believe or disbelieve.

Another is to approach a situation with an unreal idea or attitude. Nothing is more impressive than that which is not understood. To praise who or what the crowd praises and scorn what the crowd scorns, is sufficient to prove one's virtue—just as it was sufficient to prove the virtue of the crowd. Another contender is an attitude of instantaneous outraged self-righteousness. By beginning this way, one places one's self out of the reality of the ethical situation. This makes it possible and inviting to bring in many factors that conveniently support one's position despite the fact that they form no part of the present reality. Attention to the unreal will guide one right out of the context and away from the heavy chains of relevance to wherever one wants to go.

Or among all the true ideas and real things that form the context as one's means of analysis there are one or two false and unrelated ideas and one or two unreal and nonexistent things. These ideas can prove or disprove anything. These things can achieve or could have achieved anything. When the imagination enters into a context and displaces reason, the real and unreal become interchangeable. Nothing is fixed or stable. Everything is true or false interchangeably. In addition to the context of the situation and the contexts of awareness and understanding are the carefree images of the imagination. Then analysis becomes light-minded banter. Reason, reality, and common sense play no part; whatever is decided.

Any evasion of the need to be guided by evidence given in the reality of the situation for or against a decision undermines the intelligible causal sequences of objective understanding that would lead thought to a true and firm conclusion.

The classical tradition is appropriate as a way of life, but inappropriate as a bioethics. It is concerned with ethical action and bioethics with interaction. It is difficult to master and it must be possible to dwell in a bioethic from the beginning of practice. A health care professional must begin knowing what to do. The scope of ethical attention must be concentrated, and with the classic traditions it is not.

The classic tradition stresses long-term, lifetime development; a global approach and awareness; effective attitudes; and lifetime values. A bioethic has to do with dilemmas needing immediate resolution—resolutions according to appropriate standards, relevant analysis, and the vital human values of a beneficiary (a patient). Nurses and patients have a lifetime but not together.

> The classical tradition is appropriate as a way of life, but inappropriate as a bioethics. It is concerned with ethical action and bioethics with interaction.

Study Guide

1. Think about the idea of reciprocity as described by Confucius. How can this concept benefit you and your patient? How does it relate to the nurse–patient agreement?
2. What does it mean to say that something has intelligible causal sequences? What would happen to ethical decision making if this were not the case?

3. From Socrates we get the teaching method of Socratic Questioning. It is a form of questioning that allows us to delve deeply into something and do a thorough analysis that leads to a deeper understanding. Relate this idea to the study of ethics.
4. How can the context help to determine what is virtuous or not virtuous? Think of an example of this from your practice and discuss it.
5. What help does the Golden Mean of Aristotle give to nurses?
6. Think about the role of desire in human life as described by Spinoza and then relate it to your own life, personally and professionally.

References

Aristotle. *The Nicomachean Ethics* (any publication of the work).

Bahm, A. J. (1992). *The heart of Confucius*. Fremont, CA: Jain Publishing.

Spinoza, B. (1949). *Ethics*. (J. Gutmann, Ed.). New York: Hafner Publishing. (Original work published 1675)

Spinoza's Ethics and The Correspondence (any publication of the work will do).

Vlastos, G. (1991). *Socrates, ironist and moral philosopher*. New York: Cornell Press.

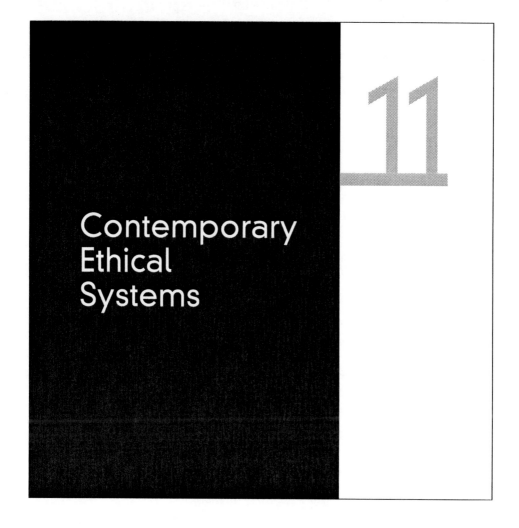

Contemporary Ethical Systems

The function of an ethical code is similar in some ways to the function of a travel agent. In order to examine that which is unfamiliar (the inner structure of an ethical code), we can have recourse to that which is more familiar (the itinerary of a vacation).

A vacation involves the time of departure—precisely when one will leave to go on vacation; the time of arrival—when one can expect to reach one's destination; the time when one will leave the vacation spot to return home; the location where one is going to spend one's vacation and the attractions and facilities that are found there; where one will stay—the accommodations one can expect and how accessible everything will be; the means of transportation to and from one's vacation spot; the cost of one's vacation; and the luggage one should take.

Would any sensible person put his entire vacation into the hands of a travel agent? Would he let the agent decide when to leave, where to go, how long to stay, when to return home, the cost of the vacation, how to get there, and where to stay?

The choice among vacation spots would be made according to the travel agent's evaluations. The traveler's desires would play no part in the planning of the vacation. No sensible person would agree to this arrangement. Yet, incredibly, many otherwise thinking people will make this arrangement with an ethical theory or the hodge podge that they have chosen, or have had chosen for them, at random. In terms of this ethical system, they plan the purpose and course of their entire life. The ethical system and their responsibilities to the role they take on in their lives may go in entirely different directions.

The demands of their ethical system may be in conflict with good judgment or a humane approach to human problems, or anything resembling relevance. But the demands are imperative; what they demand is obligatory.

If nursing and medical practice were to be patterned after the contemporary ethical systems, it would return practice to its nightmarish state of 1,000 years ago.

In our culture, at this time, two broad theories of ethics are dominant: deontology and utilitarianism.

Deontology

Deontology makes right and wrong the central ethical concepts. Ethical action consists in doing one's duty. To do one's duty is right. To shirk one's duty is wrong. The ethical agent has a duty to take the right action and to refrain from taking the wrong action. Beyond this, nothing is ethically relevant. The results of an action may be desired or deplored, but they have no ethical relevance.

The notion of duty as central to ethics arose with the Stoic philosophers about 300 BC, but its most powerful impetus was given by the German philosopher Immanuel Kant (1724–1804). The concept of duty is unrelated to our everyday concerns. Kant's duty ethic was a reaction to the social subjectivism of David Hume (1711–1776; "X is right" means society approves X; "X is wrong" means society disapproves of X [Hume, 1748/1955]).

Ought and right are both defined by a duty ethic in terms of duty. This makes a duty ethic viciously circular. The right action is that action which one ought to take (has a duty to take) because one ought to take that action which is right (that which one has a duty to take). This is to be done for no reason other than that the right action is that which one ought to take.

> The right action is that action which one ought to take (has a duty to take) because one ought to take that action which is right (that which one has a duty to take).

No deontologist has ever found the reason for duty in the demands of human life. The Stoics located it in a Platonist "World-Soul." The duties of people, the revolutions of the sun, the wetness of water are all part of the same thing—the laws that govern nature.

There is a logical drawback to this. It proves that which is doubtful (that people have duties) in terms of that which is even more doubtful (the existence of Plato's World-Soul). It is like proving that Jane will be in town at noon (a doubtful possibility) by declaring that Martians will beam her to town at noon (a much more doubtful possibility).

Kant held that the concept of duty is an innate idea. One is born knowing that he must do his duty and what his duty is (Kant, 1785/1964). This notion is also highly doubtful. In order to know the demands that duty laid upon him, a newborn would need to know of the relationships existing between himself and the world. In order to know this, he would need to know of the nature of the world. He would need to know this before knowing that there is a world. This is impossible.

Kant offered the idea that we are born with a capacity to call on a spontaneous knowledge of our duty. Kant was confident that when a dilemma arises, we are presented with an awareness of our appropriate duty through a power of internal perception or intuition.

Deontology is a duty-based ethic that directs actions taken by the agent, while ignoring concern for rewards, happiness, or any resulting consequences (Hill & Zweig, 2003). Deontology is the theory that "action in conformance with formal rules of conduct, are obligatory regardless of their results" (Angeles, 1992).

Deontology, as a bioethic, has not functioned well in the past. It is unsuited to be a bioethic in many ways.

Without the results of conduct as the measure of the rightness of conduct, that measure must be in the conduct itself. This being the case, it follows that in order for this to be possible:

> Deontology is the theory that "action in conformance with formal rules of conduct, are obligatory regardless of their results" (Angeles, 1992).

- We must not only know our duty, we must be certain of it. If we are not certain that the course of action we take is, in fact, our duty, we have no knowledge of our duty. An uncertain knowledge is not knowledge.
- We must know what certainty is to know that an innate or intuitive idea is certain.

Certainty—what circumstances call for what duties—has been a problem for deontology. The best known theories are:

- That the duty most appropriate to a circumstance is known through a storehouse of innate ideas—ideas possessed by the mind prior to birth and the onset of sense experience.
- That we possess a sort of intuitive "moral sense" which, in ethically ambiguous circumstances, reveals to us the appropriate duty to be performed.
- That our duty is revealed to us by an interplay of both of these.

This requires that we are born knowing the nature of our ethical relationship to the world. This explains the doubtful (we have knowledge before we have experience of anything knowable), in terms of the impossible (we have the ability to use the logic necessary to interpret that which is presented by the moral sense), before we know anything.

It is established by the fact that, supposedly, we do not know that it is not true. It would be impossible to adduce positive evidence for this theory. It is a groundless assumption that appears suddenly out of the imagination. It is based on the subsidiary assumptions of the existence of innate ideas and of a faculty of intuition. These assumptions have nothing to recommend them other than the fact that they are assumed. Their denial would be, at least, equally reliable for it can be based on equally weighty (or weightless) assumptions.

In all cases, the duty that is chosen must be assumed to be the appropriate duty. But if this assumption is trusted to be reliable then an assumption that it is unreliable will be equally trustworthy for it has as much (and as little) to recommend it.

> *But, strictly speaking, duties are not chosen. They are given by insight and the moral sense. To choose a duty would be to violate the spirit of duty. Duties are given to be accepted.*

Given circumstances under which conditions are not ordinary ones, she may find she has a duty not to do her duty. The problem that this inflicts on an ethical agent is that when she has the duty, if she does her duty, she does not do her duty; and only if she does not do her duty, does she do her duty. This makes the break in the connection between reality, ethics, and duty obvious, and leaves duty with no reason for being.

Duty and Justification

Deontology demands that right actions be taken without regard to consequences. A nurse cannot justify taking an action without concern for the effects they will produce. She should always be able to justify her actions in terms of their (foreseeable) consequences.

> Deontology demands that right actions be taken without regard to consequences. A nurse cannot justify taking an action without concern for the effects they will produce.

Could a nurse justify causing harm to a patient by saying "I was doing my duty?" This would not suffice legally. It surely does not suffice ethically—not if *ethically* is understood in any practical or rational sense.

If the purpose of an ethical system is to serve human life—or the efficient functioning of a profession—then deontology is not an ethical system. It is the absence of an ethical system. Consider this: The original deontologists preached the rightness of duty in action. They saw that a certain state of mind must follow these actions. The permanent possession of this state of mind was the purpose of deontology.

The Stoics called this state of mind *apatheia*, which means a state of apathy produced by living in the straightjacket of deontology. A modern name for this state is *burnout*. Apathy demands indifference to pain or pleasure, health or illness, happiness or misery. The father of modern deontology, Immanuel Kant, sings the praises of apathy in the preface to *Groundwork for the Metaphysics of Morals* (1785/1964) in a section entitled, "Virtue Necessarily Presupposes Apathy (Considered as Strength)."

The Stoics were inspired by the idea that the best thing about life is death. The best way to live is to grit your teeth and get it over with. To make this possible, they adopted a duty ethic in order to develop an indifference to the ebb and flow of fortune.

Indifference is an undesirable quality in a nurse. It is the opposite of what a nurse's state of mind ought to be. But one cannot consistently practice deontology without it. The practice of a duty ethic has never benefited patients or nursing—and certainly not individual nurses.

Nevertheless, many ethicists regard duty and morality as equivalent terms. They claim that ethics and deontology are identical. If this is true, then the only task of ethics is to list a person's duties, and, given intuitionism and the moral sense, this is unnecessary. The best a deontologist–ethicist can do is to give instructions to infallible faculties. "The idea that we are following rules when we act morally is a tired hangover from the days when the lives of people were controlled by religious and secular absolute rulers who accorded no respect or autonomy [independence] to ordinary people" (van Hooft, 1990, p. 211).

Nurses cannot escape taking the role of an ethical agent. One option open to a nurse is to answer the demands of her innate and prerational sense of duty. To do this, she must be aware of having an innate and prerational sense of duty. No one can ever be certain that an innate sense is reliable. Worse than this, no one can ever be certain that any idea is innate. An innate idea is an idea that one has not learned from experience. This means that an innate idea is an idea that one has no reason to believe. One is given a reason to accept and believe an idea by the contextual experience of the subject matter of that idea.

Dilemma 11.1

Zelda believes that she has a duty to give cardiac patients detailed information on the pathology involved in their condition. Mr. Wu and Mr. Goldfarb are two cardiac patients assigned to her. Mr. Wu is very much interested in having this information. But to Mr. Goldfarb it is terrifying. He is greatly depressed by her recitation.

Had Zelda respected the uniqueness of Mr. Goldfarb, she would have given him only that information that would have been of benefit to him and that would have caused him no unnecessary stress. She would have been motivated by beneficence rather than by her sense of duty. This would have necessitated a betrayal of the best interests of deontology. It is not difficult to see that her fidelity to duty was a betrayal of the best interests of Mr. Goldfarb. But, insofar as duty is Zelda's ethical standard, there is no significant ethical difference between Zelda's relationship to Mr. Goldfarb and her relationship to Mr. Wu.

Deontology is entirely concerned with an agent's actions. It is unconcerned with consequences (Figure 11.1). It is also indifferent to the agent's intentions, except his intention to do his duty. In principle, deontology demands indifference to individual autonomy. The recognition of autonomy would require that a nurse make choices appropriate to the uniqueness of her patient. Yet, in deontology, the demands of duty are imperative—they do not allow for choices to be made on the part of a nurse. Autonomous differences among patients call for a nurse to analyze each situation. A deontologist who analyzed contextual differences and made choices based on her analysis would have, perhaps unknowingly, abandoned deontology. A nurse who abandons her patient in order to pursue her duty has abandoned nursing.

> In principle, deontology demands indifference to individual autonomy.

Dilemma 11.2

A nurse, Ralph, is hired to care for a wealthy man, Francis, on his estate. A prerequisite of Ralph's employment is that it will be his duty not to enter the swimming pool on the estate while Francis is using it. Francis fears that someone else in the swimming pool might contaminate it and transmit a fatal disease to him—a frail, vulnerable man. Francis is extremely germ phobic. One day, while sitting beside the pool, Ralph notices that Francis has begun the unpleasant process of drowning. Ralph immediately rises to go into the swimming pool and get Francis out. But then he remembers the ethical responsibility that his duty has placed upon him. So Ralph sits back down. A flood of ideas and emotions rush through his mind. Within the constraints placed on him by duty, what can Ralph do? Has he done everything that could be done? It would be a nice gesture if he sent flowers, although, he has no duty to do so.

Utilitarianism

Utilitarianism was first formulated in terms of psychological hedonism, which means that determinism was the first inspiration of utilitarianism. Determinism is the doctrine that every human action is a response to a prior event. This prior event originates outside of the person who is (apparently) acting. The determinist holds that deciding and choosing are illusions. Determinists have described the feeling of being able to control one's thoughts and actions as a kind of dream. Psychological hedonism is a form of determinism. It is the doctrine that every action of an agent is, of necessity, a response to the experience or the expectation of pleasure or pain. It holds that one acts only to seek pleasure and to avoid pain and holds that one cannot act otherwise. It describes this tendency as being inborn.

Utilitarians claim that people cannot escape holding pleasure to be the good. Their next step was to argue for the necessity of

> the principle which approves or disapproves of every action whatsoever according to the tendency which it appears to have to augment or diminish the happiness of the party whose interest is in question. (Bentham, 1879/1962)

Then, they went on to argue, in effect, that the good of two persons is better than the good of one, the good of three is better than the good of two, and so on.

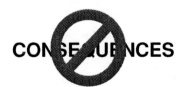

11.1

Duty rules.

✓ DUTY   CONSEQUENCES

The greatest possible good, then, would be the good of everyone, or the good of the greatest possible number. This good, they declared, ought to be the goal of every ethical agent.

Early opponents were quick to point out flaws in this reasoning. Thomas Carlyle (1795–1881) called utilitarianism a "pig philosophy." He noted that in every conceivable way, a symphony by Beethoven was a greater good than the victory of a pig wrestler. In fact, Beethoven's creativity, from every point of view, seems a greater good than the victories of a large number of pig wrestlers (Trail, 1896).

In response to this, utilitarians amended their principle to read, "The greatest (or highest) good of the greatest number." This reasoning ignores four relevant facts:

1. Let us grant that a person, through psychological necessity, holds his own pleasure to be an end in itself. This fact, in itself, gives him no reason, logical or otherwise, to concern himself with the good of others. A person might hold his good to be of value to him not because it is a good, but because it is his good. There is no logical flaw in this attitude, and any claim that it is ethically flawed begs the question.

   There is no rational reason for an agent to believe that his good is freely interchangeable with the good of other agents. His own good might be uniquely valued by him. He might hold that, if it is computed along with the good of another, it loses its motivational relevance.

   Let us imagine someone for whom this is not the case. Joe is very excited about going to a rock concert. Sally tells him that she is also going. Now, Joe is no longer excited. If Sally is going, it does not matter to Joe whether he goes as long as someone goes. Joe regards values as interchangeable. Psychologically, this does not make sense. But it is utilitarianism's view of human nature.

2. It is difficult to see how a nurse could justify actions by reference to "the greatest good for the greatest number." Her primary responsibility is to her individual patient. Her patient, in turn, has a right to choose his own goals and the consequences he seeks. He has a right to choose highly individualistic goals based solely on his own desires.

   Utilitarianism not only directs us to consider the results of an action when making moral judgments but also holds that we should look only to results. Considerations of an agent's feelings or convictions are seen as irrelevant to the question "What is the right thing to do?" (Arras & Hunt cited in Arras & Rhoden, 1989, p. 8)

   A nurse in pursuit of "the greatest good of the greatest number" would have no time to attend to her individual patients. Nor would they have any right to expect individualized nursing treatment from her. Being a nurse would not allow her to take ethical action. It would be a wall between her and the possibility of ethical action.

3. Utilitarianism collapses into deontology. This has finally been recognized even by utilitarians. To avoid this flaw, a distinction is drawn between *rule*

and *act* utilitarianism. Rule utilitarians claim that an agent has a duty to obey certain rules. These are the rules best adapted to bring about the greatest good for the greatest number. Act utilitarians declare that the value of an action is determined by its goal. This simply means that an agent has a duty to aim for a specific goal. He has a duty to act to bring about the greatest good for the greatest number. Utilitarians cannot escape deontology.

4. Utilitarianism is also an ethical theory peculiar in this: Justice is the most highly honored interpersonal virtue of our society. It is the goal of our entire legal system. Ironically, utilitarianism is a prescription for injustice.

> *One such limitation [of utilitarianism as an ethical theory] is the violation of personal autonomy... its inherent potential for discrimination, the possibility that what is perceived as "good" for the majority may be bad for the minority. (Franklin, 1988, p. 35).*

In fact, it is somewhat worse than that.

> *Utilitarianism... has fallen into bad odor, and particularly when it comes to a defense of individual rights and personal liberties... suppose... the general welfare of the community, or the greatest happiness of the greatest number, might conceivably be furthered or increased by the sacrifice of the liberty, or the well-being, or even the life of a single individual... [Would not this sacrifice be]... the moral consequence of anyone's adhering strictly to Utilitarian principles. (Veatch, 1985, pp. 30–31).*

Nevertheless, utilitarianism is today's dominant ethical trend. Many nursing ethics textbooks recommend it as a tool for ethical decision making. It is an alternative theory that a nurse might want to consider. But

> *Utilitarianism requires an agent to do that action which brings about the greatest balance of good over evil in the universe as a whole... to maximize the good of all humans... to consider all of the available alternatives and perform that act which will maximize the good of all affected parties. (McConnell, 1982, p. 14)*

This is utilitarianism. Does it not seem unreasonable to expect a nurse to know:

- What action will bring about "the greatest balance of good over evil in the universe as a whole"?
- What the nature of "the greatest balance of good over evil in the universe as a whole" might look like?
- How one might "maximize the good of all humans"?
- The precise number of "all of the available alternatives"?
- Precisely that "act which will maximize the good of all affected parties"?

Suppose that, by some miracle, the nurse could know all this. Even then, how could utilitarianism be justified in a health care system that places a high value on the individual's rights and autonomy? "No action is, in itself, ethically good or bad. Utilitarians hold that the only factors that make actions good or bad are the outcomes, or end results, that are derived from them" (Burkhardt &

Nathaniel, 2002, p. 28). Utilitarianism is a theory in which the ends justify the means (Gibson, 1993).

The utilitarian's ethical advice consists in emotionally charged, high-flying, and empty phrases urging the pursuit of the impossible. It is an impractical approach to the practical science. If an agent accepts the necessity of doing the impossible, she will become a fanatic or she will do nothing.

Dilemma 11.3

Harry is in the hospital. He is dying. Harry's very large family is unaware of the fact that he is dying. He does not want his family to know. Harry's son has been discharged from the army and is returning home. The family intends to surprise Harry with his son's return when he arrives home. What should be done?

A utilitarian would say that Harry's family should be advised of his prognosis, even against his wishes. They need to know this in order to decide what they desire to do. They are the greater number. Yet the standard of self-assertion would inspire Harry's nurse to keep her agreement with her patient. His right to control his time and effort would compel her to reveal the fact of his son's return and let Harry decide what he desires to do.

But, for a utilitarian, any claim of "the greatest good for the greatest number" is a sufficient reason to divulge anything or to conceal anything. Obviously, this is incompatible with the nurse–patient agreement as that agreement is usually understood.

The idea of modern utilitarianism was first introduced by Jeremy Bentham (1748–1832) and brought to its full development by John Stuart Mill (1806–1873). The central ethical concepts of utilitarianism are good and evil. It is the doctrine that an ethical agent's responsibility is to bring about "the greatest good for the greatest number."

Telishment

Telishment is a suggestion traditionally made to utilitarians by deontologists. *Telishment* derives from the words *telos*, the final point toward the achievement of which a process is directed (Angeles, 1992), and -*ment*, as in *punishment*.

Dilemma 11.4

Utilityville is a village run on utilitarian principles. Periodically, the town fathers randomly choose someone to serve the community. They put this person in chains in the public square and torture him to death. They inflict a punishment on this innocent person similar to but milder than that which they would inflict on a habitual criminal. This is telishment.

The death of this unfortunate benefactor serves the community in two ways:

1. Once they witness the gruesome fate of an entirely innocent person, potential criminals can imagine, in bloodcurdling detail, the horrible fate awaiting the guilty. This leads a number of potential criminals away from a life of crime and a horrible death by torture. This, in itself, brings about "the greatest good for the greatest number."

And, it has even further benefits: (kept it in, but changed but to and).

2. Many people who would otherwise be victims of crime are saved from this fate by the death of the village benefactor.

There is a drawback to this practice. The town fathers have found a very effective way to bring about "the greatest good for the greatest number." They save potential victims by making actual victims. This violates any rational conception of justice. This type of crime prevention must produce intolerable conditions. These conditions cannot be made right by more utilitarianism. There is nothing in utilitarianism to prevent any crime by a greater number against a lesser number or against an individual. Individual justice is necessary to a human form of existence and to objectively justifiable ethical action. Nothing in the principle of utility (i.e., the greatest good for the greatest number) establishes the principle of individual justice (Sarikonda-Woitas & Robinson, 2002). The recognition of individual rights must be added to the principle of utility in the attempt to prevent barbaric acts of injustice. But this is not possible.

Utilitarianism alone is not sufficient to rationally justifiable ethical interaction.

In Utilityville, the practice of utilitarianism is not necessary to effective and justifiable ethical action. Such action would be quite possible without it. Societies based on individual rights, nonaggression, and interaction through agreement flourish far better than utilitarian societies.

It is clear that utilitarianism is not necessary to rational, ethical interaction. As an ethical approach, utilitarianism is neither sufficient in itself nor a necessary addition to other approaches to bring about justifiable ethical action.

No health care setting should be a Utilityville. Utility undermines a professional's ethical awareness by directing her away from the objectives of her profession.

Under utilitarianism, reciprocity, cooperation, trust, and respect for individual rights have no ethical import since none of these serve utility. It is interesting to consider here the radical difference if the principle of utility—each serving the greatest good of the others—had been replaced with the principle of reciprocity. This would be the greatest good, by the greatest number, for the greatest number (Figure 11.2).

Triage

Triage is not a contemporary ethical system. It is an objectively justifiable ethical practice. A triage situation is generally thought of as the scene of a major fire, an

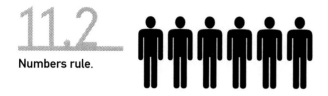

11.2

Numbers rule.

automobile or train wreck, a plane crash, or some other dramatic, emergency situation. With the exception of paramedics and emergency room personnel, few health care professionals normally face situations as tense and confusing as these. Yet, every nurse's shift has elements in common with triage situations. Patients constantly enter and leave the health care setting. The conditions and the needs of patients are constantly changing. A nurse's professional actions are best approached with these triage elements in mind. An efficient nurse must be able to meet the ethical demands of the profession with a consistent mind-set and awareness appropriate to the unpredictable.

Every triage situation, from the most catastrophic to the everyday, calls for ethical balance and proportion. Even in situations that are not so complex or demanding as a catastrophic situation, the health care setting itself is a "low-key" triage situation. Every time a professional enters the health care setting, some patients, or one patient, will have needs greater than others. A nurse masters the problem of ethical balance and proportion as she learns to locate these patients. The mastery of this art (ethical balance and proportion) can be seen in an analysis of a hypothetical situation.

We can conduct our analysis through a thought experiment: Suppose that there is a situation in which two people, Arletta and Francine, each has a stake. Their home is burning down and some of their possessions have been left inside. The possession that Arletta might lose is one she would much rather have than lose. The benefit that Francine might lose is one whose loss would cause her extreme grief. Imagine further that there is a fireman, Bill, inside the house, who has an opportunity to exercise benevolence and to act beneficently in this situation. Bill can act to assist only one person, either Francine or Arletta, but not both. In and of themselves, neither Arletta nor Francine is intrinsically more deserving than the other. Bill faces a dilemma. There is not one individual who is the center of the ethical context. Should he assist Arletta or should he assist Francine? How can he make the best decision?

There is no doubt that some possessions are more important than others. So all possible possessions can be, in effect, evaluated and numbered by Bill. He can rate them from 1 to 10 according to their importance: Class 1 possessions are those that are least in importance; class 10 possessions are those that are most important. A class 3 possession will not be prized by the person who holds it as much as a class 8 possession will be prized.

In a triage situation, the benefactor (in our case, Bill), in effect, analyzes the situation in this way:

First, Bill will ask himself, "If Arletta and Francine were not two people but only one person, what would be the best thing for me to do?" He knows very well that Arletta and Francine are not one person. But in this situation, in order for him to make the best decision, he will think of them as if they were. He will act as if they were one person with two possessions. He will rescue the possession that would be the more highly rated by this person.

If Bill can bring just one thing from the burning building, he will bring out Francine's dog rather than Arletta's wedding dress. He will judge that, if Francine and Arletta were one person, this person would rate her dog at least an 8, whereas she would rate her wedding dress perhaps a 3.

Although it is one person's dog and another person's wedding dress, Bill would still rescue Francine's dog for the same reason. He judges Francine's dog, Tippy, a living thing, to be an 8 to Francine; he judges Arletta's wedding dress to be a 3 to Arletta.

He will rescue Tippy because this is what is called for in the (triage) situation. The triage situation is an ethical situation where all the potential beneficiaries become one person. The professional commitment is not to an individual but to everyone involved taken as one person so that the most appropriate beneficiary can be discovered.

> We have been assuming that there is an equal probability of Bill's being able to salvage either Tippy or Arletta's dress. We have assumed that the risk to Bill is equal in both cases. The odds for and against a benefactor being able to bring about different benefits and the risks involved must also be factored in. If Bill could easily salvage Arletta's wedding dress, but the probability of his rescuing Francine's dog was very low and/or the peril to him was very high, then it might be more reasonable for him to salvage Arletta's wedding dress.

In a triage situation, a health care professional must sort out all the possible benefits to everyone involved in the situation—wounded soldiers on a battlefield, people injured in an airline disaster, people trapped in a burning building—regardless of whose benefits they are. She cannot make her decision according to the normal professional–patient agreement. Therefore, she must make it according to the benefits that she can bring about without encountering significant danger.

If a nurse on a battlefield finds a soldier with a broken leg and a sprained ankle, she will fix the broken leg. If she finds two soldiers, one with a broken leg and one with a sprained ankle, she will attend to the one with the broken leg for the same reason. This is the most important benefit she can bring about.

If she finds two soldiers, one with a broken leg and one with a sprained ankle, she will attend to the one with the broken leg. . . . This is the most important benefit she can bring about.

After an airline disaster, a nurse might treat the severe bleeding of a person with a broken back before immobilizing him. There is something she can do for his bleeding and little she can do for his back. At the same time, his bleeding presents a greater threat to his life than does his back. If she found two survivors, one with severe bleeding and the other with a broken back, she would attend to the one with the severe bleeding for the same reason that she would attend to an individual person's bleeding before attending to his back.

According to the triage analysis, a health care professional ought to choose her beneficiary according to:

▓ The importance of the benefit, its ranking on the scale.
▓ The probability of her being able to bring about the benefit.
▓ The risks, if any, she will encounter.

In a triage situation, she ought to regard every possible beneficiary as one person. Then she ought to direct her actions according to the most rational desires of this one person.

She ought to do this in a situation where only one person is involved because in this situation this is the greatest benefit she can bring about. This is what the rational desire of her beneficiary calls for her to do.

She ought to do this in a triage situation, where more than one person is involved, because this is what an objective reading of the situation calls for her to do. The person with the severe bleeding would recognize this action as having the greatest objective value. According to her education, training, and experience, a nurse would recognize this action as having the greatest objective value. As a member of the human race the person with the broken back would recognize this action as having the greatest objective value.

The analogy between the triage situation and the professional's everyday circumstances is obvious. So is the reasonableness of analyzing them in the same way. If the benefit to one patient is a 6 and no one can receive or lose a benefit of 7 or greater, then the professional ought to attend to this patient. If the benefit to another patient would be rated 7 or greater and providing the first patient's benefit would interfere with the second patient's benefit, the professional should act for the benefit of the second patient.

When it is possible to benefit everyone, then everyone ought to be benefited. When this is not possible, then those individuals who can be brought the greatest benefit ought to be the beneficiaries of a nurse's actions.

For purposes of analysis, ethical decision making, and ethical action, a triage situation makes every potential beneficiary one person. In the context of a triage situation, the nurse ought to bring about the greatest benefit. She ought to do this because this is, so to speak, what the rational desire of this one person would want her to do.

Suppose there had been three persons living in the home and each one, including Francine and Arletta, had wedding dresses hanging in the same closet. Triage-type thinking would still bring out Tippy. George, a utilitarian, would multiply 3 × 3, which is 9. Nine is a higher number than 8. Therefore, he would save the wedding dresses and bring them out accompanied by the screams of Tippy burning to death inside.

Social Relativism

Ethical relativism is the view that the rightness of an action and the goodness of an object depend on, or consist in, the attitudes taken toward it by some in-dividuals or groups (Runes, 1983). All of the ethical ideals that individuals have contributed to the improvement of society are available to the understanding through relativism—through that which the society accepts as an ethical ideal. Yet, if relativism is valid, these improvements were—before being accepted by the society - evil, or, at best, valueless. The problem arises: How does a flock of ideas not countenanced by the society (i.e., before being accepted), therefore ethically invalid, become ethically valid ideas that are now (since being accepted) ethical standards appropriate to act upon and to guide ethical decision making?

Another, more basic, question suggests itself: Did the society have a reason for accepting these ideas? But this question puts us in a double bind: If the answer is "no," then the acceptance had no basis and relativism is baseless as well as senseless. If the answer is "yes," this suggests a different answer for the reasons that make the society accept these ideas and not the ideas themselves, are the appropriate standards of judgment. For instance: If, at a certain time a society decides that kidnapping is evil, is kidnapping evil because of the nature of kidnapping or because the society decides that it is evil? Or, if a society believes that human sacrifice is good, is it good because society believes it is good or is it because of its intrinsic nature that sacrifice is good?

We must be able to recognize the good before we can know that this is where the sentiments of the society lead us. If we know that that which society approves is evil, then we ought to reject relativism. If we know that that which society approves is good, then the approval of society is extraneous. If we do not know, then there is no virtue in following society. We may as well follow a fortune-teller or a magician. The sentiments of society are equally superfluous.

Dilemma 11.5

Fauzuja Kassindja is 17. She is facing an arranged marriage and female circumcision (usually done between the ages of 4 and 12 but in her country it is done along with the marriage celebration). She does not want this. She was able to flee her country and come to America to ask for asylum. This brought public attention in the United States to this practice. Was she wrong it wanting to go against the practices of her country? And should she have been granted asylum? (Althaus, 1997)

Concern with what the society feels is not a way to understand anything except to understand what the society approves or what the society feels or intuits. From knowing what the society feels, one could never become aware of the significance and importance of the society's feelings. Worse than this, one might never become aware of their insignificance or the harms caused by acting on the feelings of society.

No argument for social relativism as an objectively justifiable bioethical guide can succeed. The argument would have to begin by assuming that individuals, alone or together, are incapable of judging what is good or evil in relation to them. Otherwise, there would be no need for an external guide. Then the values and feelings of society are set up as the standards of ethical judgment. It is assumed by the relativist that the sentiments of society are reliable ethical principles. This implies the following:

- The society is capable of judging what the individual cannot, what is ultimately good or evil in relation to the individual.

- The individual is capable of discovering that the ethical judgment of the society is valid, and that of the individual is not.

In order to do this, the individual must be capable of recognizing the validity of an ethical judgment in order to judge the judgment of society.

And, if the individual is capable of this, she has no need of guidance by the sentiments of society.

There is no way of knowing if the society is the source of our awareness of the good unless we have an independent knowledge of the good. If we have independent knowledge of the good then we have no need for guidance by the sentiments of the society.

> There is no way of knowing if the society is the source of our awareness of the good unless we have an independent knowledge of the good.

Dilemma 11.6

Mary and Abe Ayala have a teenage daughter, Anissa, who has been diagnosed with acute leukemia. Their physician recommends a bone marrow transplant. Neither Anissa's parents nor her brother are acceptable donors. For 2 years the family searches for an acceptable donor. Their daughter's time is running out. Finally, they face their last hope. They decide to try to have another baby in the hope that this infant will be an acceptable donor. (Toufexis, 1990).

Bars and beauty shops, radio talk shows were filled with discussions of the ethical ramifications of this. Are the parents justified in having a baby driven by these motivations? See Figure 11.3.

Emotivism

Emotivism is the theory that value terms are grounded in emotional attitudes. According to emotivist theory, ethical terms express nothing but attitudes of approval or disapproval. Emotivism arises from ethical nonnaturalism (there is no direct linkage between ethical or value judgments and facts about the world) and noncognitivism (statements about ethical judgments do not refer to any facts about the world, therefore, they cannot be described as true or false). Emotivism has nothing whatever to recommend it, but we include it here because it is general practice.

11.3

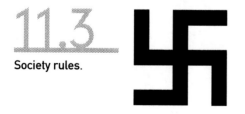

Society rules.

Emotivism arises from ethical nonnaturalism (there is no direct linkage between ethical or value judgments and facts about the world) and noncognitivism (statements about ethical judgments do not refer to any facts about the world, therefore they cannot be described as true or false).

The contemporary ethical systems quickly drive ethical agents to their feelings as standards of ethical judgment. "Emotivism claims that, in disputes about basic moral principles, we can not appeal to reason, but only to emotion. This would seem to lead to propaganda wars in which each side, unable to resort to reason, simply tries to manipulate the feelings of the other side (Emotivism, n.d., para. 5).

A.J. Ayer (1910–1989) was the ethicist who proposed to legitimize the system of emotivism. Emotivism says that moral judgments express positive or negative feelings. "X is good" means "Hurrah for X!" and "X is bad" means "Boo on X!" Since moral judgments are exclamations, they cannot be true or false. So there cannot be moral truths or moral knowledge. We can reason about moral issues if we assume a system of norms. But we cannot reason about basic moral principles (Ayer, 1936).

Some emotivists base their view on logical positivism, which holds roughly that any genuine truth claim must be capable of being tested by sense experience or logical processes derived from sense experience. Since moral judgments cannot be tested by sense experience they cannot establish genuine truth claims. So moral judgments only express feelings. Thus logical positivism leads to emotivism.

An explanation of why one comes to an ethical judgment is necessary. No explanation of why one feels the emotion one feels is possible. Unrelated memories and judgments are tied into the emotion.

Emotivism substitutes the experience of reality for reality itself. Our emotions arise from our sedimented memories at least as much as from the context. But complex memories and past judgments are not ethical decisions.

Emotivism in both theory and practice stands firmly on the subjective principle: "It all depends on how you look at it" (or, more precisely, "how you feel about it").

Let us assume, for the sake of analysis, this were true: If it "all depends on how you respond to it" (look at it/feel about it or whatever) then, before you respond to it, it is nothing. And, if it is nothing, it does not depend on how you respond to it. Nothing depends on nothing. And, if you respond to nothing, then you are seriously deluded. If the ethical quality or status of a state of affairs depends on your response to it, then before you respond to it, it is nothing. And, your responding to nothing does not and cannot bring anything into being.

Emotivism also refers to the practice of making ethical decisions on the basis of emotional responses to dilemmas. Despite what ethical agents profess, emotivism—decisions made on the basis of out of context emotional responses—is, far and away, the most widely practiced way of making ethical decisions. It has at least three drawbacks. It has nothing to do with making or ethics or decisions.

Dilemma 11.7

Evelyn, a nurse always has a feeling directing her as to what she ought to do. But these feelings are always accompanied by the feeling that she ought not do what she feels she ought to do. She has been misled by her feelings many times in the past. She has not blamed her feelings but herself for the shortcomings of her ethical decision making. How can she correct the flaws in her character that cause these unfortunate errors in judgments?

To ask: "What do I feel ought to be done?" rather than "What ought to be done?" is to miss the ethical demands of a circumstance entirely. How does one become conditioned to the point where an ethical dilemma does not draw one's attention out to it but drives one's attention back into oneself? See Figure 11.4.

Dilemma 11.8

Sometimes, when little children are very angry and they cannot express their anger, rather than holding it back they will slap or punch their own faces to express their frustration. How is this similar to adopting emotivism as one's ethical decisions making system?

Musings

None of the contemporary ethical systems will do any harm unless they are taken seriously.

Ethics is not a mere adornment to human life. It is the science of a successful human life. This has been obvious since humanity first began to consider ethical ideas. It has always been obvious in itself but not always obvious to the people

11.4

Emotion rules.

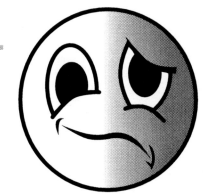

who might benefit from ethical understanding. For various reasons, ethics, while it is given much lip service, is seldom taken seriously.

The alternatives to clearly and objectively defined ethical ideas lead not toward but away from successful living. Ethical ideas appropriate to the health science professions can enormously enhance professional practice and a professional's life.

Deontology cannot offer a logical argument in its own support. Therefore, it cannot justify itself. The spirit of formalism—rigorous or excessive adherence to recognized forms—in deontology is captured in the Latin maxim: "One should tell the truth though the heavens fall." One has a duty to accept deontology is not a justification of deontology.

Utilitarianism might also avail itself of formalism. If, in a certain country, there were many rich people and very few poor ones, a Robin Hood who robbed from the poor to give to the rich would be practicing a utilitarian formalism.

If relativism can be discovered to be the source of ethical awareness, then the nature of ethical awareness can be discovered. If the nature of ethical awareness can be discovered, relativism is extraneous.

Emotivism, in presenting itself as ethical analysis, is an abandonment of concern for ethical understanding. If a nurse needs an ethic, she needs an objective ethic. If she needs a nonobjective ethic, then she needs no ethic at all. "Nurses and nursing are at the center of issues of tremendous and long-lasting impact... nurses cannot afford to limit their actions" (Milstead, 2004, p. 22).

Animals act to avoid various perils to which they are vulnerable. As rational animals we (sometimes) use our powers of reason to initiate actions to oppose the loss of our well-being. One of the ways we can do this is through ethical awareness, extending the time frame of our actions and making them more intelligible. Another is by establishing health care systems. The motivation for each of these is a reasoned desire to escape the consequences of various aspects of our vulnerability.

> When these systems, for example, deontology utilitarianism and so forth, are dominant in a health care setting they expose patients to a virulent and entirely unnecessary form of vulnerability.

Health care systems are far more efficient in achieving this than the contemporary ethical systems. Ethical systems can conflict with the purposes of the health care setting and the rational expectations of patients. When these systems, for example, deontology utilitarianism and so forth, are dominant in a health care setting they expose patients to a virulent and entirely unnecessary form of vulnerability.

Study Guide

1. Discuss each of the systems: deontology, utilitarianism, social relativism, and emotivism. Would any of these give you a sense of pride in what you are doing or enable you to think that you have done the best thing in the context for this person?

2. Think about the consequences to patients if a nurse took seriously each of these standards.

3. Discuss one of the cases in the book or from your own practice from each of these systems. Note that you may reach a similar conclusion, at times, with that of symphonology, but the process of analysis is entirely different. Thus, you may reach an appropriate decision by default.

References

Althaus, F. A. (1997). Female circumcision: Rite of passage of violation of rights? *International Family Planning Perspectives*, *23*(3). Retrieved June 4, 2007, from http://www.guttmacher.org/pubs/journals/2313097.html

Angeles, P. A. (1992). *Dictionary of philosophy* (2nd. ed.). New York: Harper Collins.

Arras, J., & Rhoden, N. (Eds.). (1989). *Ethical issues in modern medicine* (3rd ed.). Mountain View, CA: Mayfield.

Ayer, A. J. (1936). *Language, truth, and logic*. London: Gollancz.

Bentham, J. (1962). *The works of Jeremy Bentham*. (J. Bowring, Ed.). New York: Russell & Russell. (Original work published 1879)

Burkhardt, M. A., & Nathaniel, A. K. (2002). *Ethics and issues in contemporary nursing* (2nd ed.). Albany, NY: Delmar.

Emotivism. (n.d.). Retrieved from http://www.jcu.edu/philosophy/gensler/et/et-05-00.htm

Franklin, C. (1988). Commentary on case study. *Hastings Center Report*, *18*(6), 35–36.

Gibson, C. H. (1993). Underpinnings of ethical reasoning in nursing. *Journal of Advanced Nursing*, *18*, 20–27.

Hill, T. E., & Zweig, A. (Eds.). (2003). *Immanuel Kant: Groundwork for metaphysics of morals*. New York: Oxford University Press.

Hume, D. (1955). *Enquiry concerning the principles of morals*. New York: Handel. (Original work published in London, 1748)

Kant, I. (1964). *Groundwork for the metaphysics of morals* (J. H. Paton, Trans.). New York: Harper & Row. (Original work published 1785)

McConnell, T. C. (1982). *Moral issues in health care*. Monterey, CA: Wadsworth Health Science Division.

Milstead, J. (2004). *Health policy and politics: A nurses' guide*. Sudbery, MA: Jones and Bartlett.

Runes, D. D. (Ed.). (1983). *Dictionary of philosophy*. New York: Philosophical Library.

Sarikonda-Woitas, C., & Robinson, J. (2002). Ethical health care policy: Nursing's voice in allocation. *Nursing Administration Quarterly*, *26*, 72–80.

Toufexis, A. (1990, March 5). Creating a child to save another. *Time Magazine* [Electronic version].

Trail, H. N. (Ed.). (1896). *The centenary edition of Carlyle's work*. New York: Oxford.

van Hooft, S. (1990). Moral education for nursing decisions. *Journal of Advanced Nursing*, *15*, 210–215.

Veatch, H. B. (1985). *Human rights: Fact or fancy?* Baton Rouge, LA: Louisiana State University Press.

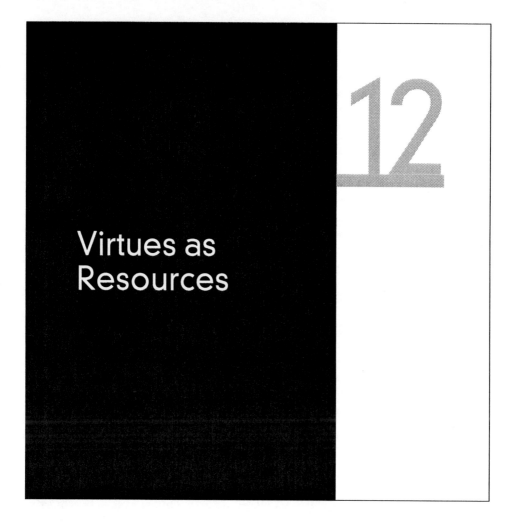

12

Virtues as Resources

The term *virtue* in its original sense meant excellence in the natural activity of a virtuous thing—a thing capable of some excellent activity or function. For instance, the virtue of a boat is its tendency to stay afloat. The virtues of a horse are its swiftness and endurance. The virtue of a physician is his ability to heal. The virtues of a wrestler are strength and skill. The virtue of a painter is the ability to portray.

In its classic sense, the virtues of a person came to mean all those excellences that arise from exercising control of one's decisions and actions through reason. This is the sense in which it will be used here.

Physicians directly serve and promote a patient's life, health, and well-being through medical interventions. This is the direct and immediate goal of a physician. The virtue of a physician is to do this excellently. For other professionals, this is a mediate goal. In matters concerning a patient's medical well-being, a physician mediates between other professionals and the

> In its classic sense, the virtues of a person came to mean all those excellences that arise from exercising control of one's decisions and actions through reason. This is the sense in which it will be used here.

patient. A physician decides what is to be done to cure a patient. "It is the physician who cures and the nurse who cares" (Nightingale, 1860/1969).

Ideally, a nurse would be one who has an immediate relationship with the person with whom she interacts. One small advance in the role that a nurse assigns to herself makes this possible. This advance makes it possible for a nurse to be more truly a professional, to provide greater benefits for her patient, and to derive the full benefits of her profession.

The nature of the health care setting and of nursing implies the nature of this advance. A nurse can make it her immediate goal to promote and serve the life, health, and well-being of her patient. She cannot do this by adopting the role of a physician. But she can do it by serving and promoting the virtues of her patient. This she does by nurturing and sustaining his power to act according to his nature—his ability to fulfill his rational desires to serve and promote his life and well-being, his pursuit of his rational self-interest. To a greater or lesser extent, many nurses already do this.

> But she can do it by serving and promoting the virtues of her patient. This she does by nurturing and sustaining his power to act according to his nature—his ability to fulfill his rational desires to serve and promote his life and well-being, his pursuit of his rational self-interest.

The virtues of a patient are identical to the virtues of a professional or to the virtues of any other human being. The virtue or excellence of a living thing is a form of well-being or power. It is the power, possessed by the living thing, to sustain its life as the kind of thing it is. Virtue, then, is a form of health. (Aristotle as quoted in McKeon, 1941).

The ethicist, Benedict Spinoza, describes virtue thusly: "reason demands...that every person... should desire everything that really leads man to a greater perfection, and absolutely that everyone should endeavor, as far as in him lies, to preserve his own being" (1949, p. 202). This is precisely what the health care setting is all about. Professionals can directly foster and nourish this aspect of a patient's virtue. A nurse, given the fact that she is with the patient over an extended period of time, can do this as no other biomedical professional can. She can be the custodian of his power to sustain his life as a human being. An effective nurse is a companion who interacts with, safeguards, and nurtures her patient's virtues.

> She can be the custodian of his power to sustain his life as a human being. An effective nurse is a companion who interacts with, safeguards, and nurtures her patient's virtues.

In addition to everything else they are, the bioethical standards are the virtues of an ethical agent. They are characteristics of a person that enable him to sustain his existence as the person he is. They are qualities of character that enable a person to develop. They enable a person to act in order to fulfill his rational desires.

The bioethical standards, as virtues, are:

1. Autonomy: The ability to sustain one's unique and rational nature—those qualities of character that enable a person to be the person he desires to be. This ability makes one an excellent human being—one able to sustain his life as the person he is.

2. Freedom: The ability of a person to project and maintain purposeful courses of long-term action is an ability that makes him able to sustain his life and identity. This ability is a form of health and a virtue.
3. Objectivity: The virtue that enables one to perceive one's path to a greater perfection and to take the actions that are necessary for him to preserve his life and health. The ability to grasp and interact with the extramental facts of reality that are relevant to sustaining one's life and well-being is an ability that is a form of health and an invaluable virtue.
4. Self-assertion: The ability to dedicate one's time and effort to envisioning appropriate courses of action is a form of power that is a form of health. This ability is a profound virtue.
5. Beneficence: The ability to envision and take actions in pursuing one's benefit or in acting to avoid harm is a power that makes one able to sustain one's life as the kind of being he is. This ability is a virtue.
6. Fidelity: The ability to maintain one's self-awareness and one's determination to continue on courses of action that serve his life and well-being is a form of ethical health, which is to say, it is a virtue.

A nurse ought to recognize these abilities as the virtues of her patient. She ought to recognize these virtues as her own. Imagine what a person's life would be without them.

Her justifiable interaction with her patient depends upon her motivating and nurturing his virtues. This is the meaning of "doing for her patient what he would do for himself if he were able." Insofar as she acts as a nurse, her actions are justified. They are also, as we shall see, invaluable to her as a person.

> *If the professional establishes a professional–patient agreement, she is, incidentally, most likely to avoid legal actions. Patients are not generally well versed on the law. Few patients ever say, "Looking back, I see where my nurse violated the law. I am going to take her to court." Patients take health care professionals to court when they perceive a violation of her ethical responsibilities—when she has made them worse off than they should have been. If she is sympathetic to her patient's virtues, the possibilities of a nurse being a defendant in a lawsuit are remote to the point of irrelevance.*

For a patient to sustain his life as the kind of being he is, two things are necessary. First, of course, he must sustain his life. It is the immediate responsibility of a physician to assist him in this. Second, he must sustain his awareness of the person he is. It is the natural and immediate opportunity of a nurse to assist him in this. The ideal health care setting will enable a patient to sustain his life as the person he is. This is the ethical ambience of medicine and of nursing. To achieve this ambience, both a physician and a nurse are necessary. Neither alone is sufficient.

The Bioethical Agreement and Its Standards

In one way or another, every ethical decision that a professional makes, every professionally justified action she takes in relation to her patient, involves the terms of the implicit (professional) agreement that establishes her dynamic relationship to her patient. Her practice is structured by it. A practice-based ethic—the ethic of this relationship—is derived from this agreement. It is based upon six noncontroversial but crucial points. These points are the bioethical standards. As noted earlier, they are presuppositions of the professional–patient agreement (and any agreement).

1. **The standard of autonomy.** In order to grasp the terms of a specific health care professional–patient agreement, a professional needs to be aware of her patient's unique nature (autonomy). Every patient is a unique personality. To interact with a patient is to interact with a unique personality.

When a nurse acts as a researcher, an educator, or an administrator, she will not be aware of the unique characteristics of any individual patient. She must, however, always be aware of the unique characteristics of patients as patients. If any professional action, however indirect, is to be justifiable, it must be an action oriented toward the welfare of unique patients.

A great actress, to be able to perform effectively in a play every night, must rehearse her role. Only by rehearsing her role, can she perfect her performance. Every night she performs the same actions with the same persons, and perfection requires rehearsal. The actress's role withers and stagnates without rehearsal.

The situation of a health care professional is completely the opposite of this. Every day she faces different ethical demands; she must take different actions, with different persons, in very different circumstances. A professional can only perfect her role if she does not rehearse it. To perfect her role as a professional, she must meet the differing demands of every patient's situation. She cannot do this before she is in the situation. The delivery of ethical nurturing, in relation to each individual patient, is a role that cannot be rehearsed.

> The delivery of ethical nurturing, in relation to each individual patient, is a role that cannot be rehearsed.

If an actress does not rehearse her role, she will never perform it other than the way it is "in general.' She will never discover the possibilities, the nuances possible to the situation, and psychological state of her role. An actress can discover why she does what she does and why she ought to do it before she does it. A nurse cannot. An actress is not given the opportunity of being (as opposed to appearing) sincere. A nurse is. A talented actress can take the role of a nurse. A talented nurse cannot take the role of an actress.

These methods of portraying feeling "in general" exist in everyone of us. And they are used without any relation to the why, wherefore, or circumstances, in which a person has experienced them. . . . True art and performing "in general" are incompatible. The one destroys the other. Art does not tolerate "anyhow," "in general," [or] "approximately". (Stanislavski, 1963, p. 108).

If a health care professional prejudges and rehearses her ethical actions, she will never make decisions and take actions toward a specific patient other than "more or less" appropriately. The life created by a playwright is entirely predictable. It is given in the play. Life in the real world is unpredictable. The two professions require, for their perfection, two completely opposed approaches.

2. **The standard of freedom.** In order to interact with a patient, a professional must interact with his freedom. Every action that a patient takes arises

from his freedom. The precondition of a professional's interacting with the freedom of a patient is that she recognizes and respects his freedom. A professional who fails to respect her patient's freedom is not interacting with her patient. She, therefore, fails to honor the agreement she has made with him.

3. **The standard of objectivity.** In order for a person to interact within an agreement, he must understand the terms of the agreement. This understanding cannot exist unless the relationship between the parties is based on a rational trust, and rational trust cannot exist unless the relationship is based on objective understanding. Except in rare circumstances, a professional who does not communicate and interact with her patient on the basis of objective awareness violates the agreement she has made with him.

4. **The standard of self-assertion.** All interaction presupposes a prior agreement between agents. An interaction that takes place through coercion of one party to the agreement is an impossible situation. If any person is coerced, there is no agreement and no interaction. A person can be coerced into doing almost anything. But no one can be coerced into making an agreement. No one can be coerced into interaction. No party to an interaction could possibly agree to be forced. If he agreed, he would not be forced. If he were forced, he did not agree.

Wherever there is agreement and interaction, there is the implicit presumption of the self-ownership and self-assertion of each person to the agreement. An agreement would be invalid if it, implicitly or explicitly, denied the self-ownership of one of the parties to the agreement. More than this, it would be a contradiction in terms. It would, in effect, leave one party to the agreement out of the agreement.

5. **The standard of beneficence.** Every agreement has a purpose. This purpose is a goal to be achieved through interaction. An agreement without a final goal would be unintelligible. It would be an agreement to do nothing and, therefore, no agreement at all. The achievement of this final goal is the purpose of beneficent action—action that achieves a benefit. Every agreement, by its nature, calls for beneficent action. A professional who fails to act beneficently toward her patient fails to fulfill the agreement she has with him. This is a profoundly unfortunate failure. In this failure, a professional fails herself.

6. **The standard of fidelity.** Wherever there is an agreement, there must be fidelity to the agreement. An agreement that will not be honored is a contradiction in terms. No professional can ever justify an ethical decision or action that violates the implicit agreement she has with her patient.

All these considerations form the ethical context of the interaction between professional and patient. The ethical effectiveness of this interaction depends upon the professional's acquisition of optimal awareness—the widest possible context of ethical knowledge—and on her bringing about, as nearly as possible, ideal conditions for what she and her patient intend.

> It takes pride to stretch beyond one's comfort zone. Comfort and pride cannot live together. Pride is a most desirable virtue in a professional.

All of this is facilitated by an increase in a professional's ethical awareness. "I urge you to be proactive in the best interest of your patients . . . and stretch beyond your comfort zone" (Meyers, 2000, p. 9). It takes pride to stretch beyond one's comfort zone. Comfort and pride cannot live together. Pride is a most desirable virtue in a professional. Comfort (i.e., stagnation) is the only alternative to pride, and it is not a virtue.

The Swan Principle

One fine day, two people sitting on a park bench fed the seagulls and swans swimming in a pond. One pointed out to the other the parallels between this scene and the health care setting, as the health care setting might be understood.

Some patients, like seagulls, are aggressive and demanding, whereas some are timid and lack self-assertion. Whereas some are annoying, others are charming; some are resourceful, and others are helpless. It is easy for a professional's emotional responses to different types of patients to lead her away from the efficient practice of her profession. It is a temptation to avoid the demands of demanding patients and to take advantage of the timidity of timid patients. On a very basic level, seagulls and patients are very much alike. But patients are infinitely more complex than are seagulls.

Soon, the seagull feeders turned their attention to the calm dignity of the swans floating in the pond. They discussed between themselves how splendid it would be if nurses in their proper setting could achieve the self-assurance and serenity of the swans. The swans appeared perfectly placid and self-contented. They were aware of their circumstances and serene within them. Fanaticism of one sort or another, until it unravels, can produce an ethical assurance and certainty. But fanaticism is not a virtue. Only ethical competence can produce a reliable attitude of confidence and resilience. Without ethical awareness, professionals can be caught by surprise, and then their serenity and confidence are gone. Ethical serenity and confidence can only arise from a professional's awareness of herself and her professional role. This awareness must produce a constant attitude, arising from, in Aristotle's words, a firm and stable character.

> *A great nurse is one who is not a mere instrument. A great nurse is one who (given the context of her knowledge and the situation she faces) interacts in a way that accomplishes all that can be accomplished. A great nurse is vital and active agent engrossed in her profession. She is part of a team, but not a mere functionary. (Fedorka & Husted, 2004, p. 52).*

Living her role makes it imperative that her attitude be focused on her patient. As a professional, her role is that of the agent of her patient doing for her patient what he would do for himself (through the exercise of his virtues) if he were able.

Every health care professional needs a framework to guide her professional practice. The clearer her state of professional consciousness, the more effective her competence. A framework will clarify her consciousness. This framework is the ethical aspects of her role as a professional. The framework of her role, ideally, will be explicit—an ever-present thought she can clearly express to herself. It ought to provide her with a constant, driving, motivating strength. Her explicit awareness of her role will take and keep her out of her comfort zone. It will bring her to a calm, swanlike, and reality-based dignity.

It will proceed somewhat as follows: "My patient's virtues (autonomy) are such that he is moving (self-assertion) toward this goal (freedom) in these circumstances (objectivity) for this reason (beneficence). My virtues (autonomy) are such that I must act with him (interactive self-assertion) to assist him (his freedom) within the possibilities (of beneficence) in his circumstances to achieve every possible benefit that can be discovered (by objective awareness)."

Awareness of this framework for those professionals who are aware of it, unites and integrates their thoughts and actions, and makes their actions an extension of their thinking.

A topic to reflect upon: Through her life, every professional is the agent of a patient, motivating and inspiring her patient to a state of agency, and guiding her patient's actions. That patient, of course, is the professional herself.

Dilemma 12.1

Marilu is caring for an 82-year-old woman, Lillian. Lillian has been quite active in charitable affairs. One day while delivering food for Meals on Wheels, she slipped on a patch of ice. Lillian fractured her clavicle in the fall. She was taken to surgery and the fracture repaired. Her postoperative orders included 10 mg. of valium and oxycodone/acetaminophen (5/325 mg.). Lillian became very confused and within 2 days did not know her name. Her physician diagnosed her as senile. He began making plans for her to be transferred to a nursing home. He contacted her daughter, who lived in a different state, to get her permission. Her daughter gave her consent and decided to wait to visit until her mother was transferred to the nursing home. Marilu is convinced that Lillian was not senile, but the physician refused to consider the reasoning that she is very elderly and is overmedicated. Marilu believes that if Lillian is taken to a nursing home she will never again return to her normal life. She has every reason to believe that Lillian would not want to go to the nursing home until all other avenues are tried.

Professionals, Patients, and Caring

Helen Keller, the famous lecturer and author, remarked that "Life is a great adventure or it is nothing." Every professional comes into her profession expecting that it will be a great adventure. But sometimes, under the pressure of caregiver strain, professionals, especially nurses, become burned out. When this happens, their profession stops being a great adventure and becomes meaningless.

A professional who suffers from burnout has lost her enthusiasm, her strength, and her endurance. She has stopped caring. Perhaps, from the beginning, her caring was flawed (Nelson, 1992). She may have never defined *caring*.

"Caring is the essential fuel of a nurse's interaction with her patient. It is an essential means of understanding the needs and purposes of her patient. Without this, nothing can produce a successful chain of cause-and-effect interactions between them" (Husted & Husted, 1997, p. 17). Caring is the moral integrity of a nurse's [or any professional's] practice (Hartman, 1998).

> "Caring is the essential fuel of a nurse's interaction with her patient . . ." (Husted & Husted, 1997, p. 17)

Caring can open the way to understanding the needs of a patient. It cannot produce understanding of the ways to effectively meet these needs. Exclusive attention to caring assumes that there are only simple bioethical dilemmas and that professionals can deal with these dilemmas instinctively. It further assumes that ethical dilemmas do not occur in the external world of the patient but only in the mind or the emotions of the professional. This is false. To experience caring is a virtue, to concentrate on caring is a flaw; in the same way, to concentrate on a standard rather than on a patient is an error and a flaw.

A caring perspective can replace an interactive relationship with a mere response. Caring, in and of itself, does not provide guidance. Guidance must be produced by an intellectual understanding and emotional understanding of the patient in his circumstances. This understanding must be guided by logical consistency.

There is no reason why logical consistency cannot coexist with compassionate caring. In fact, each perfects the other. Caring without logical consistency—caring for the wrong reason, in the wrong way, or to an illogical extent—will produce, as those who denigrate caring in favor of justice claim, injustice. Injustice to the patient, to the health care professional, or to both cannot be justified. On the other hand, logical consistency without caring will distort the whole reason for being of a health care system in an ethically healthy society. This will, by that fact, produce injustice.

Caring can mean different, and even opposed, things, including:

1. Sharing the values and motivations of another because they are values and motivations for this other. For instance, sharing a patient's struggles to regain his lost well-being through empathy for the patient.
2. Being concerned with and attending to something or someone. For instance, sharing a patient's struggles to regain his lost well-being simply because he is one's patient.
3. Undergoing mental suffering or grief. For instance, feeling overburdened from sharing a patient's struggle and struggling with a patient as a burden.
4. Being under the power of one emotion and devoting oneself to strengthening an opposed emotion. For instance, feeling overburdened from sharing a patient's struggle and struggling to feel a concern that one does not feel for a patient.

Ways of Caring

"Caring is a concept central to the nursing profession. Although references to caring in the literature are abundant, there is little clarity about the definition and process of caring" (Scotto, 2003, p. 289). "Caring" therefore, is in need of rectification.

Let's examine different ways of caring: *Theatrical caring* is the way that one feels for a character in a movie or on a TV program. It is not a caring for a person. It is a type of play-acting. One rejoices at the success of a character-type—a patient. Or one is distressed at his failure. But it is not the patient as a person for whom one cares. It is a character in one's personal soap opera. At best, theatrical caring is an exaggeration of common courtesy. At its worst, it is an unpleasant affectation.

Another way of caring might be called *reaction formation caring*. This is when a professional tries to produce caring when she does not care—because she does not care. She is unwilling to admit to herself that she does not care, and so this kind of caring becomes a mask to cover her indifference. She cannot face the fact that she is indifferent to her patient, so she sees this mask as herself. Reaction formation caring does little to nourish a patient and, for a professional, it is a process of self-deception and self-destruction.

A third way of caring is *codependent caring*. This consists of a nurse trying to find her sense of ethical worth by working to make herself and her patient mutually codependent (Armstrong & Norris, 1992; Summers, 1992). It begins with self-sacrifice on the part of a professional. She escapes the need to think and understand by neglecting herself and focusing exclusive attention on her patient. When she finds her patient's response insufficient to fill her needs, she begins to feel victimized, resentful, and still dependent. Then "compassion may disappear and a hardened facade may cover the nurse's . . . feelings of powerlessness, fear or shame . . ." (Summers, 1992, p. 70–71). Through this way of caring, a health care professional may attempt to find herself by abandoning herself. She attempts to fulfill herself by a course of action that destroys her (Morris & Trigoboff, 1996).

Another way of caring might be called *affinity caring*. It is that which a professional feels when she shares the desires and purposes of the person for whom she cares. She cares for this person because he is a person and because he is this person. She cares for him because she values what he values and because she shares an adventure with him. This is the health care professions' great adventure.

> Another way of caring might be called *affinity caring*. It is that which a professional feels when she shares the desires and purposes of the person for whom she cares.

Affinity caring is genuine caring. It nourishes a professional and her patient. It is caring for a person. This is the way of caring that health care professionals can be and ought to be noted for. "Nursing is about interacting with people . . . in a meaningful way that can make a real difference in their lives" (Trossman, 2000, p. 8).

Caregiver Strain

The problem of caregiver strain arises because of ethical dilemmas. What these dilemmas are is not important because caregiver strain itself is a dilemma. It is a dilemma that none of the contemporary ethical theories will solve. In fact, it is a dilemma that any contemporary ethical theory will exacerbate.

There is a process that can increase the emotional strength and staying power of a caregiver. If anything can solve the problems of caregiver strain and

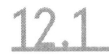

Burnout.

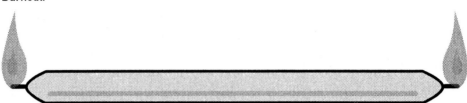

burnout, this increase in strength and staying power can. For burnout is the loss of emotional strength and staying power (Figure 12.1).

Under ideal circumstances, a professional will want to give care. A professional will want to see her patient's pain and suffering decreased through her efforts for a very personal reason. Pain and the loss of self-assertion are both forms of suffering. Ideally, a professional hates suffering in general and specifically hates it as it affects each patient. A professional gains a deep sense of personal satisfaction simply by taking part in decreasing the pain and loss—the suffering—of another person, the person for whom she cares. "Compassionate fatigue", thought to be a form of burn-out, is brought on by health care professionals coming in almost constant contact with suffering (Gentry, Baranowsky, & Dunning, 2002).

What follows is given as an antidote to compassionate fatigue and a preventive of the consequent burnout.

Objectified Ethical Abstractions

Caring and a dedication to beneficence do not require a professional to lose sight of herself or the facts of her life in order to share her patient's suffering. Ideal circumstances in the health care setting will increase a professional's self-awareness and strengthen her attachment to her life. She can create ideal circumstances through the technique of orienting herself emotionally onto an objectified ethical abstraction.

> *Objectified means thought of as "existing in a context independent of the perception of a perceiving subject." For our purposes, objectified will be thought of as "existing as a reality in itself apart from the concrete contexts in which it is found." For a practice-based ethic, ethics means "a system of standards to motivate actions taken in pursuit of vital and fundamental goals." Therefore, we use ethical to mean "pertaining to vital and fundamental goals."*

Abstract means mentally derived from individual instances. Tom, Dick, and Harry are individuals. By taking them together, the abstraction *men* can be formed. Tina, Doris, and Harriet are individuals. By taking them together, the abstraction *women* can be formed. By taking the (individual) abstractions *men* and *women* together, one forms the abstraction *persons*. This action does not add anything to the external world. It simply adds to the mind's power of dealing with the external world. Therefore, by *abstraction* we will understand "that which can only exist in and for the mind, but which can be thought of as if it existed outside of and apart from the mind."

Forming the Objectified Ethical Abstraction

In order to form the objectified ethical abstraction, a professional begins by observing her patient's suffering. Then, through an act of abstraction, she turns her awareness to many instances of suffering—perhaps her own suffering and the suffering of all her patients. She looks upon this abstraction, *suffering*, as if it were a concrete thing in itself. From here she broadens her abstraction to include all suffering—suffering as such. Finally, she looks upon this abstraction—suffering as such—as if it were an independently existing thing.

Ordinarily, to do this would be to commit the fallacy of personification. This fallacy consists in attributing existence in external reality to an abstract idea. Examples of this would be: "History tells us that..." History tells us nothing... historians tell us things. "Medicine has come a long way..." There is no such being as medicine. *Medicine* is not a thing that moves from one time or place to another. The "long way" is a figure of speech meaning that medical professionals now have more skills and instruments than they had in the past. "Society demands." *Society* is not a kind of thing that demands. Only individual people demand various things.

Here, in forming the objectified ethical abstraction, one is not guilty of the fallacy because one knows that suffering is not the kind of thing that one might bump into or meet face to face in reality. One only takes suffering to represent a concrete reality in order to generate the emotional attitude that enables a professional to avoid or overcome caregiver strain.

Now she has her objectified ethical abstraction—suffering. Suffering is an abstraction because it is taken (abstracted) into the mind from every individual instance of suffering and exists as an individual thing only in the mind. Suffering is objectified because it is treated as a concrete thing existing apart from the mind.

> One only takes suffering to represent a concrete reality in order to generate the emotional attitude that enables a professional to avoid or overcome caregiver strain.

Suffering, as an abstraction, is an ethical abstraction. For the realm of values and disvalues is the realm of ethics. Suffering is the one supreme human disvalue the health care system was created to combat.

Interacting With the Objectified Ethical Abstraction

By interacting with the objectified abstraction, as well as with her patient, a professional's attitude is focused on more than the concrete present moment. The objectified abstraction gives the present moment a new and wider meaning. It enables a professional to relate to her patient without alienation on the one hand or codependence on the other.

By regarding this abstraction as concrete, her actions are motivated toward an almost visible entity. Her hatred of suffering and her consequent desire for the well-being of her patient are given a new strength and endurance.

It is impossible for any human to function without an awareness of abstractions. It is impossible to deal with Ethel's suffering, George's suffering, and Frank's suffering, as well as one's own suffering without being aware of the reality of that which is signified by the term *suffering*. If a professional is not spurred on by antagonism to the existence of suffering, her actions will be hindered and weakened by her unacknowledged awareness of suffering's vicious presence.

The entire purpose of the health care system is to help patients overcome suffering, recover their well-being, or attain a peaceful death. Any professional who is not motivated by a hatred of suffering is out of sync with her profession—and her own nature. The absence of this motivation is not appropriate to a health care professional or a human being.

If one is enmeshed in the concrete, one cannot act effectively. One loses sight of the reasons for one's actions—the end result that is one's purpose. One's actions and one's purposes are made easier if one knows why one is doing what one is doing—if one has a firm idea of the end result being pursued. If a professional knows what she wishes to accomplish in general and what she can accomplish here and now with this patient, the means to accomplish this become less tedious and stressful.

In one way, she is keeping her attention directed on her patient, for she is combating her patient's suffering. In another way, by keeping her thoughts on the defeat of suffering and the victory of freedom from suffering, she is keeping her attention directed toward the abstraction of suffering. This unites a professional and her patient by giving them a common enemy and a common goal. At the same time, it puts a psychological distance between them. This distance frees them from an unhealthy dependence on each other and does this in such a way as to bring them closer together.

This seems a strange, paradoxical result. But, before the professional formed her ethical abstraction—before she objectified suffering—she regarded suffering as a concrete object and took it instance by instance, up close. She was focused on her patient, who, in turn, was focused on his suffering. By focusing her attention on the abstraction, she places both the patient and his suffering back into perspective. Then she can see the health care setting in relation to her role and purpose and her role and purpose in relation to this patient's situation.

> By focusing her attention on the abstraction, she places both the patient and his suffering back into perspective.

Through this, the professional and her patient are closer. At the same time, she has a defense against caregiver strain. She has an emotional defense. She is not meeting this strain head on. She has distanced herself from the caregiver situation without distancing herself from her patient.

This distance, instead of hindering and sapping her action, gives her an abstract experience of the meaning and purpose of her action and gives her action long-term strength and endurance.

Dilemma 12.2

Tyler, a 65-year-old known alcoholic, is admitted to the intensive care unit of a tertiary care hospital with renal complications. He is semicomatose and is unable to communicate or give indication of his wishes. He has been noncompliant with his physician's medical directives for years, has lost his job and his wife, and his children have no communication with him. He currently lives in a one-room apartment over a bar. His mother and sister visit the intensive care unit and communicate with the physicians regarding his care. He does not have a living will and his family indicates that he has never communicated his wishes regarding medical care. The physician plans aggressive treatment of the kidney problem and believes that the patient has a 10% to 20% chance of returning to his prior level of functioning and lifestyle posttreatment.

The patient's mother and sister communicate to the physician that they want no aggressive treatment for him. They refuse to authorize intravenous antibiotic therapy for the kidney problem. Without this treatment, the patient will most likely worsen and die. What should be done?

What Goes Around . . .

Most occupations or professions offer benefits peculiar to themselves. For instance, an architect can design his own home. Plumbers can avoid the (allegedly) exorbitant prices charged by plumbers. Surveyors are able to get out into the outdoors. Accountants are able to stay in, out of the outdoors. Teachers have a wonderful opportunity to learn. Clowns are able to enjoy the enjoyment of children.

One occupation said to have a notable side benefit is that of the horse groom. There is an ancient saying to the effect that, "The outside of a horse is good for the inside of a man." This saying arose, supposedly, because horse grooms—those who care for the well-being of race horses—must give painstaking care to the horses in their charge. In addition to this, they have much time for themselves. Yet they are unable to travel far from the stables on any given day. This puts them in the habit of taking care of themselves. Notoriously, they tend to live a long life in good health.

There is also a notable benefit to be found in nursing. There is an approach to the profession that makes nursing one of the most rewarding of all occupations. This approach offers a benefit that is as great as any benefit offered by any other occupation on earth.

> Throughout her entire life, a nurse is the nurse of a nurse. She is a nurse to herself. She gives counsel to and serves the virtue that is her own.

We have defined a nurse as, "The agent of a patient, doing for a patient what the patient would do for himself if he were able." A nurse must give counsel to her patient. She must also, as everyone must, give counsel to herself. As a nurse, she must inspire action in her patient. As a person—as an ethical agent—she must inspire action in herself. Throughout her entire life, a nurse is the nurse of a nurse. She is a nurse to herself. She gives counsel to and serves the virtue that is her own.

Dilemma 12.3

A donor heart became available and there were two heart-transplant candidates in the same hospital who were a match for a donor heart, Mr. X and Ms. Y. Mr. X had been on the waiting list a long time and he was near death. He is 64 and has suffered from a heart condition for years. He has had two angioplasties and two bypass operations to correct a blockage of the heart's blood vessels. He still smokes, eats fatty foods, and is very overweight. He has been warned each time after a procedure, but says it is too hard. Ms. Y has just been put on the list and could be sustained with medication for some time until another heart became available. She does not smoke and is not overweight. She tries to watch her diet. Who should get the heart? (Heart Transplant, 2000)

Virtues and Happiness

A health care professional ought to nurture and safeguard the virtues of her patient. Even more so, she should act to nurture and sustain her own virtues. If she does, she will enhance her patient's life. She will enhance the performance of her professional role. She will enhance her own life.

Ethics has to do with action and interaction. People have a purpose in interacting: to maximize the power of their action. They interact because they can accomplish more through interaction than they can by acting alone. If people did not enhance their lives by interacting, they would not interact. They would have no reason to interact.

> People have a purpose in interacting: to maximize the power of their action.

People also act alone in order to enhance their lives. There is no such thing as a human action that does not make a difference. Nearly every human action either benefits or harms the actor. Every action, properly so-called, is an action toward a goal. Because of this, there is another reason why a nurse should nurture the virtues of her patient.

In recognizing and respecting the bioethical standards, a nurse safeguards the abilities of her patient's agency. To act freely, to make himself aware of the facts of his circumstances, to pursue benefits—these are abilities a patient shares with every human being. In safeguarding the abilities of her patient's agency, a professional honors her patient's rights. To be the person he is, to initiate action, and to control his time is every person's right. In honoring her patient's rights, a professional nurtures the virtues of her patient. In nurturing the virtues of her patient, she helps him to help her to succeed. She achieves virtue—professional competence—and excellence as a health care professional. These are one and the same. In safeguarding and nurturing the virtues of her patient, in acting as the custodian of her patient's virtues, a professional creates and strengthens her own character.

First, she observes in her patient that a certain ability—a certain virtue— is needed. She does this by observing why that ability is needed. To observe that it is needed and why it is needed is the same observation. These are two perspectives on the same fact. These observations are the bridge between a professional and her patient. The ethical virtues are the bioethical standards— the standards of a professional's ethical action.

Dilemma 12.4

Mrs. C is a 52-year-old woman with metastatic ovarian cancer who is hospitalized with a bowel obstruction and pain. She has undergone multiple therapies including surgery and chemotherapy, but now her disease has progressed. She is not a candidate for surgery to relieve bowel obstruction. She has no advance directive but has expressed a desire to be kept pain free, even if this requires her to be sedated at the end of life. She was started on IV morphine. This affords her good pain relief until, 3 days later, her condition deteriorates and she lapses into a coma. Her family requests that the morphine dosage be decreased so that she can be more alert and interactive. The family also asks that total parenteral nutrition (TPN) be started so that she does not "starve to death" (Maxwell, 2000, p. 57). What should be done?

Musings

The experience of attending to her patient's virtues allows a nurse to experience and to exercise her own. A professional looks into herself for her awareness of the virtues she must motivate and nurture in her patient. She will find these virtues in herself because, in filling her role as a professional and in working within the framework of her profession, she will have put them there.

This is the professional role a nurse, in particular, can make uniquely her own: to motivate, safeguard, and nurture the virtues of her patient. A professional can help a patient sustain his development and remain the unique being he is. She does this by maintaining her fidelity to her agreement with her patient and, through this, her fidelity to her patient.

In nurturing her patient's uniqueness, she sees the value of uniqueness and accepts herself as unique. She sees the value to her of those who are different from her. She sees her value to them. She teaches herself reciprocity. In nurturing her patient's freedom, in practicing fidelity to her profession, she sees the value of freedom and teaches herself courage—the courage to accept and encourage her patient's freedom. In nurturing her patient's objectivity, she sees the value of objectivity and embraces it as her own standard. She achieves wisdom. She teaches herself to rely on all the knowledge she has gained through experience and to accept the fact that her knowledge is limited. This is the virtue of wisdom. In nurturing her patient's self-assertion, she sees the value of self-ownership and teaches herself integrity—a sense of unthreatened control over her time and effort. In approving her patient's striving for his benefit, she deals with him on the basis of beneficence. She sees the value of beneficence to him and to herself, and, prompted by reason, she teaches herself justice. In seeing the value to her patient of his fidelity to himself, she learns the value of fidelity and teaches herself pride in her profession and in herself. Pride in herself produces fidelity to herself.

She becomes aware of the value of the virtues to her patient. She sees his grim struggle to regain them. She learns the value of the virtues to herself. They are valuable to a person because of what it is to be a person. Virtue is the ability to be a human being. More than this, it is the ability to be a human being successfully.

By learning the value of the virtues, she learns the value of character. For a person's virtues are her character. From her patient's struggles, she learns the importance of destiny. From being a nurse she learns the matchless value of life.

> By learning the value of the virtues, she learns the value of character. For a person's virtues are her character.

When she comes to understand the value of life, she comes to understand the importance of destiny. When she comes to understand the importance of destiny, she comes to understand the value of character. By coming to understand the value of character, she gains an understanding of the virtues. No occupations on earth can facilitate this understanding and the acquisition of these abilities more perfectly than the profession of nursing.

The French novelist, Balzac, warns us that an unfilled vocation draws the color from one's entire existence. Those who look for the glory of nursing in the right places will find it; those who do not, have looked for it where it is not to be found.

Study Guide

1. Give some thought to your own virtues—your excellence as a professional. Describe yourself to yourself; it is a great exercise in self-understanding.
2. Not all nurses or health care professionals are excellent. Some by virtue of not knowing, but some by not caring. How can you mentor others in, of course, a caring way that would help them?
3. Observe caring behaviors in others—affinity caring—and note how patients respond. Give your colleagues some positive feedback regarding this—what goes around comes around.
4. What is the point of the swan principle?
5. How might you use objictified ethical abstraction? Try it and see if it helps ward off feelings of burnout and fatigue.

References

Armstrong, J., & Norris, C. (1992). Co-dependence: A nursing issue. *Focus on Critical Care, 19,* 105–115.

Fedorka, P., & Husted, G. L. (2004). Ethical decision making in clinical emergencies. *Topics in Emergency Medicine, 26,* 52–60.

Gentry, J. E., Baranowsky, A. G., & Dunning, K. (2002). The accelerated recovery program for compassion fatigue. In C. R. Figley (Ed.), *Treating compassion fatigue* (pp. 123–137). New York: Brunner-Routledge.

Hartman, R. L. (1998). Revisiting the call to care: An ethical perspective. *Advanced Practice Nursing Quarterly, 4(2),* 14–18.

Heart Transplant. (2000). Bioethics case studies. McGraw Hill.

Husted, G. L., & Husted, J. H. (1997). Is a return to a caring perspective desirable? *Advanced Practice Nursing Quarterly, 3*(1), 14–17.

Maxwell, T. (2000). Ethical decision making at the end of life: A series of case studies. *Patient Care for the Nurse Practitioner, 3*(11), 57–61.

McKeon, R. (Ed.). (1941). *The basic works of Aristotle.* New York: *Random House.*

Meyers, T. A. (2000). Why couldn't I have seen him? *American Journal of Nursing, 100*(2), 9.

Morris, M., & Trigoboff, E. (1996). Co-dependence. In H. S. Wilson & C. R. Kneis (Eds.), *Psychiatric nursing* (5th ed., pp. 776-815). Redwood, CA: Addison-Wesley.

Nelson, L. N. (1992). Against caring. *The Journal of Clinical Ethics, 3*(1), 8–15.

Nightingale, F. (1969). *Notes on nursing.* Toronto, Canada: Dover. (Original work published 1860)

Scotto, C. (2003). A new view of caring. *Journal of Nursing Education, 42,* 289–294.

Spinoza, B. (1949). *Ethics.* (J. Gutman, Ed.). New York: Hafner Publishing. (Original work published 1675)

Stanislavski, C. (1963). *An actor's handbook.* New York: Theatre Arts Books.

Summers, C. L. (1992). Co-dependence: A nursing dilemma. Revolution. *The Journal of Nurse Empowerment, 136,* 68–79.

Trossman, S. (2000). Health for all: RN fights to level the playing field. *American Nurse, 200,* 8–9.

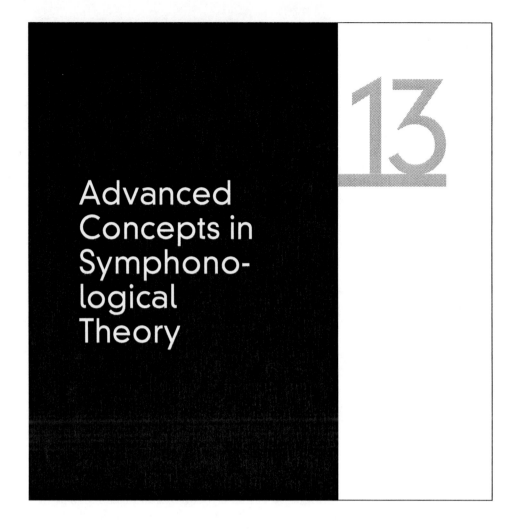

13

Advanced Concepts in Symphono- logical Theory

We all live in the same world. We all have the same world to understand and a human way of understanding it. We are all faced with the need to act to achieve happiness (a state of success with ourselves) and to avoid unhappiness (a sense of ourselves failing as humans). This involves the need to make decisions. Our life is made possible by appropriate decisions. Our life is tremendously enhanced by agreements. Ethics is the science of making and acting on these decisions and agreements.

Symphonology is a bioethical theory. In being a bioethical theory, it takes as its subject matter the decisions and agreements that structure the health care professions. The essential aspects of nursing and health care have to do with the ethical practice of the health care professional and her relationship to her patient. A nursing and health care theory is one that should direct its practitioners to appropriate ways of practicing.

> Our life is tremendously enhanced by agreements. Ethics is the science of making and acting on these decisions and agreements.

Every person has a philosophy of life, whether or not the person realizes it. This philosophy impacts the person's professional philosophy and guides the approaches she takes to her role as a health care professional (Gaberson & Oermann, 2007). That philosophy is more than ethics. A person's ethic is, so to speak, surrounded by her view of the world—the nature and the possibilities offered by reality, and a notion of what is and what is not possible to know, how one comes by knowledge, and what makes knowledge reliable.

Metaphysics

Metaphysics is the study of the nature of and what is possible to existence and existing things.

The universe we live in is structured in such a way that the processes that existents act or interact to produce on a broad, even infinite, scale are replicated on very small scales. The Aristotlean tradition pointed out a fact on which all of our experience and our belief in the order of the universe are based. *Actio sequiteur esse* (action follows on identity). This is the fact that the characteristic action of every existent arises from the nature of the existent. In consequence of this, the characteristic interaction of several existents follows on their natures in relation to one another. These different sorts of processes are sufficiently similar in their form and functioning to justify inclusion under one highly abstract concept—the concept of *agreement*. Agreement and disagreement are found in all interaction; therefore, they also follow on identity.

The concept of agreement signifies, on every level, a propensity or formal potentiality in existents to behave in specific ways when they are interacting, based on the nature of each existent. On each level, agreement consists in their interacting in a form necessary to that level.

The agreement between existents is a relationship between their natures, arising by virtue of their identities or formal structures and producing specific interactions through offers and acceptances characterizing that level of existence. The levels of agreement particularly relevant to symphonology are the:

Natural agreement—An agreement among things that they will interact according to the nature of each. For instance, a leaf will be carried by the wind. The nature of the wind is such that it has a propensity to carry light objects such as leaves. The nature of a leaf is such that it will allow itself to be carried by wind.

> *Hopefully, it will be understood that on this level of agreement there is no suggestion of conscious awareness motivating or accompanying interaction.*

Natural agreements arise through the nature of each existent. Their natures produce intelligible and predictable interactions. Natural agreement is the objective foundation of purpose in purposive beings. A purpose always involves rearranging and redirecting things according to the possibilities afforded by natural agreements.

Instrumental agreement—A natural agreement compatible with a purpose. It is the agreement of an instrument to serve a purpose. This type of natural agreement arises in the same way as any other natural agreement—according to the natures of the things that affect each other—but according to human or animal purposes. Specific instances of this agreement are hammer and nail, screwdriver and screw, a boat on water, bees building a hive with the material that makes this possible, and beavers using trees to build a dam.

Vital agreement—An agreement between the life of a living thing and the organic and physiological conditions necessary to its survival and flourishing. It is life's agreement with itself. The vital agreement is the subject matter of medical knowledge. It is the interaction of an organism with itself; a form of natural agreement based on a most fundamental level of purpose—the organic level. The vital agreement exists on that level of purpose from which conscious purpose is an outgrowth. Nonpoisonous food, climates compatible with life, the existence of medical science and systems, and the means of protection from enemies are, in effect, instruments assisting the organism in sustaining its vital agreement. The circulation of blood and the process of respiration are some examples of the organism acting to sustain its vital agreement with itself.

Finally, there is a living organism's capacity and propensity to pursue or prolong pleasure and avoid or escape suffering.

Cognitive agreement—An agreement of the understanding with the object that is understood; the agreement between a knowing mind and its known object. It is a propensity of consciousness in its act of being conscious. Examples of this type of agreement are a dog and master recognizing each other, grasping the existence of instrumental agreements, the awareness of temporal and spatial relations, recognition of the meaning of words, and the identification of a spruce tree.

Ethical agreement—An agreement to interact in order to pursue vital (related to the preservation or enhancement of life) and fundamental (preconditional, necessary to the vital) goals.

Formal agreement—An agreement between agents to interact on the basis of complementary motivations. It is perfect or imperfect insofar as it involves the character structures and virtues of those who interact. Formal agreements produce interaction based on trade and formulated in a meeting of the minds. The formal agreement is an outgrowth of cognitive agreements and is made possible by the ability of conscious beings to achieve a meeting of the minds. A familiar example is the health care professional–patient agreement. The objectivity and rationality of formal agreements depend, in every instance, on their harmony with the more basic levels of agreement.

The objectivity and rationality of a formal agreement depends on its harmony with the more basic levels of agreement.

> The objectivity and rationality of formal agreements depend, in every instance, on their harmony with the more basic levels of agreement.

In each case, agreement (or disagreement) is a propensity of existents to behave in specific ways when they are interacting, based on the nature of each existent. When one takes note of how the different levels of agreement intertwine, how each level is dependent on the lower levels, and how it is not possible to put concrete examples of agreement into one isolated level, the relationship of dependence between the levels of agreement becomes clear (Table 13.1).

Epistemology

Epistemology is the study of the origin, nature, and extent of truth and knowledge.

The two most plausible epistemological theories are conceptualism and moderate realism. Different epistemologists place different shades of meaning

13.1 Agreements and Clarification	
Agreements	**Clarification**
Natural agreements	The relationship between the natures of things that cause them to interact as they do.
Instrumental agreements	The ability of things that form natural agreements to serve agents in achieving their purposes.
Vital agreements	Harmony between a living thing and the conditions of the organism that support the continuation of its living and its flourishing.
Cognitive agreements	Harmony between the nature of a thing known and the knowing of it.
Ethical agreements	An agreement between agents that they will interact in the pursuit of vital and fundamental goals.

on the two terms. For our purposes. Conceptualism is the theory that concepts (retained mental impressions) are formed through the similarities of similar things, the nature of an individual thing cannot impress itself on (or cannot be grasped by) the mind, and the mind is not capable of discovering the nature of an isolated individual thing. We will limit moderate realism to the theory that concepts are formed through the abstract sameness of things and the source of human knowledge is its discovery of the nature of individual things. It presupposes that the mind is capable of discovering the nature of an individual thing. The theory most appropriate to the health care setting is moderate realism.

Conceptualists claim that one can form, for example, the concept *round* by virtue of the fact that round things are similar in being round. Moderate realists claim that insofar as two things are similar in being round, they are, abstractly, the same. In her earliest years, a learner will learn in the way conceptualism describes but when she becomes competent she adopts realism.

In the health care setting, a very common, implicit, and undetected error—a mind-set—is to understand a patient in the manner of conceptualism. "This patient is sick because he has what that patient has and that patient is sick. Everyone who is similar in having this condition is sick. This is what makes him a patient." A conceptualist viewpoint brings health care professionals to understand patients through the fact that patients are similar. This implies that an individual patient can be understood in terms applicable to all patients—without being understood as an individual. Additionally, a certain course of action is ethically appropriate to this patient because it is ethically appropriate to that patient and that patient's context is similar to this patient's context. Conceptualism is dreadfully inadequate as a theory to guide professional inter-action.

Moderate realism would hold that this patient is sick because his present physiological or psychological state is inadequate to his normal vital function. A moderate realist approach brings a health care professional to understand a patient through the fact that, one by one, patients are who they are. This implies that an individual patient must and can be understood through his unique character structures, or a certain course of action is beneficent in relation to this patient because this course of action would best nurture and strengthen his character structures. This is the symphonological approach.

Truth

The two most plausible theories of truth are the coherence theory and the correspondence theory. Coherence is the theory that a belief is true if it is logically coherent with the collection of one's other true beliefs. This perspective is pandemic in the health care system and nearly everywhere else. It dovetails neatly with conceptualism. It is, in effect, conceptualism applied to beliefs. "This belief is true because it is coherent with (does not contradict) that belief and that belief is true." And so on into a whirlpool of subjectivism.

With the emotions as the source of truth the emotional state is spontaneous and all encompassing. In the emotivism that dominates much ethical decision making in the health care setting, the process goes as follows: "This assumption must be true because it coheres (does not conflict) with my emotional state. Assumptions that cohere with my emotional state are true. More than this, they are good, right, and justified."

The correspondence theory holds that a belief is true when it arises from, is formed according to, and corresponds with the state of affairs that is the object of the belief. The alternatives, as ethical perspectives, are:

- For coherence: "This dilemma arouses in me a specific set of beliefs and feelings. These beliefs and feelings do not contradict beliefs I presently hold, and do not disturb my current emotional state. Therefore, these beliefs and feelings constitute a valid judgment."
- For correspondence: "Given my examination and analysis of this dilemma, I have formed the following belief that I hold to be adequate to explain its nature and to suggest appropriate responses."

It must be obvious that an effective professional cannot make decisions appropriate to dilemmas in the health care setting based on an examination of the ideas, beliefs, and attitudes preexisting in her mind and brought to her attention by a superficial experience of the dilemma. It must be just as obvious that an effective professional must make decisions appropriate to dilemmas based on an adequate understanding of the dilemma achieved through the acquisition of beliefs corresponding to the nature of the dilemma.

A decision maker must:

- Work with clues that could mean many different things.
- Pay attention to clues that are important.
- Ignore clues that are not important.
- Integrate apparently random data into a meaningful pattern.
- Work with data that cannot easily be explained.

▓ Carry intelligence from the mind into the circumstance through in-dwelling in the circumstance,
▓ Recognize a coherent pattern among clues.
▓ Perform feats of integration without being aware of what one is doing.
▓ Tacitly integrate clues into meaning.
▓ Move from clues or parts to wholes (Polanyi, 1974).

Polanyi proposed that understanding is derived from awareness of the entirety of a phenomenon, that the lived experience is greater than separate observable parts. Tacit knowledge, that which is implied, is necessary to understand and interpret that which is explicit. "These concepts, the uniqueness of the individual and the extension of reason and rationality with insight and discernment to create true understanding, are the foundations of symphonological method" (Scotto, 2005, p. 587).

Only moderate realism and correspondence make this possible.

Health and the Virtues

Many health care professionals embrace either a traditional ethical system or a contemporary ethical fad. Many others, discouraged by these ethical outlooks, either become calloused in relation to their profession and their patients or they, haphazardly, become benevolent. They give no explicit attention to the ethical underpinnings of their interactions. They lose concern for an understanding of what it is about their profession that makes it a worthwhile endeavor.

A practice-based bioethic must serve to keep a professional and patient on intelligible, cause-and-effect courses of interaction. This requires direction toward a state of affairs taken as a final cause and an objective principle of judgment. For the health care professional, it is the life, health, and well-being of sick and disabled individuals.

There is no absolute disability without a weakness of the virtues. There is no perfect health without their strength.

Ethical agents are never more useful to one another than when each is strengthening the virtues—the power to survive and flourish—of the other. To do this is to meet the demands of justice—a causal relationship, the purpose of which is to benefit one another, enrich each other.

This is the invigorating and mostly undiscovered essence of nursing. Like the picture that is worth a 1,000 words, demonstration is the best form of teaching. It teaches the patient. Even more so, it teaches the agent—the health care professional. It is an ancient truth that the best way to learn is to teach.

The Remarkable Nature of the Bioethical Standards

Nothing can assist the nurse more in the accomplishment of her profession than the bioethical standards. The bioethical standards are not guidelines to action imposed from outside. They signify properties inherent in the nature of every human person. These properties are the innate and defining properties of a human life. As guidelines, they prevent *contradictions* (actions or interactions) that conflict with a person's power to act (his agency).

The bioethical standards are not conventions. They become objects of awareness through discovery. They signify internal and external realities that are essential to human development, fulfillment, and flourishing.

Rules are, in the end, only rules. Mathematical schemes are, finally, only schemes. But the bioethical standards are:

> The bioethical standards are not guidelines to action imposed from outside. They signify properties inherent in the nature of every human person.

> The uniqueness of a human individual's nature is expressed in her exercise of the standards as character structures.

1. A blueprint of an individual's human nature. The uniqueness of a human individual's nature is expressed in her exercise of the standards as character structures.
2. Descriptions of the ways one experiences oneself as human.
3. Descriptions of the way one experiences another as human—what it is to be human in an interpersonal context.

The bioethical standards describe the psychological preconditions of thought, choice, decision, communication, agreement, action, and interaction.

4. Resources through which one is capable of making and retaining decisions.
5. Assets making one capable of maintaining and controlling a directed state of awareness within oneself and together with others.
6. Objects of awareness through which each person is able to communicate with and understand the internal states of others.
7. Taken for granted by everyone who enters into an agreement.

Anyone who makes an agreement with another person is, at least implicitly, aware that the person with whom he makes the agreement is self-controlled and seeking benefits. This is why we make agreements with people and why we do not make agreements with rocks, trees, snakes, or breezes.

8. Implied by the existence of individual rights because they are the necessary and sufficient preconditions of individual rights.
9. Virtues of an ethical agent—one's excellence as an agent; qualities of character that enable one to form and accomplish purposes.
10. Natural instruments that enable agents to sustain and enhance their lives.
11. Subjective conditions of an agent's relation to every aspect of the external world.
12. Critical indicators of ethical thought and of everything of which ethical thought is a precondition (e.g., ethical decision/agreement/interaction/justification).
13. Avenues not only to the thinking of others, but also to introspection—to the psychological location where one meets oneself.
14. Basic reasons that rationally motivate ethical agreement and interaction.

15. Instances of (implicit) decisions or agreements that are necessarily included in every explicit decision or agreement.
16. Standards of decision and action through which ethical decisions and actions are justified.
17. Preconditions of all thought and knowledge and the benefits humans pursue by thinking and acquiring knowledge.
18. Purposes that are realized through action.
19. Preconditions of the enjoyment of any value, including the value of life.
20. Sinews connecting the individual to his life.
21. Objects of personal awareness that enable one to enter an ethical relationship—a relationship based on possession of these character structures by oneself and another.
22. Constraints on an agreement.

The standards set the parameters of what is necessary in an agreement and what is and is not objectively appropriate.

23. Instruments to evaluate one's ethical decision-making process.
24. Objectives of ethical action. Values that are gained through the exercise of ethical action.
25. Principles of human nature and development.
26. Principles of human action.
27. Indispensable ethical principles.
28. Necessary means to bioethical expertise.
29. Instruments to analyze dilemmas and to guide decision making.

These then are the beginning and end of human life.

Musings

It is a mind-set that makes a nurse a nurse. This mindset is the resolve that she will place no responsibility before her obligation to her patient. When she accepts her profession, she establishes her professional obligation to recognize, accept, and act on her professional agreement with her patient.

The ethical aspects of her profession require that she acquire as complete an understanding of her patient's human situation and as complete an understanding of her individual patient as circumstances permit. In the health care setting, the analysis of the majority of ethical dilemmas she faces will require little more than an understanding of her patient. In order to act as the agent of her patient, her first and nearly only need is the ability to understand her patient and to know what to do with her understanding.

The existence of a formal agreement establishes the parameters of her *obligation*. If the professional/patient agreement does not establish her sense of obligation to her practice nothing will. That a health care professional has no ethical obligation to honor her professional/patient agreement implies that she has no ethical obligations at all. If she has no ethical obligations at all, then the idea of a professional ethic involves a contradiction in terms. This would make the nurse/patient agreement a very strange pheno-menon.

The First Agreement

The first agreement that people ever form is the agreement that agree-ments are possible. This agreement is formed on some occasion such as when a baby is hungry and cries, and mommy comes and feeds the baby. The baby comes to understand that this consistent event is the product of an agreement that Mommy has formed with her baby. The implication being that there are such things as agreements. Her baby's implicit understanding of the nature and existence form the agreement between them that agreements are possible.

The Worst Agreement

There is such a thing as a bad agreement. **Among the worst agreements a person, especially a nurse, can make is that agreements can be impossible to make.** Here is one example of what might motivate this and how it comes to dominate the person who makes it. It can be formed over time as a nurse's opinion of herself, her abilities, and her character rises to a level too high to be supported. She begins to find that others do not agree with her illusory evalua-tion of herself. Motivated by resentment, she makes a decision whose purpose is revenge against an unappreciative world. She forms an agreement which she offers to everyone–patients, marriage partner, children, colleagues, and friends–that she will offer them none of the comfort and reassurance that can be found in an agreement. This means that an agreement with her will be impossible. The purpose of her interaction with them will be not to nurture but to injure and they have no alternative but to accept this agreement.

- Deeply thoughtful and concerned, a nurse will keep her patient looking on the dark side of things. Her patient will leave the health care setting not upbeat and forward looking but downbeat and uncertain about the future.
- The agreements that could strengthen the relationship between marriage partners will never be forthcoming. Every offer of an agreement will be most with a painful apology or rigid 'honesty'. Every offer of an agreement will be met with the description of a problem that must be solved before the agreement can even be considered.
- Boys who seek agreement and reassurance from their mothers as to how masculine and intelligent they are find that their mothers see only prob-lems with their masculinity and intelligence. Mother is certain that sonny will outgrow this, so it is nothing to worry about. Girls who seek agree-ment and reassurance of their attractiveness and intelligence from their fathers find that their fathers can only find problems with their daughters' femininity and intelligence. Both mother and father find flaws where, like Tartuffe in Moliere's play, "no one else would even think to look."
- Colleagues who seek confirmation through discussion and agreement do not find confirmation but rather an attitude of doubt and distrust of their competence when they propose topics for agreement. They have

proposed this agreement to one whose sole and unbending agreement is that agreements are not possible.

■ Friends who ought to be expected to strengthen and encourage their friends with the comfort and reassurance of agreements will find discouragement in their discussions.

Much value is produced by interactions based on agreements. Much misery and destruction is produced by the psychological effects of the agreement that no agreement is possible.

A patient is afraid and a nurse allays his fear. A patient looks forward to a dismal future and a nurse shows him that his future contains many bright possibilities. A patient feels abandoned and all alone and a nurse shows him that there is someone who understands him and wishes him well. In none of these cases will the result be a patient overflowing with gratitude and admiration for his nurse. It is an extreme folly for a nurse to expect this. In the first case, his mood will change from fear to courage. In the second case, his outlook will change from despair to hope. In the third case, his feeling of isolation will be replaced by a feeling of being supported.

This nurse was so disoriented by her desire for admiration, that she was attempting to put the effect (the admiration of her patients) before the cause (the joy her patients experienced by passing from a lesser perfection to a greater perfection). The joy he expressed in his change from a negative to a positive attitude should have been her reward. It was the sign of her success. But she nurtured an expectation that her patient would forget himself, his values, his motivations, and direct all of his attention to her. This was the effect she was striving for in her interaction with him. She was initiating the right cause but expecting the wrong effect. Let us x-ray this:

If a boy's parents give him a bicycle for Christmas and he is thrilled with the bicycle, his joy will not be directed toward his parents. (If it could be, then, his joy at receiving the bicycle was not strong enough to evoke a powerful emotion.) The pleasure of his gratitude toward his parents comes later. It comes as a result of his joy, and his manifesting of the joy, at receiving the bicycle. (This is, of course, assuming that the value of the bicycle to the boy was the bicycle itself, and not its significance as a proof of their love for the boy.)

No nurse who looks to others to create pride in her character has a right to pride in her character. Only the nurse whose joy at her character is generated by herself alone has a right to enjoy her character. Much value is produced by time and effort devoted to a genuine and dynamic agreement. Much value is sucked out of life by time and effort devoted to trying to gain an agreement where nothing but confusion and frustration is possible. Fortunately for patients, very few nurses devote their professional efforts to the nonproductive task of winning universal admiration or carry resentment for what they are obligated to do for their patients. **Most nurses find their motivation and their rewards in their own growth and in what they are able to achieve for their patients.** This is the most important aspect of a rational self-interest.

If a health care professional believes that her rational self-interest is achieved, through the pursuit of her professional obligation, she is logically compelled to honor the ethical implications of her agreement. In this case, her agreement is not a flimsy thing and it will support her stable ethical obligations.

She is practicing, at least, a primitive form of symphonology whether or not she knows it.

Study Guide

1. Think about your day—what kind of agreements have you encountered? Think about how these agreements have helped you to function, to be in a world that you can understand, and, perhaps, some of them have even enhanced your life.
2. What are the metaphysical and epistemological foundations of symphonology?
3. Think of some examples for each of the agreements—just have fun with it— be creative. See the chapter by Dr. Scotto for details on how the theory was formed, descriptions of the metaparadigm, major assumptions, and so forth.

References

Gaberson, K. B., & Oermann, M. H. (2007). *Clinical teaching strategies in nursing*. New York: Springer Publishing Company.

Polanyi, M. (1974). *Personal knowledge: Towards a post-critical philosophy*. Chicago: University of Chicago Press.

Scotto, C. (2005). Symphonological bioethical theory. In A. M. Tomey & M. R. Alligood (Eds.), *Nursing theorists and their work* (6th ed., pp. 585–601). St. Louis: Mosby.

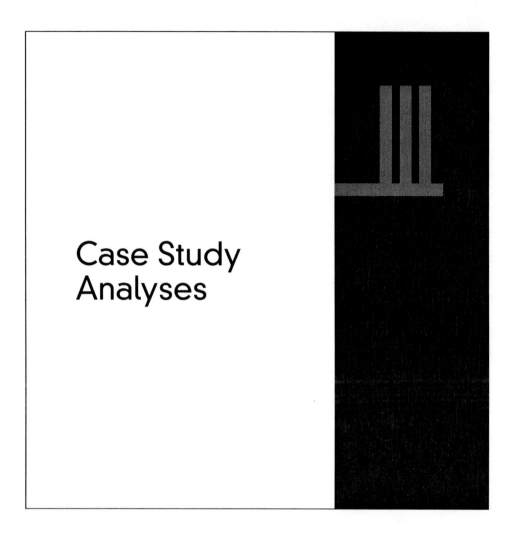

Case Study
Analyses

Analyses of Dilemmas

A Note to the Reader

In reviewing these dilemmas, the reader should recall that they are abstract case studies. In abstract case studies, of course, it sounds as though the nature of the case is very clear and the responsibility of any health care professional is equally clear and rigid. In the context of a real-life situation, however, a health care professional seldom enjoys this clarity.

It is possible that for one or more dilemmas, a reader may come to a different resolution than the resolution given. This is not surprising. There is no real-world context to which to refer. Everyone approaches a dilemma from the perspective of recent experiences, ideas, and attitudes. A nurse may unconsciously rewrite the dilemma from her perspective. Or it is possible to add something to the context that is not given in the dilemma. A different perspective or context may, very logically, result in a different resolution to this new and different dilemma. The reader is asked to perform a thought experiment: Without changing anything of the dilemma as it is given, form a different perspective of the dilemma in your mind—one that suggests the resolution given. This will significantly sharpen your understanding of ethical decision making.

A simple example of this: John is in the hospital. The hospital is notified that John's wife has died. John's nurse, Emma, is elected to tell him of his wife's death. One possible resolution: Emma should tell John at this time. Another possible resolution: Emma should not tell John at this time. If one assumes that John would suffer no harm by being told at this time or might be benefited in some objective way, one would come to the first resolution. If one assumes that John might suffer harm by being told at this time and would not be benefited, one would come to the second resolution. Not all dilemmas will be this simple. But many will be. Even in this dilemma, background information is necessary to its justifiable resolution.

There is a very large difference between a real-life context and a case study. Nothing that follows should instill a feeling of ethical incompetence in the reader. Many of the following dilemmas are highly context dependent. In addition, some are quite difficult. Several are dilemmas nurses or other health care personnel meet in their interactions with physicians. These usually are more difficult to resolve than dilemmas that only involve patients.

Whereas most of the dilemmas only involve nurses, not all of them do. Some involve other professionals, such as physicians, pharmacists, physical therapists, social workers, dieticians, psychologists, and so forth.

The final resolutions of some of these dilemmas can be discovered only in the actual context in which they arise. All that can be done in a case study analysis is to make the nature of the dilemmas clear. In some cases, we will offer only broad suggestions as to the direction the resolutions one might take.

The purpose of these analyses is to make the reader stronger and more knowledgeable. Many ethical agents do not allow themselves to know when their response to an ethical situation has been inadequate. Without knowledge, there is no growth. Without growth, there is no possibility of consistently appropriate ethical decision making. It is a nurse's responsibility to know. The purpose of these resolutions is to enable the reader to orient her or his thinking about bioethical matters and to develop competence and confidence at ethical decision making.

Analyses

Dilemma 3.1, page 35

What should be done about a woman who says she wants to quit going to dialysis, but continues to get on the bus?
When we are faced with two unpleasant alternatives we often complain bitterly about the one we find the least undesirable. In effect, Mrs. B changes the alternatives from what they are to stopping the dialysis or not having the condition to contend with at all.

Here the problem is to determine what Mrs. B wants. There is evidence that she wants to stop the dialysis. She has told everyone within hearing that she hates it and does not want to live this way. On the other hand, when the physician describes the risks of not having it, she continues to board the van that takes her to dialysis. The evidence that she wants to stop the dialysis is much less compelling than the evidence she wants to continue it.

When she has to choose between the actual alternatives she faces, she chooses to continue the dialysis. The old platitude "actions speak louder than words" is true. Her actions are sufficient to resolve the dilemma.

Dilemma 3.2, page 40

Is the use of "deception" to protect a patient's pride justified?
First off, Dee did not tell Anna, "Everyone does this." Anna's right to be different ought to be explicitly recognized. It was.

Dee accepted Anna's autonomy and she resolved the dilemma through indirection. Dee asked Anna, as a favor, to taste a batch of pigs-in-the-blanket that she had made. She told Anna that she made them for her in-laws and she wanted them to be perfect. She induced Anna to try them and give her suggestions on how she might improve them. She told Anna that she had made several unsuccessful tries and asked Anna to show her how they are made. She brought the makings to Anna's home—enough so that Anna had to freeze some.

The message that Dee delivered to Anna was unmistakable: "Anna, after all the nice things I have done for you, how can you refuse to do this for me?" The dam was broken. Anna assented with some degree of joy and gratitude, knowing full well that Dee's actions had been a ploy. They shared a joke at Anna's expense. Autonomy always points to the right direction. Sometimes, the direction it points to is indirection. A practice-based ethic, based on beneficence, does not require that people bump heads or argue in endless circles.

Dilemma 3.3, page 44

What is the nurse's obligation to herself in this difficult situation?
Lori could give Paul CPR.

If a nurse has a responsibility to prevent harm from coming to a patient, it is radically misguided to imagine that she has no responsibility to prevent harm from coming to herself.

On what basis might Lori conclude that her life is less important than Paul's? There is none.

In order to be an adequate nurse, one must have three qualities:

- One must be capable of making rational and objective decisions.
- One must have some concern for human well-being.
- One must realize that one is human.

We will not argue for this. It is certainly self-evident.

If Lori would give CPR to Paul without a mouthpiece, this would establish that she is, at least sometimes, capable of making irrational and nonobjective decisions. And this to a point where she could not be trusted to make a decision for anyone.

What Lori ought to do in this case is call 911 for help.

In the meantime, there are a number of things she can do, short of giving mouth-to-mouth resuscitation. In this way she is keeping the agreement she has with her life and taking the necessary steps to help Paul. At the same time, she is meeting the responsibility she has to her life by not putting herself in harm's way. She is keeping the context and functioning as a nurse.

Dilemma 3.4, page 47

Should a patient in a persistent vegetative state be allowed to die?
All four arguments given in chapter 3 are misleading:

- The unique individual that he once was does still exist. The state of being that he once enjoyed, however, no longer exists. Even if it were true to say that, "The autonomous individual no longer exists," nothing would follow from this. If anything ought to be done, this can only be because an autonomous individual does exist. If an autonomous individual does not exist, then there is nothing that must be done.
- There is no way that anyone can benefit this patient. What should be done cannot be determined by beneficence. There is no way to exercise beneficence in relation to this patient.

■ Life is not precious to him. Nothing is or can be of any value to him. If a tribute can be paid to him and to his life, that tribute might be his death as well as his continued existence.

■ The notion of autonomy involves three notions—uniqueness, rational animality, and ethical equality.

As a rational animal, the patient is specifically identical to every other human individual. Therefore, he is ethically the equal of every other human individual. Autonomy also involves ethical equality.

It is true that no one has a right to terminate the life of an autonomous individual. This is not because an autonomous individual is unique. It is not because, when he is observed, he appears different from other people. An autonomous individual acquires the right to life through the fact that he is a rational animal.

Every person and the context of every person is unique. Certain general principles, such as the individual person's independence, must guide every action in any context similar to this. Consideration must also be given to the actual differences that exist in the context.

In this person's context, there are four relevant differences:

■ He has requested that he be allowed to die.

■ He is now permanently dependent on the efforts of others.

■ None of the elements of human autonomy now characterize him. He is conscious of no desires; he is totally out of touch with the world. He engages in no reasoning processes, nor will he ever.

■ His life consists in basic physiological processes; this is not autonomous. He has no purposes. He has no power to exercise agency. Allowing his life to terminate is not the same as terminating his life.

The recognition of this patient's autonomy does not speak against allowing him to die. The bioethical standards do not demand that he be kept alive.

Dilemma 3.5, page 51

Can the agreement be broken for a once in a lifetime opportunity?

Jeffrey, a young child, is your patient. You have an agreement with him to stay until his parents arrive. If you break this agreement, why would you have any reason to keep any agreements? There is a serious implication behind a decision to break your agreement with Jeffrey. That is an assertion that you are not a professional nurse. If there is ever a reason to break an agreement there must be a cutoff point where one side, which is breaking the agreement, is acceptable and the other side where it is not. For instance, you get a call that your own child has been in a terrible automobile accident and is on his way to the ER. Your agreement with your own child in this situation is prior to your agreement with Jeffrey. The cutoff point would be where keeping an agreement would necessitate breaking a prior and more basic agreement. The concert is well over on the other side of the cutoff point.

Dilemma 4.1, page 60

What should the health professional do when a patient delays life-saving treatment to protect the life of her unborn child?

The fact that Mabel is lying to herself has great ethical relevance in this context.

Autonomy: By lying to herself, Mabel has closed off her autonomy to Sharen. In refusing to consider one or more relevant factors, Mabel takes herself out of any objective context. She has broken the connection between the context of knowledge and the context of her situation. She has broken the connection between Sharen and herself. Mabel presents no autonomy and no objective context with which Sharen can deal.

Mabel has not considered the fact that the two outcomes open to her are opposed to each other. She cannot have the child and fight her cancer. Mabel can establish an objective context only by considering all the alternative possibilities and choosing one.

The fact that she is unwilling to consider every possibility makes it difficult or impossible for Sharen to communicate with her.

But Sharen, in approaching the problem directly, is making it difficult for Mabel to communicate. Indirection might be a better direction to take. If Sharen asked Mabel as a hypothetical or rhetorical question, "Mabel, if you had to make a choice between saving the life of this baby or your own life, what do you think you would choose?" Or, "Mabel, if a woman had to make a choice between saving the life of her baby or her own life, what do you think she would choose?" "What do you think she should choose?" Or, "Mabel, when a woman gets pregnant she makes certain agreements with the baby. Do you think she makes an agreement to (three or four agreements), for instance, keep the baby safe?" Then in discussing this relatively, nonthreatening question about her thoughts, Mabel might finalize a choice, begin to discuss it, and come to a decision.

Freedom: Mabel is unwilling to make an objective judgment based on every alternative open to her. Under these circumstances, she cannot engage in free action. She has bound herself. Sharen cannot try to influence her freedom. Mabel has given up her freedom. But if she is not free to decide she might be free to analyze it as a hypothetical question. Instead of a momentous decision she will deal with an interesting discussion.

Objectivity: Sharen owes Mabel the truth. A patient also has some responsibility to give truthful communications to the health care professionals caring for her. Mabel is violating this standard. This gives Sharen no basis for effective ethical action. Another approach is in order; Sharen's duty is no resolution.

Self-assertion: Mabel is using her self-assertion to protect herself against the reality of her situation. She is defending herself against the value of the counsel that Sharen could give her. No doubt defending herself against much more than that. But, in defending her feelings she is attacking her life.

Beneficence: Mabel is walled off from the influence of Sharen and other health care professionals. Under the circumstances, beneficence is not possible. Except the beneficence of indirection.

In order for Sharen to benefit Mabel, Mabel will have to analyze her situation and apply some level of reason to the course of action she decides. Mabel seems entirely unwilling or unable to do this. She may be willing if she does not have to face it head-on.

Fidelity: In this narrow aspect of their relationship, there is no communication between Mabel and Sharen. Since there is no communication, there is no agreement other than the most arid basic nurse/patient agreement. This is, however, enough agreement to base some small talk on.

Dilemma 4.2, page 62

Should a dying patient remain full code because of his family's optimism?
Autonomy: If the desires of Edgar's family are given priority, his autonomy is obviously violated since his desires and theirs contradict each other.

Freedom: Not to honor Edgar's wishes is obviously a violation of his freedom. The more so since there is no possibility of his achieving freedom in the future.

Objectivity: The family's optimism is a subjective feeling in conflict with the facts. Subjective feelings, except those of a patient, have no weight in a practice-based ethic.

Self-assertion: Assertion of one's values for another is not an example of ethical analysis nor a valid application of the standard of self-assertion.

Beneficence: It is not beneficent to take over a patient's right to self-assertion in order to indulge a formalistic and malevolent whim. It is not beneficent to take over a patient's right to self-assertion in order to indulge a formalistic and benevolent whim. It is not justifiable to violate a patient's right to self-assertion for any reason. No motivation can justify this.

Fidelity: The physician's agreement with Edgar does depend on the attitude of Edgar's family.

Dilemma 4.3, page 64

Should a nurse be held to her promise of secrecy?
This is not a dilemma that a nurse is very apt to find. However, the dilemma presented in this extreme case points to the principles involved in any dilemmas of this kind.

Autonomy: The patient is unique. The nature of his desire is determined by this uniqueness. How his desire is shaped by his uniqueness in the situation cannot be known. The nurse must go on the knowledge she has. But the dilemma assumes that she has very little knowledge.

Freedom: If she reveals what her patient has told her, she will, at least apparently, be taking action against him. If she informs the physician, she will also be taking an action for him. She will be helping him to continue acting on the purpose he had in entering the hospital. This purpose inspired his original agreement. If his nurse keeps her later agreement she will have broken her earlier and more basic agreement. This would imply that agreements are to be broken. In fact, it is implicit in the original agreement—that the hospital would function as a hospital—that no contrary agreements would have any status. This alone, in and of itself, would free the nurse from any responsibility to keep her promise.

Objectivity: In order to meet the demands of the standard of objectivity, a nurse must be guided by beneficence. Does objectivity call for her to keep her promise to the patient? Or does it call for her to inform the physician so that he can take the best possible action? In order to discover the demands of beneficence, she has to know the probable outcomes of different courses of action given her patient's ultimate purposes.

There is no way the nurse can know what direction beneficence takes. But all of this takes place in a health care setting and when there is any doubt, the nature of the health care setting must determine action. There is no way to interpret the patient's revelation to his nurse as anything more than a joke. If it was a matter of any seriousness, she is entitled to believe he would not have revealed it.

Self-assertion: We also find some assistance in the standard of self-assertion. The nurse does not take over the ownership of her patient unless she does something for him that he would not do for himself. If she does something for him that he would do, then she is simply acting as his agent.

In considering the dilemma from the vantage point of self-assertion, it is possible to see one important fact: Silence maintains the patient's self-assertion and self-governance only if he would be willing to harm himself.

Perhaps he would. Perhaps his reason for wanting to keep his condition secret is important enough that he would be willing to endure this harm. The nurse must ask herself, however, why he would have told her if this is the case. If secrecy here is important enough for him to endanger himself in this situation, why would he have told his nurse? Consideration of the case under the standard of self-assertion tends to indicate that the nurse should tell the physician what the patient told her.

Beneficence: Contextually, it seems as if beneficence calls for telling. But the harm of telling is not known. Action is behavior arising from knowledge. An agent should always prefer to act on what she does know rather than on what she does not know. The harm of not telling is known. If this harm is at all serious, then that which is known must override that which is not known. Beneficence, guided by reason, suggests that the nurse break her promise of secrecy.

Fidelity: Fidelity requires the nurse to make a choice. She must exercise fidelity either toward her promise or toward her patient. Her promise, of course, was a promise to her patient. All the same, she owes fidelity not to one aspect of her relationship to her patient, but to the entire relationship and to the destiny of her patient. In the context of a purposive ethic, she owes fidelity to her patient and to what she knows.

A ritualistic ethic would demand that a nurse keep her promise, but very few nurses would. A purposive ethic would demand that a nurse keep her attention on the purpose that brought her patient into the hospital.

When a patient tells a secret to a nurse, he should not forget that the first purpose of the health care system is his health and well-being. Secrecy for the sake of secrecy must give way to health and well-being.

Dilemma 4.4, page 65

Should a dietitian provide TPN to a dying man against her better judgment because it is what the physician wants?
Autonomy: Very few people would want TPN under these circumstances. Therefore, we must conclude that it is unlikely that Luke would. We have no

reason to believe that his desires would be different from the great majority of people.

Freedom: We do not enhance Luke's freedom by giving him the freedom to suffer.

Objectivity: The physician has an ethical obligation to those he asks to assist him, in this case, Betty and the nurse. His obligation is to provide some objective reasoning in support of this course of action.

Self-assertion: We have no reason to believe that Luke would act to do this for himself. Therefore, we have no justification for doing this for him.

Beneficence: To prolong a patient's painful dying process is not beneficent. If it were, there would be no such thing as a maleficent course of action.

Fidelity: Many times, when we give fidelity to our powerful enthusiasm, we practice a fidelity to ourselves and our own feelings of well-being. We never have a right to choose our enthusiasm over the welfare of our patient.

Dilemma 4.5, page 67

As the agent of the patient, what could the nurse have done?
Autonomy: It is difficult to understand what motivated the physician. But whatever unique character structure would cause him to encourage Sarah to continue useless treatments rather than taking this vacation with her family, is entirely inconsequential. The autonomy of each member of the family would be enriched more by spending some memorable time with Sarah before her death rather than buying her a few more days or weeks of suffering.

Freedom: All of Sarah's freedom will be lived according to her decision on what she wants to do right now. This is a decision for the rest of her life. It is a decision that will also affect the rest of her family's life.

Objectivity: The physician was "playing a part" and was disconnected from Sarah's desires and the reality of her situation.

Self-assertion: What self-assertion would motivate Sarah to decide, would motivate anyone who was aware of the context to decide. And, in all cases, this would be the best decision to make.

Beneficence: There is nothing beneficent in the physician's prescribing futile care. There would be nothing beneficent in Sarah's taking this advice without question.

Fidelity: Sarah owes fidelity first to herself. And then to her family. And not at all to the physician.

The nurse should help Sarah and her family and suggest to them that they get their mother a second opinion.

Dilemma 4.6, page 71

Is it ever right to tell lies from benevolent motives?
Autonomy: Whatever the nature of their autonomy, it is inconceivable that Robin's parents would take a calm and disinterested view of Robin's death.

Freedom: Obviously, the power of Robin's parents to move into the future was truncated by the nurse's actions.

Objectivity: When Robin's parents heard the details of their daughter's death, this did them no good and could not fail to do them harm. It did nothing to help them assimilate this event into their lives and to begin to move on.

Self-assertion: No one's agency was increased by this. The experience they underwent at the hands of Robin's nurse will, predictably, interfere with Robin's parents getting on with their lives. They will always carry this picture in their mind.

Beneficence: Robin's nurse harmed the parents emotionally and forever. It did nothing to increase their ability to reason. Robin's nurse acted dutifully, but she failed to act beneficently. She did not fail to act irrationally.

Fidelity: Obviously, no rational purpose was served by this action. The nurse cannot justify her action by appealing to fidelity.

Dilemma 4.7, page 74

Should heroic measures be used to keep alive a dying patient who is in excruciating pain?

Autonomy: If heroic measures are not taken and Martha is allowed to die, then, certainly her uniqueness will be lost along with her life. Her uniqueness will pass out of existence. This fact, however, has no ethical relevance. The ethical concept of autonomy is not the uniqueness of a person that the outside world gazes upon. It is the uniqueness of a person as the person lives it. It is the person's self-identity as he or she experiences it. Not to allow Martha to die would not preserve her autonomy. It would violate her autonomy. Not to allow Martha to die is not the same as allowing her to live. It is forcing her to continue dying.

Freedom: If it is Martha's desire to die and health care professionals have agreed to act as her agent, then in applying heroic measures they would violate their agreement. They would take an action for her that she would not take for herself. Any claim that they violate her right to freedom in not applying heroic measures is one of the extreme points of ethical absurdity.

Objectivity: As far as making her decision is concerned, Martha has all the information she needs. Her excruciating pain and the fact that she is terminal provides this. The standard of objectivity does not enter into the picture beyond this. In her physical state, her body is reasoning for her.

Self-assertion: When a person makes an agreement with a health care professional, he or she makes it from the perspective of self-governance. Martha made her agreement on this basis. If someone has a right to force Martha to live in these circumstances (for instance, a legislator who passes a law), then this person has taken over the ownership of Martha. This is true despite the fact that Martha has never given up her self-governance.

It is absurd to say that Martha's self-governance is not violated under these circumstances. If another person takes over control of Martha's actions, this person certainly violates her right to self-assertion.

Beneficence: In dilemmas involving passive euthanasia, people have widely differing views as to what constitutes beneficence. Ultimately, it is up to every individual to determine what constitutes "doing good or at least doing no harm." What a person believes and what a person can justify are often very different things.

Staying in the bioethical context, let us try to clarify the question of justification through a thought experiment: Try to imagine that to end Martha's life and suffering would be to harm her. Imagine that to keep her alive and suffering would be to bestow some good upon her.

Now that you have seen this in your mind's eye, let us take it one step further. Imagine a patient, Marian, who is dying a peaceful and painless death. The technology to keep Marian alive is available, but is excruciatingly painful. Assume that Marian ought not to be kept alive under these circumstances, and then try to devise some justification for keeping Martha alive. Is it not absurd to keep a patient in unendurable pain alive while permitting a patient who is not in pain to die?

Suppose that ethics demands that patients such as Marian, as well as patients such as Martha, be kept alive. This supposition implies that every health care setting ought to become a combination cemetery and torture chamber. If a person can believe this, nothing more can be said. If a person can justify it bioethically, he or she will have transformed the nature of bioethics and of modern biomedicine—not necessarily for the better.

Fidelity: The demands of fidelity, of course, depend upon the agreement. If health care professionals agree to act as Martha's agents, and they agree to act toward her with beneficence, then they agree to act toward Martha as she would act toward herself. Martha would not act to keep herself alive. If health care professionals keep her alive in these circumstances, they break their agreement with her.

Euthanasia, even passive euthanasia as discussed in Martha's case, is a very complex and controversial subject. In order to illuminate the analysis we have made through the bioethical standards, we will analyze it through the elements.

Desire: It is inconceivable that the desire of a terminal patient in unbearable pain to continue living as long as possible could be a rational desire. The element of rational desire calls for allowing Martha to die.

Reason: To paraphrase the philosopher Benedict Spinoza: Reason demands nothing contrary to nature and nature demands nothing contrary to reason. If a person wages a war on his existence (a war that he cannot win), and if he denies everything that he knows to be true, he turns his back on reason, on everything he is. Reason demands that a person accept the facts of his existence and the reality of his world. If reason demands anything, then it demands that a person accept that which he knows to be true.

For a person to accept that which he knows to be true is for him to act in harmony with his own nature. It is for him to act in harmony with the reality of the world around him. Reason and nature demand nothing less than this.

The reality of Martha's existence calls for the exercise of reason. It calls for the biomedical professionals who are her agents to exercise reason and beneficence.

Life: Martha is alive only in the sense that an irrational animal is alive. Martha is not an irrational animal. The best promise life offers her is death. If Martha's life is allowed to speak for itself, then Martha ought to be allowed to die.

Purpose: Analyzing Martha's situation from the vantage point of purpose shows that Martha ought to be allowed to die. This is not surprising. In the context of the bioethical standard, it is an ethical purpose. It is a rational purpose. And, not least, it is Martha's purpose for herself.

Agency: Every ethical agent in exercising agency should exercise it with courage and clarity of vision. If biomedical professionals are given the power to decide Martha's fate, they should decide with courage and clarity of vision. For they are her agents.

Both the bioethical standards and the elements suggest the ethical propriety of allowing Martha to die.

Dilemma 5.1, page 82

Are there circumstances under which a nurse is justified in discontinuing home visits?

Martin is a biomedical professional. As such, he has a professional role. He has a responsibility to care for Frank as long as Frank needs him. But has he? We have run into a contextual kink. There is an ambiguity on the word *needs*. Frank's health is such that he needs Martin to help him change his self-destructive habits. But insofar as Martin has no influence on Frank, insofar as Frank will not change his self-destructive habits, Frank has no need for Martin. If Martin had, more or less, 20 such patients and with each one he lived up to his professional role, perfectly filling his responsibility, he would be perfectly useless as a biomedical professional.

Sometimes the best direction is indirection; the best way to straighten a kink is to put a kink in it. Suppose Frank had the services of a home health nurse who encouraged his heavy smoking and his dietary habits. From what we know of Frank, he would be no better or no worse off with or without visits from this home health nurse. These visits would change absolutely nothing. And, Martin's visits have precisely the same influence. Likewise, Frank would be no worse off without visits from Martin. And he is not better off with Martin's visits. Another patient might be considerably better off.

Dilemma 5.2, page 83

What is the relative importance of protocol versus patients?

Nearly always when a context is distorted and misread, it is because it has been widened beyond its relevant contours. The situation can also appear problematic if the context is narrowed too stringently. On the one hand, the patient needs attention that she cannot be given in Ron's location. On the other hand, hospital policy and practice requires that an attending physician sign a transfer order. Looking at it from the narrow perspective, then, is no way to resolve it.

But the context of the situation is formed by purposes that are to be accomplished in the health care setting. And that is not possible here. A wider context must be sought. It must be sought in the context of knowledge.

The primary elements of the context of knowledge are formed by the nature and definition of the roles of those engaged in seeking to achieve the purpose. In this case, it is the definition of a physician, a nurse, and a patient.

However a physician is defined, the purposes of the physician that do not involve the welfare of patients are far less important than the purposes that do.

These latter are the defining purposes of the physician and the entire health care system.

The ethical course for Ron to follow is to transfer Mrs. Allison to the other hospital. And then depend on the calm, modest, rational objectivity of the physician. This attitude of the physician is the only ethical attitude possible to her. The ethical responsibilities of any professional are set out in the definition of her profession.

Dilemma 5.3, page 92

Should homeless men without relatives be considered organ donors?
The right of a person to make decisions for himself, dispose of his property, and so on, is firmly established in law. The facts that John Doe is deceased and could not express his wishes, that there was no family or friend to express what he would want, and that he was an excellent candidate for organ donation are all entirely irrelevant. What can be gained in minor violations of rights justified by rationalizations is very far outweighed by the consequent threat to rights. Rights is the product of an agreement among rational beings. Whoever breaks this agreement on whatever pretext, proves himself not to be among the class of rational beings. John Doe changed. He moved from life to death. The hospital personnel choose unilaterally to benefit from this change in John Doe's condition. There was no voluntary consent on his part. This violated John Doe's rights.

Autonomy: A human person does not have rights because he is alive. He has rights because he is a human person. The prenatal right to inherit and the postmortem right to bequeath are recognized even by the law. The rights of the living continue even when they are no longer living. This includes the right to dispose of or not to dispose of that which was theirs as they wished.

Freedom: It is not the case that what one did not explicitly forbid, he tacitly consented to. On the contrary, that which he did not consent to in the disposition of his values, unless there are compelling arguments from his perspective that can be made, it must be assumed he tacitly forbade.

Objectivity: To violate any implication of the rights agreement is to violate the rights agreement.

Self-assertion: It is not possible to properly analyze this dilemma without understanding. And, it is not possible to understand it without seeing its comic dimensions. The only principle on which they can justify their action is some version of, "If you believe that it is so, then it is so." This reveals much more about them than about the dilemma. A safer conclusion than that their actions were justified, would be the conclusion that, "If they believe that it is so, then it very probability is not so," since their only reason for belief is the fact that they want it to be so.

Beneficence: To assume that a drowning person would want to be saved is justified. To assume that a person would want to be an organ donor without any immediate evidence is not justified. Therefore, it is not an exercise of beneficence.

Fidelity: The only way to exercise fidelity would be to recognize the absence of an agreement.

Dilemma 5.4, page 93

Should a physician order beneficial surgery against a patient's wishes?
Autonomy: Harold is unique. His motivations for refusing the amputation of his gangrenous leg must certainly be unique. But they are his motivations; it is his leg and his life. The physician, apparently, did not ask Harold why he was refusing the operation. Or, if she did, Harold's answer did not satisfy her.

Harold's motivations and values are unique. So are the motivations and values of the physician. In order for Harold's answer to satisfy the physician, their motivations and values would have to be harmonious. If Harold's answer must satisfy his physician, then Harold's physician has the same rights in relation to Harold's life as Harold has. In fact, this would give the physician not only the same rights but greater rights than Harold.

As one human to another, the physician has a right as a health care professional to exert gentle coercion. But since Harold is an autonomous individual, by right he has no ethical responsibility to satisfy his physician on a decision concerning an operation that he does not want.

Freedom: The physician's action is an attack on Harold's freedom of choice in the matter of his own life. If this freedom is taken away, Harold has no freedom left. Without freedom, there is no possibility of Harold acting ethically. There is no possibility of Harold acting at all. Because Harold cannot engage in ethical actions, he cannot engage in ethical interactions. And, therefore, Harold's physician cannot be engaged in an ethical interaction with Harold.

The ethical choice that the physician is forcing on Harold is not a choice. Harold cannot choose because Harold cannot think and decide for himself. It is not possible for any person to think, decide, or choose when a course of action is forced upon him.

Harold's physician believes that her course of action is best for Harold despite Harold's disagreement. The course of her ethical development was arrested too soon. A higher level of ethical development would produce the belief that no interaction can be justified unless that interaction is chosen by free ethical agents with an equal ethical status and, in her case, on the basis of a professional agreement.

Objectivity: This dilemma does not involve the standard of objectivity:

1. It does not involve Harold's physician attempting to deceive him.
2. Harold has no ethical responsibility, in this context, to give his physician any objective information. Harold's physician has no right to expect Harold to tell her any truth that would assist the physician in her aggression against Harold's rights.

Self-assertion: A health care professional does not protect a patient's right to self-assertion by destroying it.

Beneficence: To destroy a patient's individual sovereignty is not to act beneficently toward him. There is no such thing as acting beneficently toward a person by giving him a benefit he does not want.

H. G. Wells wrote a story called "The Richest Man in Bogota." This is the story of a man whose airplane crashes in a valley among the mountains of Columbia.

In the crash, the man loses sight in one of his eyes. The valley where he crashes is filled with diamonds. The brilliance of these diamonds has made everyone who lives in the valley blind. When the inhabitants of the valley discover what has happened to the airplane pilot, they decide that they must put out his other eye. They are all very happy not being sighted. They do not suffer the glare of the diamonds. They believe that anyone who can look out upon the valley must suffer from the glare. So they decide they will blind the pilot, out of beneficence, for his own benefit.

Coercive beneficence cannot be beneficence.

Fidelity: Ask yourself if you would enter into an agreement with a physician if one of the terms of that agreement allowed the physician unlimited freedom to do anything she wanted.

Analysis through the bioethical standards does not justify the physician's actions.

Dilemma 5.5, page 94

What are the rights of a gay couple?
Autonomy: Cal and Art have been living together for 10 years. The meaning of this is quite clear. There is no reason to doubt that Cal would want Art to make his health care decisions. In order to make a valid decision, it would be necessary that someone have knowledge of Cal's situation. Art has this and the family does not; they want everything done to keep him alive.

Cal's dying process cannot be reversed. This is a sufficient reason to go against the family.

Freedom: Cal is dying. He has no ability to exercise freedom, but we can exercise it for him. The family's only reasonable course is to accept this.

Objectivity: It may be that the family deeply loves Cal and cannot bear to lose him. There is not sufficient evidence on which to base this. Another supposition, equally tenable, is that the family wants to keep Cal alive in order to punish him. The health care system cannot cooperate in this.

Self-assertion: After Cal and Art have lived together for 10 years, the family wanting to forbid Art from coming into Cal's room brings the benefits of self-assertion to a halt. They have no right whatever to do this.

Beneficence: Beneficence could not be expressed without the dismissal of hysterical resentment. The health care system, hopefully, has tried to establish beneficence into Cal's last days and will not stop that effort now. Art being with Cal would make for a beneficent ambience. Spite and beneficence do not fit well together.

Fidelity: Cal spent a great deal of time with Art. Art was a very important part of Cal's life. Fidelity to Cal must definitely include the recognition of what Cal would want.

Dilemma 5.6, page 97

Should a person be forced to do what is in her own best interest?
Autonomy: This woman is, as all persons are unique; this means that she acts on her own values and ideas for her future. She has the absolute right to do

this. Her husband and the surgeon acted on an implicit belief that they have the same rights over the woman as she has. This is an assumption that their right over her is more authoritative than her own rights. If assumption is a standard, then everybody has this right.

Freedom: The action of her husband and the surgeon entirely took away her freedom. Without freedom, she cannot take ethical action or interactions. The action they took was not an ethical action open to analysis and debate but rather an act of aggression.

Objectivity: So long as she is capable of evaluating the facts of the situation and knows the possible consequences of her actions she is exercising her objective awareness. This is not even a case in which they are not sure what she wanted, such as in cases involving incompetent patients. They could not even say that she was in extreme pain, and there is not evidence that her fear has made her unable to meet situations in a rational way. She had no opportunity to act on her objective awareness in this circumstance.

They had an intuition from right up front, face to face with the dilemma. She also had an intuition and a little more than an intuition. After a period of analysis she made a decision—an objective and reasoned intuition. If their intuition is on a par with her decision then there is no point to consult with a patient.

Self-assertion: This has to do with self-governance and being able to choose what she does and does not want to do. This has been taken away from her. Her power of self-assertion has been taken away. She has to determine how she will use this time and to what she will put her efforts. This has been denied her when she is put under an anesthetic and all decision making power is taken away.

The woman's power of self-assertion would be lost during the operation. For all intents and purposes her right to self-assertion was lost. No doubt her husband and the surgeon would claim that after the operation she would regain her right to self-assertion. Then it would be incumbent upon them to explain the process by which someone loses her rights and then regains them. If they cannot, the implication is that she now lost rights forever.

Beneficence: Nonobjective beneficence is not beneficence. In her case it is coercive. Coercive beneficent is not beneficent even though they did it in her own best interest from their perspective.

A young man's father sent him to college on a football scholarship so his son could follow in his father's footsteps. This was very beneficent, save for the fact that his son wanted to be a ballet dancer. In this case, it is nonobjective.

Fidelity: If you have an agreement with someone, in order for it to be an objective and ethical agreement, it has to respect the rights of those involved to decide on his or her own course of action. If one is not faithful to this, then the agreement is violated.

Our emotions may tell us to do this since the evidence for a good outcome is overwhelming and, oh well, she will be glad afterwards. I, myself, might be powerfully pulled to follow the course taken by the husband and surgeon—especially if it was my wife or husband whom I loved. However, the woman made an implicit agreement with the surgeon that he would not take the action he did. He did take this action. The implication is that the surgeon had an agreement do to anything he wanted to do. This would mean that the woman relinquished all her rights. But no one can assume this, except through a criminal action.

But there is no reason why the husband, surgeon, nurse, and others should not use gentle coercion. It is really persuasion with a view to her own rational nature.

Dilemma 5.7, page 100

In the case of an in vitro fertilization and subsequent divorce, who owns the embryos?
Peggy wants to be a mother. There was an agreement between her and her husband that this would be for the purpose of procreation. John donated his sperm—an almost inexhaustible resource. Peggy donated her eggs—a very limited resource. This gave John a way to punish Peggy that she could not use against him. In order to evaluate John's concern for the fate of his sperm, one must have recourse to one's sense of humor.

Peggy owns the eggs. And, unless John's sperm can be extracted without harm to the eggs, they are hers.

Dilemma 6.1, page 114

Should a young girl be told she is dying despite what the mother wants?
Autonomy: There is little doubt but that Bonnie does want to discuss her dying. Research supports the fact that when a patient asks directly, "Am I dying," they really want to know and consequently, should be told. She is telling her mother about her uniqueness with her questions.

Freedom: Bonnie's mother has blocked every expression of Bonnie's freedom. We have no reason to believe that she does not mean well. Nor do we have reason to believe that she does mean well. But, she is not thinking of what is best for her daughter in this situation. It is up to a health care professional to inform the mother of this and help her deal with it so that she can truly help Bonnie.

Objectivity: Since Bonnie has expressed the fact that she knows she is dying, wants to know how much time she has left, and wants to talk about it, the path is clear. She is objectively aware of the situation.

Self-assertion: Bonnie's mother is making this even more dreadful than it is. She is confining everyone including Bonnie and her father. Bonnie is blocked from taking control of the little time she has left and doing what she wants to do with it.

Beneficence: Bonnie's mother seems unwilling to accept the fact that what she is doing is not the beneficent thing for Bonnie. It is necessary that someone should deal with the mother, if possible, in a kind way. If there is anyone that Bonnie's mother would relate to best, this person should be found. If not, it is up to Carrie, the hospice nurse, to do this.

It is possible that Bonnie's mother is thinking of the times after Bonnie dies when she can discuss this with her friends from her point of view. She can describe her role in a way calculated to gain the admiration of her friends.

Bonnie knowing and being able to talk about the fact that she is dying, will enhance the dying process for her, it will lighten her load by sharing it with others.

Fidelity: Her mother is taking from Bonnie something that she will never be able to make up to her. Time is of the essence.

Although one can have empathy with the mother, the primary empathy must go to Bonnie. Someone has to tell Bonnie what she already knows and help to give her some peace.

Dilemma 6.2, page 117

Should the wishes of a daughter to be an organ donor be honored now that she is dead?

Autonomy: To many lay people, the desires that Kim expressed would be entirely alien. To her father, it is inconceivable. The fact that Kim's ethical intent is alien or inconceivable to many is completely irrelevant. Ethics is not a matter of approval or disapproval.

Freedom: To donate her organs would be Kim's last action and the last, but very real, exercise of her right to freedom. There is no justification for violating this right. She had this right throughout her whole life and if it is violated her life is violated.

Objectivity: Kim's desire to donate her organs does not violate any ethical standards. There is no objective reason to come in conflict with this. A nonobjective reason would be no reason whatsoever.

Self-assertion: Kim's self-assertion should be interrupted if it can be shown that someone will be harmed. This cannot be shown. Quite the contrary. The feelings of the father, although important, are not ethically relevant. It is Kim's body, her organs, and her self-governance.

Beneficence: The harm that would be done to someone who would otherwise receive one of Kim's organs and to Kim herself would be far greater than the harm to Kim's father.

Fidelity: To help Kim act on her value motivations would be to help her serve her fidelity to herself.

Kim's nurse has a professional responsibility to help her father through this crisis. To help him in a gentle way to understand and come to terms with the fact that this was his daughter's last wish is the best thing the nurse can do for Kim.

Dilemma 6.3, page 117

Should a young girl be informed that her physician has discovered the condition of testicular feminization?

Autonomy: There is no question that informing Amelia of her condition will be an assault on her self-image. There is no question that it will have negative effects on her (developing) autonomy. An analysis of the effects on Amelia's autonomy of being told of the condition reveal these reasons why she should not be told. It reveals no reasons why she should be told.

Freedom: It is certainly the case that Amelia will enjoy less freedom by knowing of her condition. Thus, at best, the standard of freedom does not support informing her of her condition.

Objectivity: It is hard to see how Amelia would be better off knowing of her condition. Benevolence does not call for her to be informed. The effect that being informed will have on her autonomy is an excellent reason for her not to be informed. The standard of objectivity does not justify informing her.

Self-assertion: The act of informing her would surely be an invasion of Amelia's self-assertion. She has not invited, and it is probable that she would not invite, Dr. Richmond to inform her.

Beneficence: There is no question that not informing her is the more beneficent course of action.

Fidelity: The agreement between a patient and a health care professional is an agreement that the health care professional will try to make a patient's state of well-being better and not worse.

What Dr. Richmond can do immediately will make Amelia's state of well-being better, although Dr. Richmond is not the only surgeon in the world who can do this.

On the other hand, the long-term detriment of being informed will vastly outweigh the benefit that Dr. Richmond will bestow on Amelia through his immediate action. Once Dr. Richmond does this harm to Amelia, there will be no one who can undo it.

Despite the bioethical standards, many contemporary ethicists would call for Amelia to be told of her condition. Because of the complexity of this situation, let us examine it in terms of the elements of Amelia's autonomy.

Desire: Most 17-year-old girls would not want to be informed. It cannot be known with certainty whether Amelia would want to be informed, but it can be known with certainty that she probably would not.

Reason: Knowing of her condition will make it more difficult for Amelia to think positively of herself and her life. The element of reason calls for Amelia not to be told. Knowing would do Amelia more harm than good. There is a slight suggestion, in reason, that she not be told. If reason is to be beneficent, then there is a powerful demand that she not be told.

Life: No part of her life is threatened by not knowing. Therefore, there is nothing at all in the element of life to suggest that she should be told.

Purpose: None of Amelia's purposes would be served by her being informed. At the same time, it cannot be doubted that some of her purposes would be hindered by her knowing. The element of purpose counsels that she not be told.

Agency: Amelia's agency would be hindered by her knowing. Her self-image would be damaged. Her approach to the world would change.

Amelia has a right to know. She also has a right not to know. She has a right not to be harmed.

Contemporary ethicists offer two arguments as to why Amelia should be told:

1. Amelia will probably find out anyway.

This is a contextual factor that must be taken into consideration in an actual context. It is, however, a factor that can be taken into consideration only in an actual, real-life context. It is a logistical factor and, as such, it is not one of the ethical aspects of the context. If there is any way that it can be brought about that Amelia will not find out about her condition, then this way should be discovered.

That Amelia will find out anyway is a rationalization. It is a health care professional's excuse for doing his duty when he knows he should not.

2. It is suggested that Dr. Richmond has a responsibility to Amelia's relatives. Amelia must be informed so that she can discuss this condition with them. It might be advantageous to them to be aware of the recessive disorder that may run in their family.

Let us examine the ethical strength of this argument. Dr. Richmond may believe that he has a duty to inform Amelia's relatives. As we have seen, duty is an entirely inappropriate bioethical standard, so he cannot justifiably act on this feeling. Perhaps, however, Dr. Richmond reasons that Amelia has a duty to inform the members of her family. There is no reason to believe that Amelia has any such duty. Claiming that Amelia has a brother (and she may have a brother) does not prove that she has a brother. Claiming that Amelia has a duty does not, logically or ethically, establish the fact that indeed she does have a duty. Every bioethical standard implies that she does not.

It is probable that Dr. Richmond's reasoning, strictly speaking, is not deontological. It is not based on a declaration that either he or Amelia has a duty. His reasoning, probably, is at least partly utilitarian. He is probably motivated by the belief that by informing Amelia, "the greatest good for the greatest number" will be served. But it can be seen that this too involves a duty. We have also seen that utilitarianism is as inappropriate to a biomedical context as is deontology. The utilitarian standard will also fail to justify Dr. Richmond's action.

The difference in this context between a symphonological ethic and utilitarian ethic is this: According to a symphonological ethic, Amelia is at the center of the ethical context. Dr. Richmond must expect nothing of Amelia but that she pursue her own welfare and the welfare of those whom she values. A utilitarian ethic, on the other hand, allows Dr. Richmond to expect Amelia to pursue the welfare of the larger number of people simply because they are the large number rather than whether she values them. Her well-being must be sacrificed to their benefit.

If Dr. Richmond was motivated by a symphonological ethic, he would choose among contextual alternatives. Then he would decide according to rights and responsibilities. He would try to make his decision intelligible in relation to cause and effect. He would try to bring about ethical proportion and balance. Such a decision would call for Amelia to take on the burden of knowing about her condition only if she chose to do this. If Amelia knew all the facts, she might, out of beneficence, wish to inform her relatives.

Let us subject Dr. Richmond's position to a rational ethical analysis. Amelia should value her relatives only if she has some rational reason to value them. For instance, if they are abusive or contemptuous of her, she lacks a rational reason to value them. If she values them in spite of this, she has no ethical reward to offer those who are not abusive or contemptuous of her.

Amelia should choose in favor of her relatives only if she has a rational and objective reason to value them. This reason would have to be sufficient to make her willing to bear the burden of knowing of her condition. She has this objective reason only if her relatives, in turn, place a high value on her.

Let us see where this leaves us. If Amelia's relatives place a high value on her, they will be concerned with the effect of knowing about her condition on Amelia. If her relatives would be unconcerned with the effect of her knowing of her condition, then Amelia has no objective reason to value them.

If Amelia does not have an objective reason to value her relatives, then to inform her of her condition so that she can inform them is simply to sacrifice her to the greater number. To inform her, Dr. Richmond would have to assume that Amelia is or ought to be motivated by self-contempt.

If her relatives place a high value on Amelia, they would not want her to undergo the trauma of knowing of her condition. They would regard the detriment to Amelia as out of proportion to the benefit to themselves.

In the context of a symphonological ethic, Dr. Richmond would have to conclude that: If Amelia has no objective reason to value her relatives, then, in the context of a symphonological ethic, beneficence will not be a rational motivation for her to be informed.

If Amelia does have objective reasons to value her relatives, then her relatives will not want Amelia to know of her condition. Their balanced and proportioned desire would not be to place Amelia's benefit above theirs. Rather, they would consider Amelia's benefit to be of greater benefit to them.

Amelia's relatives have reason to value Amelia only if she respects their desires. If Amelia respects their desires, then she ought to accede to their desires for her welfare to be protected.

It is not difficult to understand that Amelia's increased happiness and self-confidence throughout her life would be more prized by her relatives than their increased convenience.

Suppose that one of Amelia's relatives is a nurse. Should a nurse place this high a value on her convenience? How would she relate to her patients? Could you, as a nurse, place a high value on this nurse?

In the context of a symphonological ethic, there are no ethical circumstances calling for Amelia to be informed of her condition.

Nurses and the Physician's Dilemma

This is a dilemma that falls on a physician to resolve and not on a nurse. However, in the health care system, very often a physician resolves a dilemma but a nurse must deal with his resolution. Quite often, it is a nurse who must explain the physician's resolution to the patient and, perhaps, spend the better part of a day with the patient and/or the patient's family answering questions. These situations can be very frustrating for nurses.

Nurses should be able to analyze even the most difficult dilemmas. Knowing how to analyze difficult ethical dilemmas makes it easier to analyze simple dilemmas. It might also enable a nurse to win the respect of her colleagues in the health care system. It might make it possible for her to negotiate with them and, one hopes, to become involved with them in the decision-making process.

The implication of Dr. Richmond's duty is that his satisfaction at feeling right, which lasts for 1 hour, is of greater overall importance than Amelia's feeling of being wrong, which lasts for 60 years. This implies that in Dr. Richmond's ethical world, he lives there all alone.

Dilemma 6.4, page 120

Does a terminally ill patient have a right to expect something from a nurse that might be injurious to his health?
This is several dilemmas in one:

- Whether a patient in these circumstances has the right to something he wants if it may be injurious to his health.
- Whether a physician is justified in refusing him.
- Whether a nurse has a right to disobey the physician's orders.
- Whether a nurse has an ethical agent obligation that overrides the physician's order.

Obviously, a dilemma of this complexity can be resolved only in the context. But analysis will reveal something about it.

Autonomy: Rodney's autonomy is expressed in this desire. This desire is very short range. But, in fact, Rodney has no long-range desires. His desire is the expression of his autonomy in his present circumstances.

Freedom: If it is probable that the drink of water would not increase Rodney's suffering or if his increased suffering could be alleviated, then we must consider the following: When Rodney entered the health care system, he was better able to act for himself. As time passed, he sank into a more helpless state. To refuse Rodney's dying request while he is in this state is to violate his right to freedom. Had Rodney known that he would be subjected to this violation, it is, in principle, possible that he would not have come into the health care system. In light of the fact that Rodney cannot recover, the physician's action is an action entirely lacking ethical balance and proportion. It was a callous violation of Rodney's freedom.

If it is probable that the drink of water would increase Rodney's suffering, and if his increased suffering could not be alleviated, then the violation of Rodney's freedom is not outside of the agreement between Rodney and the professionals in the health care setting.

Objectivity: Lynetta owes Rodney an explanation of what might happen if he does take the water.

Self-assertion: Lynetta has a responsibility to the physician. She enjoys a position of trust in relation to the physician. It would be understandable if she did not find the position particularly enjoyable in this situation.

Lynetta has an agreement with her patient. If there is a low probability that the water will increase Rodney's suffering, then in failing to give him water Lynetta would be failing to act as her patient's agent. This would be a violation of the nurse–patient agreement and of Rodney's self-governance.

If there is a high probability that the water will increase Rodney's suffering, then in not giving him the drink of water Lynetta would not violate his self-governance. Beneficence is one of the terms of the agreement. The agreement is an agreement to spare Rodney from suffering.

Beneficence: What is and what is not beneficent at every step of the way must be determined in the context.

Fidelity: Lynetta is Rodney's agent. She is also an agent of Rodney's agent—the physician. If the drink of water would increase Rodney's suffering, then Lynetta really does not face a dilemma. If it would not, then she must determine where her greater loyalty ought to lie. She must also decide what she is willing to risk. On the one hand, she risks retribution from the physician. On the other hand, she risks committing a senselessly cruel act.

Dilemma 8.1, page 141

Should an individual with dementia be medicated against his will to make him "easier to handle"?

Fred is aggressive, and no one has a right to be aggressive. Therefore, this is not a right that a nurse, acting as Fred's agent, must protect. Nonetheless, an attempt should be made to reason with Fred at a very basic level. This could be done somewhat as follows: "Fred, you are not insane. You are not even stupid. Taking this medicine does not mean that you are insane. Insane people eat eggs. Insane people take aspirin. Is this a reason for you not to eat eggs or take aspirin? When you take this medicine, you feel better and live better. Isn't that the only thing that is important?" If this does not succeed, then the antidepressant ought to be given to Fred by whatever means are possible, but the less invasive, the better.

The motivation for giving Fred the medicine is not utilitarian. It is simply to protect the rights of the people who have to deal with him. Analysis by extremes quickly shows that this is the right thing to do. For instance, it is obvious that it is better that Fred should have no right to aggress than an unlimited right to aggress. It is right that Fred should have no right to aggress than an unlimited right to aggress.

Dilemma 8.2, page 142

Is a health care professional right in attempting to compel a patient to make decisions regarding his treatment?

- It is true that, in delegating responsibility to the health care professional, a patient is exercising his freedom. The health care professional is an agent acting for his patient.
- In a health care setting, a patient's power of choice and decision are weakened. The knowledge he might act on is limited. The most rational exercise of his freedom might well be to delegate responsibility to a health care professional. This is constantly assumed in emergency situations. In these situations, the health care professional goes about his task with no questions asked.
- A patient's relationship to a health care professional, or any type of professional, does always involve a delegation of responsibility.

On the other hand:

In delegating his right to freedom, the patient is not refusing to exercise it.

- In recognizing the nature of his autonomy, the patient is not abandoning it.
- It is ethically desirable that a patient assume responsibility for himself and delegate as little as possible. But what is as little as possible for one person in one context will not be as little as possible for another person in another context.

Dilemma 8.3, page 143

Should a dying patient be told of his condition if the information will terrify him?

Ken and Rachel are friends. Nonetheless, Rachel does not know which alternative—knowing or not knowing—Ken would choose, and she cannot directly ask him. This adds a complication to the dilemma. Because of this complication, the best way to analyze the dilemma is through the elements rather than through the standards.

The dilemma arose because Rachel is unsure of how to interact with Ken in this situation. She must analyze the elements of his autonomy as they function in this context.

Desire: Ken would desire to get his affairs in order, but he does not want to be made aware of the seriousness of his condition.

If Rachel is noncommittal (by *noncommittal*, we mean Rachel should say something like, "If you do not recover . . ." rather than, "Ken, you are dying and therefore . . .") with Ken, it allows him to either deny the seriousness of his condition or accept it internally without having it thrust at him from the outside.

If Ken cannot be motivated in this way to get his affairs in order, then his desire is obvious. Ken, above all, does not want to know the seriousness of his condition.

Reason: A noncommittal approach on the part of Rachel can help Ken exercise his reason much better than can Rachel's thrusting the details of his condition at him.

Life: Only Ken can compute the importance of his terror in the present, as opposed to his desires for the future.

Purpose: Ken's purposes are in conflict. No one but Ken can tip the balance.

Agency: His agency is involved in getting his affairs in order. His condition precludes agency. As a long-term factor, the element of agency cannot enter into Rachel's deliberations. But, in the time left to Ken, Rachel's responsibility is to strengthen Ken's agency, to do for him what he would do for himself if he were able.

Dilemma 8.4, page 144

What is to be done when intrafamily coercion is suspected?

Autonomy: Their relationship is unique. It is uniquely complex and troubled. It will not be a simple matter for the biomedical team to adequately evaluate their relationship and advise them. Two unique personalities interacting together produce a state of affairs much more complex than a single individual. Out-of-context moralizing should be avoided.

Freedom: Rick and his mother both have a right to freely arrive at a decision and act on that decision.

Objectivity: The consultation between Mrs. Raymond and the biomedical professionals ought to go into exhaustive detail. Mrs. Raymond, quite probably, has a long time to live. Rick's future is very uncertain at best. Rick is trying to preserve his life. At the same time, Mrs. Raymond's reasons for donating her kidney may not be well thought out. Her questions should be elaborated on until she has related the new information given to her to the entire context of her knowledge and the situation.

Self-assertion: No attempt should be made to interfere with Mrs. Raymond's exercise of her time and effort in donating her kidney to Rick. Every effort should be made to enable her to make a decision that reflects her actual values.

Beneficence: No one owes Rick any specific beneficence beyond performing the operation and advising him on a health regimen. No one owes him assistance in deception. Mrs. Raymond is owed the beneficence of clarity of vision. She deserves to know what she is doing. The biomedical team can help her gain this clarity of vision. She also deserves to know why she is doing what she is doing. This knowledge she must gain for herself and from herself. Skill on the part of the biomedical team might help her in this.

Fidelity: Biomedical care comes in various forms and degrees of excellence. Hopefully, fidelity toward the Raymonds will possess a high degree of excellence.

Dilemma 8.5, page 146

Should a comatose Jehovah's Witness be given a blood transfusion?
Autonomy: There is no way to have certain knowledge of this patient's autonomy.

Freedom: As his agent, his nurse ensures his freedom by acting for him. But she has no way of knowing what actions he would take if he were free, that is, if he were conscious. The fact that this patient belongs to a particular religious sect does not necessarily mean that he accepts every practice of this religion. If he were conscious and declared that he did not want a transfusion, then, in the context of the bioethical standards, that would end it. But he is not conscious, and the direction that his freedom would take if he were is not known.

Objectivity: The standard of objectivity offers no guidance in this case.

Self-assertion: The patient is unable to express his ideas and desires. Therefore, there is no way to know what his self-assertion would consist of.

Beneficence: It is impossible to know what would be beneficent in relation to this patient.

Fidelity: This situation offers no grounds for an agreement.

This is a case a biomedical professional must decide for herself without any help from the bioethical standards. Because the nature of this patient's autonomy also is not known, the elements of autonomy offer little guidance. The decision would need to be made on the basis of the commonalities that all humans share. The element of life offers what may be little more than a suggestion: A person's religion is, to a greater or lesser extent, an important part of his life. But every whole is greater than any one of its parts. The patient's life is more than his religion. The best decision that can be made in this situation is that he be given the blood transfusion. This option will allow him to pursue his autonomous purposes for his life. Otherwise he will die, and all the options of his life will be closed off.

Dilemma 8.6, page 147

How does a nurse deal with a patient who makes demands on her that interfere with her attention to other patients?
The center of Irene's attention cannot be Henry alone; she has other patients. She cannot make an agreement with Henry that would violate the well-being of her other patients. Therefore, her dilemma cannot be resolved by analysis through the standards or the elements. Irene must analyze this as a triage situation.

Dilemma 8.7, page 147

Does a parent's right to know override the right of a child to have his parents not know?
This is a very simple dilemma. It is resolved by the fact that Marilyn has an agreement with Bobby.

Marilyn, of course, also has an agreement with Bobby's parents. But Marilyn is a nurse. A nurse is a professional. As a professional, Marilyn's agreement with Bobby is superior to any agreement she may have with his parents. This agreement overrides any pleasure Marilyn might derive from unguarded small talk.

Many times it will happen that Bobby's health and well-being will require that his parents be given certain information. In that case, Marilyn should give them the information. But this is not because of her agreement with Bobby's parents. It is because of her agreement with Bobby.

Let us assume, for the sake of argument, that Bobby's parents have a right to know of his bedwetting. Even in this (questionable) case, they have no right to expect Marilyn to tell them. Marilyn's only responsibility in this case is to Bobby. Their knowing will not increase Bobby's health or well-being. Bobby desires Marilyn not to tell his parents. In most cases, a nurse cannot know whether a patient's desire is as well-reasoned as it might be. In this context, there is no reason to believe that Bobby's is not a perfectly rational desire.

Marilyn could very well say to Bobby, "I won't tell them, Bobby. Why don't you tell them?" This is a loaded question. Bobby may feel a greater need to defend his request than to explain it. He may give Marilyn information she needs to make a more informed assessment of the situation.

Marilyn might reply to Bobby's parents, "Bobby is a little boy in a scary situation. Why don't you take some comfort to Bobby?" This is also a loaded question based on the fact that if Bobby's parents are motivated by factors they are unwilling to reveal, they will probably respond with righteous indignation and reveal information that Marilyn ought to have. If they agree without indignation, the problem is probably solved.

Somewhere along the way, this course of action should reveal if Bobby has a problem he should not have.

Dilemma 8.8, page 149

Should a nurse give out information on the phone if this information might help or might harm her patient's best interest?
Lotte's only responsibility is to Ray. Her only agreement is with Ray. This agreement does not include taking the word of a caller and informing the caller of Ray's condition. It might seem as if Lotte is interfering with Ray's freedom. She is not. Ethically, Lotte cannot interfere with Ray's freedom unless he expresses a desire.

It is reasonable to assume that if Ray had expected a call or regarded it as important, he would have expressed a desire to her. He would have asked her to give the caller the information he wanted. It is also reasonable to assume that if the matter was important, the lawyer would have sent someone to the hospital. Lotte has no responsibility to assist Ray's lawyer in his failing to act as Ray's agent.

Before she gives any information to the caller, Lotte ought to talk to Ray. Ray might be unable to talk to her. If Ray were unable to talk to Lotte, then he would be unable to talk to his lawyer.

Perhaps the caller is Ray's lawyer. In this case, it would have been better had Lotte given him the information. But Lotte could not know this. She can only justify acting on what she does know. In this context, Lotte took the only justifiable action she could.

If she gave him the information, she would have done the best thing for Ray. But she would have done the best thing by accident. It is not possible for an accident to justify an action.

Dilemma 8.9, page 149

Should a feeble and elderly patient be let out of restraints to freely walk around?
Every possible consideration should be given to Margaret. Let us grant this without argument.

There are two facts in conflict with each other:

1. Sandra should not assist Margaret in actions that will predictably injure her. To do this would be contrary to the nature and purpose of the health care system.
2. Aside from this, Margaret has a right to freedom of action.

These two facts can be brought into harmony if Margaret is allowed to walk around when she can be watched and assisted. When she cannot be, gentle coercion (persuasion) should be exerted to keep her in the safety of her wheelchair.

Sometimes a dilemma can be resolved by not choosing one possibility over another. An agent can meet both demands of the dilemma. She can do two things at different times and according to changes in the context.

Dilemma 8.10, page 150

Should a nurse interfere with a patient's activities if these activities threaten his well-being?

Autonomy: Charlie cannot leave his identity and his life situation behind.

Freedom: Ingrid deals with one aspect of Charlie's life. He deals with every aspect of his life. He has a right to be free to do this.

Objectivity: The standard of objectivity will extend as far as gentle coercion but no further. Once Ingrid has related the facts to Charlie, he has a right to do whatever he wants to do.

Self-assertion: Ingrid ought to warn Charlie. If it is possible, she should exert gentle coercion. But Charlie is a private individual and he has a right to decide and act for himself.

Beneficence: Strictly speaking, for Ingrid to do nothing is neither beneficence nor a failure of beneficence. If she interferes, this is against Charlie's freedom. Actions she takes against Charlie's freedom are not acts of beneficence. Beneficence is central here.

Fidelity: Fidelity to their agreement requires Ingrid to look after Charlie's health and well-being without violating the bioethical standards. The bioethical standards are the terms of their agreement.

An indirect course of action that might be more effective would be for Ingrid to explore the reasons why their conversation should not continue to Charlie's business associate. If the business associate seems unconcerned, this might cause Charlie to be put off and discontinue the conversation knowing that the business associate is taking advantage of Charlie's condition. Or, the business associate may himself bring the discussion to an end.

Dilemma 8.11, page 151

Should a nurse give sensitive information to a family member before she has discussed this with her patient?

Karen and her nurse have an agreement. The bioethical standards are the terms of this agreement. The agreement provides Karen's nurse with no preexisting knowledge of what she ought to do in this situation.

Let us see if we can analyze the situation in terms of the elements of autonomy.

Desire: Only Karen knows what she desires. So this is no help to Karen's nurse.

Reason: It is up to Karen's reason to deal with this. Her nurse's only obligation is not to make it more difficult for Karen.

Life: It is up to Karen to integrate this situation into her life. Obviously, her nurse cannot help her with this.

Purpose: Karen's nurse has no purpose to serve and no right to try to guess Karen's purpose.

Agency: Karen's nurse cannot act as her agent in this situation.

The elements of autonomy provide no more direct guidance in this circumstance than the bioethical standards. The elements, however, do imply a principle by which the dilemma can be resolved. This principle calls for

Karen's nurse to evade the question and get away. We will now turn to that principle.

Awareness and Ethical Action

Contextual action is action taken on the basis of objective judgment. Contextual action requires an awareness of the context of the situation. It also involves an agent's awareness of the context of his or her knowledge.

Awareness is not simply desirable for effective ethical action. It is absolutely essential to it. In circumstances like that of Karen and Steve, we would suggest to the reader this overarching ethical principle: *If you do not know why you are going to do what you are going to do, do not do it.* This principle is not always easy to apply. It must be applied in a context according to the nature of the context. But it is directly implied by the elements of an ethical agent's autonomy.

Desire: An agent can be motivated by either his or her own desire or that of a beneficiary to whom the agent is responsible. If, on the other hand, an agent is aware of no desire, then the agent has no basis for action and no responsibility to act.

Reason: Not to act when one does not know what one is doing is the essence of practical reason.

Life: When you do not know why you are doing what you are doing, you cannot effectively guide your actions. You cannot know what effect it will have on your life or the life of your beneficiary. Under these circumstances, it is irresponsible to take action.

Purpose: To act without knowing what you are doing is to act purposelessly. This cannot be justified. The purpose of an action is its ethical justification.

Agency: To act without knowing what you are doing is to act without agency. It is not acting at all. It is a behavior that is not guided by awareness. It is a violation of your agency.

Dilemma 8.12, page 152

Should a nurse tell a patient's wife that a symbolic agreement the patient and family member had was not realized?
Not telling Denise does not violate the standard of objectivity. If there is any dilemma whose resolution is given right along with the context, this is it. Only a formalism utterly inappropriate to nursing would counsel Lucy to inform Denise that she had not succeeded. We can be quite certain that Lucy would not do this.

Dilemma 8.13, page 152

What should be done about a conflict between what a family needs to know and what a patient does not want his family to know?
This dilemma does not involve the relationship between Ike and Joan. The dilemma involved in this case involves the relationship between Joan and Helen.

This dilemma must be resolved according to an objective view of the demands of their rational self-interest. Any other resolution would create chaos.

There are legal entanglements to this dilemma. Joan and her colleagues might be sued by Helen if Joan does not give Helen the information she needs to get her affairs in order. This being the case, Ike has no right to place Joan in jeopardy. He has no right to expect an agreement with Joan when she does not know the background facts of this agreement, when the agreement has nothing to do with the regimen of his health care, and when this agreement would place Joan at risk.

Let us examine Joan's situation in terms of the elements.

Desire: No one would reasonably choose to pursue an occupation in which they would have no way to avoid periodic lawsuits. Ike has no logical right to assume that nursing is such an occupation. The law may be unclear in situations like this. This lack of clarity would not prevent Helen from suing Joan and the hospital. Joan desires to pursue an occupation that is not potentially destructive of her rational self-interest. Helen desires to avoid a mountain of problems.

Reason: If Joan were to keep Ike's confidence in this situation, it would be irrational on her part. It is irrational for Ike to expect this. People in the biomedical professions have no implicit agreement with a patient to expose themselves to lawsuits and they a responsibility not to behave irrationally.

Life: Joan's life would be greatly diminished if her patient's whim could place her in jeopardy or if she had to serve as a weapon against a patient's unsuspecting enemy.

Purpose: Joan's purpose, as a nurse, is to provide some value for her patient. She would have no motivation for this unless she had purposes for herself. If she acceded to Ike's wishes, Joan's purpose would be purposeless. Joan could allow herself no long-term purposes. Her future would be, at best, entirely un-predictable.

Agency: Joan's agency, as a nurse, should be devoted to the health and well-being of her patients. What Ike asks of her has nothing to do with her role as nurse. Joan can and ought to talk to Ike, and if necessary, explain why she cannot keep his condition a secret from Helen. She does not have this agreement with Ike.

Dilemma 8.14, page 153

When should a nurse report a case of suspected child abuse?
It will be seen that the elements best illuminate this dilemma.

Desire: Shawn's desire for help is rational. Doris's desire for secrecy is not justifiable.

Reason: Shawn needs Alice to help him achieve the benefit of reason. Doris is not acting on reason if Alice is right in her suspicion.

Life: Shawn has a right to a better life if he is being abused.

Purpose: Shawn's purpose is justifiable. Doris's is not.

Agency: Alice is Shawn's agent. (If Shawn is a battered child, a great deal of good can be done. If he is not, no great harm will be done if the investigation is done in an ethical manner.)

Dilemma 8.15, page 154

Are there limits to patient confidentiality?
Autonomy: This certainly seems a unique, even bizarre attitude on Dan's part. If Dan will not divulge the information to his children, a health care professional ought to. How doing this might be a violation or betrayal of some aspect of Dan's character structure is difficult or impossible to understand.

Freedom: Telling his children would be a violation of his freedom if, and only if, their knowing would interfere in some way with legitimate actions Dan wants to take. This is a question that his nurse ought to discuss with him.

Objectivity: So long as the nurse remains open to the reasons why Dan does not want his children to know of his condition, she does not fail the responsibility of objectivity. If Dan will not give his nurse a justifying reason—a reason to leave the children ignorant of information they ought to have—he violates objectivity. He has an implicit agreement with his children to act in their best interest.

He tells his nurse that there is a reason but refuses to tell her what the reason is. He is, apparently, not willing to expose his reason to analysis. This does not relieve the nurse from a responsibility as a fellow human being to provide the children (the children's mother) with the information. (This can be done postmortem.)

Self-assertion: It is difficult to see how telling the children the facts would compel Dan to take undesirable actions—even in the broadest sense of actions. Dan ought to offer some justification on this score.

Beneficence: The nurse has no reason to believe that telling Dan's children of their father's condition would involve a failure to provide a possible benefit or cause possible harm to Dan.

Fidelity: The nurse–patient agreement does not call for a nurse to act on blind faith. If Dan revealed his reasons to his nurse, it could possibly harm him. But, given what we know of the matter, there is no reason to believe this.

One ought to strive not to interfere with the efficient enjoyment of the self-governance of another. Dan has a right to self-governance. He does not own and he has no right to frivolously disrupt the lives of his children.

Dilemma 9.1, page 159

How should a nurse counsel a patient who must decide on whether to gamble on a long-shot treatment?
This is a situation that Vladimir very well might want to discuss with his nurse. If he does, it is desirable that she understand the vital and fundamental factors influencing his decision. Vital and fundamental factors, in a purposive ethic, are ethical factors.

Here the bioethical standards are irrelevant. This is not, in its most important sense, a case of a nurse dealing with a patient. Nor is this a case of a nurse helping a patient deal with another person. This is a case of a nurse acting as a sounding board in order to help her patient think and make a decision for himself. Vladimir needs self-awareness. His nurse can help him to analyze his situation by reference to the elements of his autonomy.

Desire: Vladimir will have to decide whether his greater desire is to play again or to retain the gross motor movements of his hand. Then he must examine the strength of these desires against the probabilities of realizing each one.

Reason: Vladimir must assess the benefits and detriments of each course of action. Then he must decide on what his most reasonable course of action will be in light of his rational desires.

Life: Vladimir must try to ascertain what his overall lifestyle will be if either operation succeeds or fails. Then he must decide whether he is willing to take the risks of one course of action or be content with the results of the other course.

Purpose: In assessing all the possibilities, Vladimir will have to decide on the purposes that motivate him.

Agency: When Vladimir has made a decision, he ought to think about whether this decision really reflects his character and values.

There is no question of a nurse making the choice for a patient in a case like Vladimir's. Even if she is asked, it is obvious that she ought to refuse. But, if she is skilled, her consciousness can be a mirror in which her patient can see his ideas and values reflected.

Dilemma 9.2, page 162

Is a nurse ever justified in not following a physician's orders?
The fact that Mr. Judd cannot speak for himself and Amanda is speaking for him ought to lead Amanda to analyze the dilemma from the elements of autonomy. If Mr. Judd did argue for himself, he would argue from his autonomy.

Desire: Mr. Judd's life functions—even though this is desire at its lowest level—are still active. This, in and of itself, provides some evidence that Mr. Judd wants to live. The physician has no reason to believe that Mr. Judd would want to be taken off food and fluids. There is, at least, some evidence against the physician's position, and there is no evidence for it.

Reason: It is too soon to know whether pleasure or pain will prove the major factor in Mr. Judd's future. Mr. Judd could not make an objective decision for himself based on the knowledge available to him. If he cannot, certainly the physician cannot.

Life: Mr. Judd's life has changed. Life is constantly changing. The mere fact that it is changing, when there is no way to know what direction the change will take, does not justify withdrawing food and fluids.

Purpose: The physician proposes to take over Mr. Judd's purposes—to exercise Mr. Judd's time and effort. The physician has no right to do this in these circumstances.

Agency: The physician efforts would not increase Mr. Judd's agency. They would entirely nullify it.

Amanda ought not condemn the physician to Mr. Judd's family. But she is certainly justified in advising them against withdrawing food and fluids.

Dilemma 9.3, page 163

How should a nurse deal with a young person in exceedingly difficult circumstances?

Bioethical dilemmas are among the most complex and difficult that any human being ever faces. Wally's case is certainly among these. It will be difficult to resolve this dilemma with optimum beneficence—in such a way that Wally is done some good and no harm. If she handles it badly, a nurse can do Wally much more harm than good. A nurse who can handle this beneficently must be able to exercise a sort of ethical artistry.

Autonomy: Wally is in the health care system. The health care system has its own specific structures and purposes. The health care system is responsible for the health and well-being of everyone who enters it. On the other hand, Wally is young. He did not come into the health care system on his own. He was not even brought in after discussion. He is suddenly thrust into a strange environment.

Taking Wally for debriding without his consent suggests that Wally's body can be taken for treatment and his consciousness can be left behind. This interaction between Iris and Wally would be truly inhuman. Iris's momentary reflection on her own nature would show her that such interaction is ethically undesirable. Whatever its benefits, and they are obvious, compelling Wally to go for treatment at this time would violate his autonomy.

Freedom: It is part of the implicit agreement that is the basis of human rights that the young shall be protected. What are the right and wrong things for Iris to do depends on the context of her relationship with Wally. It may be necessary for her to establish a rapport with Wally very quickly. There are overwhelming reasons why Wally ought to go for debriding. Nonetheless, if Iris were to take him by coercion, this would be a violation of his freedom.

Objectivity: If Iris is to deal with Wally on the basis of objectivity, she will have to tell him that his mother is dead. The absence of ethical value in this is obvious. For Iris to put both burdens on Wally at one time would be fiendish. She would increase Wally's objective awareness in a context where this would decrease Wally's ability to act on objective awareness. She would abandon her own objective awareness of the nature of the health care system and the meaning of her role in it.

Self-assertion: Wally now has some self-governance. He has the potential for full self-governance. Badly handled, the overwhelming adversity he faces can stunt this potential. A nurse never knows how much good or harm in a person's life she can do. Her pride ought to compel her to do the best she can.

Beneficence: Beneficence calls for Iris to do as much good and as little harm as possible. Ideally, this would consist of finding a way to get Wally to treatment without inflicting force on him. It would involve telling him of his mother's death under optimum circumstances.

Fidelity: The nurse–patient agreement begins with an exchange of values. This may be the best way for Iris to proceed in order to do good and avoid harm to Wally. It may be best for her to continue this exchange. Iris needs to hang loose. She needs to bargain with Wally, to find some way to trade values with him. This will avoid the trauma to Wally that a violation of his autonomy and freedom would involve.

A skillful and effective nursing intervention here calls for Iris to treat Wally not as a "big boy," but as a human person. Although Wally is legally a minor, this is a very fine place to avoid paternalism.

Analysis under the elements of Wally's autonomy might clarify even more what is to be done.

Desire: Wally's desire to wait for his mother is rational. Force is irrational. Force would be a psychological assault on Wally.

Suppose Wally had been treated at the scene of the fire. He probably could have been treated without a prior discussion and without psychological harm. But his hospital room takes him away from the noise and stress of the disaster. It suggests that now there is a chance to think and to discuss. The situation calls out for Iris to bargain with Wally. Iris should not tell Wally that his mother is alive. Aside from this, truth is the last thing to be considered at this moment.

Reason: In Wally's context, it is perfectly reasonable for him to want the comfort of his mother's presence. Effective and skillful communication and trade will have to be carried out at this level. There is probably no way Wally can reason on a more abstract level than this.

Life: Wally ought to be treated with the highest consideration. With the loss of his mother, he is at a point where he must begin to build his life again.

Purpose: In order for Iris to trade with Wally effectively, she must discover the nature of Wally's most rational (practical) purposes. She must discover what she can do to make Wally see his most desirable purposes under these conditions of his life.

Agency: The purpose of exchanging values with Wally is to enlist his desire for some purpose, to motivate his agency, and to increase his cooperation with Iris.

Dilemma 9.4, page 166

How should decisions be made for a premature infant with Down's syndrome?

How a context involving a retarded child with a severe heart defect can be analyzed.

We are assuming that nonaggressive treatment in this situation is a real possibility. The neonatologist has asked the mother and father if this is what they desire. They have not rejected this alternative. We also assume that nonaggressive treatment is not a question to be answered entirely at the direction of the parents. Maureen, the infant's mother, does not approach it as a question requiring only her arbitrary decision. Some (but very few) ethical dilemmas are not much more than questions of etiquette. Others involve the deepest values of human life. This dilemma is one of that type. It is very difficult and, outside of the actual context, it would be improper to approach it dogmatically. But analysis in terms of the elements will shed some light on it.

Desire: If meaningful answers could be evoked from people born in the condition of Maureen's baby, then the desires of these people could be known. The question cannot be asked. The answers can only be inferred.

There is a school of thought that holds that infants in this condition should never be treated aggressively. There is another school of thought that holds that infants in this condition should always be treated aggressively. In the context of a symphonological ethic there would be two major ethical considerations:

1. The reasonable desires of the infant's parents. What is reasonable in this context is determined by the benefit the child will bring to their lives in contrast to the detriment it will bring to their lives.

It is very easy to make a moralistic analysis of the situation and ignore the rights and values of the parents. But the process of analysis ought to be realistic. The answers derived from analysis ought to be appropriate to the real world.

2. The desires of the individual person the infant will become, insofar as these desires can be inferred. The best possible estimate of this should be made and put into the analysis.

Reason: Reason demands that the decision be made in context. Analysis against the background of a symphonological ethic would preclude a judgment made on the basis of preexisting beliefs. A symphonological ethic would hold that the only relevant beliefs are those that are gained from an examination of the infant and his parent's context.

Life: A proper ethical decision, in the context of a symphonological ethic, would depend upon an interweaving of:

- The effect the infant will have on the life of the parents. This aspect of the dilemma can be used to justify nonaggressive treatment only if caring for the infant would be significantly detrimental to the life of the parents. A matter of simple inconvenience to the parents cannot justify nonaggressive treatment. (It must be observed that if the parents have carried the analysis this far, they are not motivated by simple convenience or inconvenience.)
- The decision the infant would make in the future for or against his life, if he were capable of making such a decision.

Purpose: Purpose ought to be analyzed from two sides. The future purposes of the infant ought to be a powerful consideration. The only other consideration ought to be the purposes of the infant's parents.

Agency: At some point, life without agency is not a full human life. It is not necessarily an undesirable life either.

Dilemma 9.5, page 167

Does a child's rights protect him against a procedure he does not desire?
The concept of rights is very difficult to deal with here. For purposes of bioethical analysis, rights as we have discussed is

the product of an implicit agreement among rational beings, by virtue of their rationality, not to obtain actions nor the product or condition of actions from others except through voluntary consent, objectively gained.

- In the same way the rights' agreement arises, among all people everywhere, another agreement arises. This agreement arises by virtue of the reasoning power of a parent, the undeveloped state of a child's reasoning power, the naturally dependent state of the child, and the bonds of love that exist between parent and child. It is the agreement that a parent will protect and nurture the child. It is a bond of benevolence uniting parent and child. This agreement calls for a parent to decide for a child in a situation where the child is incapable of deciding for himself. Sandy's mother does have a moral right to sign the consent form.
- Sandy's nurse has a moral right to give him the preoperative medications. She is acting as the agent of Sandy's mother. She is doing what Sandy's mother would do if she were able.
- The surgeon is also acting as her agent. He also is doing what Sandy's mother would do if she could.
- Sandy will acquire the rights that would protect him against this procedure when there is no longer a need for the parent/child agreement.
- Sandy's mother, the surgeon, and the nurse have rights that would protect them from undergoing this procedure involuntarily. With maturity, they have acquired this right.
- Sandy's mother, the surgeon, and the nurse acquired the rights that they possess when they acquired the experience and the rational capacity to decide for themselves.
- Sandy will acquire the rights that his mother, the surgeon, and the nurse possess when he acquires the experience and the rational capacity to take over his parent's role in making his vital and fundamental decisions.
- Sandy will acquire the right to decide for his children when his reason becomes more powerful than his emotions.
- Sandy's desire is not a rational desire. It is the short-term whimsical desire of a child. It is true, and Sandy knows it to be true, that his desire must give way before the parent–child agreement.
- Sandy's uniqueness cannot protect him. It will begin to protect him only when it becomes a rational autonomy. Until then, it is not sufficient for the exercise of rights. No irrational autonomy will protect Sandy's short-term urges only against his rational self-interest. He becomes ethically autonomous only when his autonomy is strong enough to protect Sandy against his whims.

Dilemma 9.6, page 169

Does a physician have the right to compel a patient to undergo a procedure that she believes the patient ought to undergo, against the patient's wishes?
Even assuming that this is a procedure that he ought to undergo, Roger's physician and the court were not justified in the course of action they took. Roger's reasoning and decision might not have been the best, but they are not entirely irrational. Sometimes, the rights of others prevent us from doing that which we very much want to do. If this were not the case, there would be no reason for the existence of rights. Roger's rights should have prevented the physician from doing what she wanted to do.

A health care professional's role cannot give him extraordinary rights. These extraordinary rights would be a right to violate the rights of others. There cannot be such a thing as a right to violate the rights of others. If there were such a right, there could not be any rights at all.

The nurse's role in this situation would be to counsel Roger, to apply gentle coercion, and to offer no encouragement to Roger's physician.

Let us assume that the method by which the judge declared Roger incompetent became a method common in the legal system. It is obvious that this would make the legal system an all-powerful tyranny where no one would have any rights whatsoever. The purpose of the judicial system would no longer be to protect rights. Its purpose would be to arbitrarily establish rights for some people and to violate the rights of others. If this were permissible in this case, one would be hard pressed to establish a point at which it is no longer permissible.

There are several significant differences between Roger's situation and Sandy's:

- There is no parent–child agreement between Roger and his physician. There is no basis for such an agreement between them.
- Because of the parent–child agreement, Sandy's rights were not violated. Roger's rights were violated.
- Sandy does not have the rational capacity nor the experience to decide. Roger has. Sandy is immature. Roger is not immature or even senile.

At his age, Sandy's situation speaks for itself. Roger's does not. Sandy's mother has a right to speak for Sandy. Roger has a right to speak for himself.

Dilemma 9.7, page 179

How should one go about "turning around" a patient who has lost hope?
Negative thoughts and emotions have overwhelmed Mrs. Smith's autonomy. The task is to overcome these negative emotions with positive ones. This can be done, if at all, through the elements of autonomy.

Desire can be used to inspire positive thought processes to increase her desire. It is important that the positive values that are possible to her—given a state of living that she can enjoy—overcome the influence of her immediate negative experience.

The elements of her autonomy, if she is to put her life back together, will strengthen her desire to act, her objective awareness, and her fidelity to the life that is still hers for the taking. Despair is best combated through the elements.

To inspire Jody to meet the challenges life presents and regain the possibilities her life offers would be a splendid ethical achievement. Nonetheless, there is a vast difference between achieving this entirely for Jody's sake and achieving it for the sake of others.

Dilemma 9.8, page 181

Is it ever justified to sell one's organ?
There are a number of reasons why one might want to sell an organ. A person with masochistic tendencies might find it a gratifying means of self-mutilation.

Under extraordinary circumstances, a parent might sell an organ as his only means to feed his starving children.

Reason: To give up a greater value, such as a family member's life, when it could be saved at the cost of a lesser value, a piece of one's liver, is irrational. To condemn one for giving or selling an organ to save a loved one's life, is to make an arbitrary and indefensible judgment. To satisfy a desire for self-mutilation is disproportionate in the other direction. It would be an action that could not be justified.

Desire: When one possesses that which one desires, it becomes a value to one. One's values exist on a hierarchy. One gives up one's value in favor of another for many complex reasons. The values are one's own and the reasons are one's own. When federal and state laws are passed, the state claims ownership of the value it has taken under its control. Today the state prohibits the sale of what it owns. Tomorrow, it may find this property a valuable source of state income.

Life: We only live once and life has meaning for us. This meaning is given to life by things we value. If we value nothing or nothing very much, then we do not value life or we do not value it very much. If we are not allowed control of the things we value, we are not allowed control of our lives. And, along with this, goes our liberty and the pursuit of our happiness.

Purpose: Sometimes when the beams of a bridge shift and the bridge threatens to collapse, a bridge worker's foot will be caught between two girders. To save his life his foot must be amputated. Should this be illegal? Perhaps not. No one benefits but the worker himself. Though why this should make a difference is puzzling.

Agency: When we analyze a situation, when we choose a option, when we decide on a course of action, we do all this for the purpose of protecting or maximizing our agency. What process of analysis, choice, and decision could have inspired one law covering this vast spectrum of human dilemmas?

As for Ms. Sparrow, to be so determined to sell a kidney in order to pay back the hospital was a very questionable motivation—a drastic step. It is certainly giving up a greater value for a lesser value. It would be unethical to become involved in this. The appropriate person, who is not the nurse, should get involved and help her to solve the dilemma with a payment plan.

Dilemma 9.9, page 184

Is this a case in which the living will should not be respected?
"One can never know if a person's life can be a happy one until the moment of death for if they live in success and luxury their entire life, but die in a condition of misery and squalor, theirs was not a happy life" (Aristotle).

Autonomy: The probabilities are very high that Beth would want to be rescued and given the news of her son.

Freedom: There is no doubt that this will make Beth's life a happier and more successful one and, if she could, she would use her freedom in this way.

Objectivity: The objective fact is that she is dying. Nothing is going to change that. Another objective fact is that she may live days, weeks, or, who knows—the will to live may be very strong now because her son has been found.

Self-assertion: She used her self-assertion to ask for a DNR order. Now the context has dramatically changed. Now she cannot exercise her self-assertion, so the nurse must do it for her.

Beneficence: No demand of beneficence would be violated. By rescuing her, it would be the opposite—it would be the beneficent thing to do.

Fidelity: In counteracting the results of the drug and restoring her, if possible, you are being faithful to her and to yourself.

Dilemma 9.10, page 186

Should a psychiatric patient who is brought into the hospital against his will be forcibly medicated?
There is a strong tide of opinion that supports the idea that, "Every human being of adult years and sound mind has a right to determine what shall be done with his own life..." (President's Commission for the Study of Ethical Problems in Medicine and Biomedical and Behavioral Research, 1982, p. 20).

Everyone has the right to be free of outside interference. The acceptance of a person's right to determine what will be done with his or her life ought to be part of the mind-set of every person involved in making ethical decisions for others.

Competency is very difficult to assess. According to the President's Commission of 1982, the assessment of competency depends upon values, goals, choices, life plans, and purposes. The assessment of competency, then, is an ethical assessment. Ethics is concerned with values, goals, choices, life plans, and purposes. It is not surprising that the issue of competency makes many ethical abuses possible. The criteria for assessment that the President's Commission has set down are ethical criteria. The criteria are ethical in the framework of a symphonological ethic. The President's Commission (1982, pp. 57–60) proposed three elements of competency. To establish competency, a person must:

1. Possess a set of values and goals that are reasonably consistent and that remain reasonably stable so that they do not radically conflict.
2. Have the ability to understand and communicate information so that it can be known that this person can appreciate the meaning of potential alternatives.
3. Have the ability to reason and deliberate about choices in light of values, so that he or she can compare the impact of alternative outcomes on personal goals and life plans.

A person's decision-making capacity is impaired if it fails to, at least, minimally promote his or her desires and purposes.

It is very difficult to determine incompetency. A patient who does not want to do what a nurse or physician wants him to do or what they think is best for him to do, is not necessarily incompetent. It may be that this patient has a better outlook on the context of his life than either the nurse or physician. With this better outlook, his judgment may be superior to that of the nurse or the physician.

On the other hand, it is not necessary to regard every statement a person makes as reflecting his desires and purposes. A child's vision is not sufficiently long range to always express his real desires and purposes. The same may be true of a patient in extreme pain, one in shock, or one with brain metastasis, mental retardation, or psychiatric problems. He may be able to act, at best, only on urges. The difference between desires and purposes, on the one hand, and urges, on the other, is that the latter are short-term motivations whereas the former are integrated into a person's life.

The desires of the truly incompetent patient are not the result of an objective reading of the facts facing him. In this sense, they are not desires at all. The expression of his desires is the product of a type of free association.

If a person is unable to express his desires and purposes, this, in itself, does not establish that someone else has a right to do it for him. The best that another person can do is to help him establish a longer range outlook. Ideally, a health care professional, when dealing with an incompetent patient, would ally himself with that patient as he is when he has a clear vision of his life purposes.

The situation of an incompetent patient is very much like the situation of a child with one major difference: The child is in this situation a very long time; the patient, it is hoped, will be in this situation a very short time.

For different reasons, neither an incompetent patient nor a child has the rational capacity to make decisions. The relationship between a health care professional and an incompetent patient is the most delicate of all bioethical relationships. It may be that this relationship calls for an agreement very similar to the parent–child agreement.

When acting for an incompetent patient, a health care professional must attempt to do for the patient what the patient would do for himself if he were able. The health care professional must try to put himself in his patient's shoes. In order to do this, he must obtain some familiarity with a patient's situation and values. If he cannot obtain this understanding of the patient's context, then perhaps he should act toward his patient as he would act toward the naked comatose stranger. This requires that he protect his patient against himself and other health care professionals. A health care professional can look upon the treatment of a psychiatric patient either from the perspective of utilitarianism or as a triage situation.

From the utilitarian perspective, the professional's viewpoint will be "extensionalist." He will be interested in the effect of his action on the group—on the patient's family, the rest of the hospital staff, and so forth. His goal will be the greater good for the greater number, not the welfare of his patient. This cannot fail to narcotize his concern for his patient.

If he looks at the situation as though it had the same form as a triage situation, his viewpoint will be "intentionalist." He will be interested in the effect of his action on his patient. This will make the welfare of his patient the center of his attention. This is where the center of his attention belongs.

The legal and ethical positions of the incompetent patient are very often in conflict. Ideally, ethical decisions would be made for the incompetent patient only within the following parameters: For a health care professional to assume responsibility, make ethical decisions, and take actions for a patient, there ought to be some implicit or explicit invitation for him to do so. Otherwise, there is a violation of the patient's self-governance. With the violation of the patient's self-governance, there is coercion. Coercion is not ethically justifiable.

The only exception to this would be in a situation strongly analogous to that of the naked, comatose stranger. But, even here, there is a kind of implicit invitation. There are times when the psychiatric patient is in virtually the same state as the naked, comatose stranger. Then the same conditions for treatment would hold. A radical ethical differentiation should be made between the patient who comes into the health care setting voluntarily and the patient who does not. The patient who comes in voluntarily makes an implicit agreement with the people in the health care setting. The patient who does not enter voluntarily makes no such agreement. His self-assertion is violated. If he has a right to self-assertion, he has a right to refuse to make an agreement. He has a right to have this refusal accepted.

This is the only course of ethical action consistent with the bioethical standards. This course of ethical action is very much at odds with the laws presently governing these situations. The current laws provide the patient some protection; however, they provide much more opportunity for exploitation.

There is a very old saying, to the effect that, "Where there are many laws, there is much tyranny." This is because where there are many laws, people do not concern themselves with ethical thinking or ethical analysis. They come to follow the letter of the law and, beyond this, they do whatever is convenient. It goes without saying that this only holds when the patient has not threatened or committed any criminal action. If he has, then of course the ethics of the situation are very different.

Bioethicist Morris Abram, head of the President's Commission for the Study of Ethical Problems in Medicine and Biomedical and Behavioral Research (1982), stated:

> ... while recognizing the important role that the law has played in this area, the Commission does not look to the law as the primary means of bringing about needed changes in attitudes and practices. Rather, the Commission sees "informed consent" as an ethical obligation that involves a process of shared decision making based upon the mutual respect and participation of patients and health professionals. Only through improved communication can we establish a firm footing for the trust that patients place in those who provide their health care. (p. 32)

Everyone, whatever his or her condition in life, possesses individual rights and ethical status. People possess rights by virtue of their rationality. This does not mean that someone who is irrational does not possess rights. The possession of rights is species wide. Everyone, regardless of physical or psychological conditions, possesses the right to ethical treatment. Suppose it were possible to pick and choose which members of the human species would have their rights recognized. Obviously, under these circumstances, there could be no trust among ethical agents.

Without the possibility of trust among ethical agents, no one could possibly possess rights. For this reason, the possession of rights must be enjoyed by every member of the species. When making a decision for an incompetent patient, it is especially important to make the decision according to the values and goals of the patient. Otherwise, the bioethical standards have been violated.

Throughout history, the treatment of psychiatric patients has been the scandal of medicine. Every health care professional ought to remain fully aware of the right of an individual to make decisions for his or her own life. When it becomes necessary to force a patient to do something or to restrain the patient from doing something, a health care professional should never take the situation as the status quo.

The difficulties of dilemmas involving psychiatric patients are very complex. They cannot be captured in a case study. In Jason's case, it certainly appears that his agency is impaired. In all likelihood, if he were in touch with his life, he would want to recover from his present condition. If it is justifiable to treat him against his expressed desires (or urges), the person who does treat him should not lose sight of the fact that the purpose of treatment is to return Jason's agency to him.

Dilemma 11.1, page 211

What should be done when a patient's right to know conflicts with his desire not to know?

There are times when a patient must be told the details of his condition. This is necessary in order that he can understand and make decisions concerning his course of treatment. For Zelda, it is a rule that a patient has a right and a responsibility to know the details of his condition. When Zelda relates all this to Mr. Wu, she obeys the rule and satisfies Mr. Wu. If Zelda had informed Mr. Wu, not on the basis of a rule but on the basis of analysis and the realization that this action on her part was appropriate, there is no way in which Mr. Wu could have been worse off. The fact that she did it on the basis of its being a rule in no way increased its benefit to Mr. Wu. It is quite conceivable that had she taken the action on the basis of analysis, she might have done it more effectively and she might have guided her actions more skillfully. But a practitioner of duty has no reason to be concerned with the skills that might be developed through analysis.

Let us see if we can find a bioethical standard to justify Zelda's relating this information to Mr. Goldfarb.

Autonomy: Mr. Goldfarb's nature is such that he does not desire this detailed information. Having this information does not do him any good. At the same time, it does him some harm.

If a patient's primary reason for entering the health care system is to receive information, then perhaps Mr. Goldfarb's autonomy would have a lessened relevance. In entering the health care system, it might be said that he consents to receive the information. If a patient's primary reason for entering the health care system is to receive information, the majority of patients who come into the hospital would discover the details of their condition and leave. Such is not the case. The primary reason for a patient's entering the health care system is to regain his physical or psychological well-being. Zelda violated Mr. Goldfarb's autonomy.

Freedom: Mr. Goldfarb has a right to know. A patient has the right to know because knowing enables him to take informed action. If knowing does not enable him to take informed action, then knowing has little value. Knowing has no value for Mr. Goldfarb. His right to take action is prior to and logically more important than his right to know. His purpose (health and well-being) is more important than information for its own sake.

In addition to his right to know, Mr. Goldfarb has a right not to know. This right ought to especially be respected when his not knowing assists his freedom of action and his well-being better than his being informed. Zelda's exercise of complete freedom takes away all of Mr. Goldfarb's freedom. There are others, not so morally fastidious, who could tell Mr. Goldfarb what he needs to know and no more. Zelda is taking the place of a nurturing nurse.

Objectivity: Every truth that a nurse relates to a patient should be treated like a wild horse. It should always be controlled by beneficence. The detailed truths that Zelda related to Mr. Goldfarb were not motivated by maleficence. However, Zelda should have been guided by beneficence and she was not. She was guided by nothing but rules. The standard of objectivity offers her no justification.

Approaching the question of objectivity through Zelda's eyes utterly undermines objectivity. In the health care system, objectivity is not simply having information but being able to act effectively on the information one has. It is much better that Mr. Goldfarb's course of action be guided by objectivity rather than have it undermined by information.

Self-assertion: In order that people in their interactions do not aggress against each other, there must be an agreement between them to respect each other's self-governance. Ethically, no one can be involved in an interaction unless he has given his consent. One person cannot influence the action of another person without the consent of that other person unless he takes over the ownership of that other person. Try to imagine someone controlling the action of a pair of scissors without controlling the pair of scissors.

Between Zelda and Mr. Goldfarb, as between every nurse and patient, there is an implicit agreement that each will respect the self-governance of the other. Zelda violated that agreement. In his condition, Mr. Goldfarb needs the power to exercise self-assertion.

Beneficence: Zelda did Mr. Goldfarb harm for the sake of doing that which did no good. Perhaps Zelda did not know the effect that her action would have on Mr. Goldfarb. If she did not know, she should have known. She cannot appeal to the standard of beneficence.

Fidelity: Zelda was faithful to the standard of fidelity only in case the nurse–patient agreement involves a nurse's taking particular actions regardless of their consequences. The nurse–patient agreement, of course, does not involve this. Zelda can find no support in the standard of fidelity.

Dilemma 11.2, page 212

Which is more important, duty or saving a life?
This dilemma is certainly extreme. But, it reveals the serio-comic nature of deontology in the sick room.

Picture this: A platoon of soldiers in basic training is in formation and being trained to march. Sergeant Austin is drilling them. They are beginning to look sharp. As they are marching, Lieutenant Brown steps over and says to one of the soldiers in the marching line, "Private Jones, I have a duty for you to perform.

Report to Sergeant Smith for kitchen police duty." Note carefully, that the lieu-tenant did not tell the private he was giving him a duty to continue marching. That would not have made any sense. Private Jones was already marching. In order to do his duty, Private Jones had to leave the column of marchers, go somewhere else, and do something else.

When a nurse goes into a patient's room, it is not possible to know what she is going to find. But, whatever she finds, if a duty were placed on her, she would have to leave the room and go to where it would be possible to perform that duty. Even in the unlikely scenario where she did not have to leave the room and abandon her patient spatially, she would have to abandon him spiritually. Does this make for efficient nursing? Does this make for any kind of nursing?

The duty that is placed on a nurse especially violates a patient's freedom and self-assertion and it violates the nurse's fidelity.

Dilemma 11.3, page 215

Should a dying patient's desire for confidentiality override his family's plans for a pleasant surprise?

The bioethical standards are principles of the nurse–patient agreement. The standard of freedom requires Harry's nurse to reveal the fact of his son's return and let Harry decide what he desires to do. Nonetheless, we will analyze the dilemma in terms of the bioethical standards.

Autonomy: Harry's nurse must keep her agreement with her patient. If she could know that Harry's character structure was such that he would prefer his family's knowing in order that he might enjoy the surprise, then perhaps she should inform his family. This would not be for utilitarian reasons, but for Harry's benefit and in keeping with their agreement. At all odds, it is very unlikely that Harry's nurse could have any certain knowledge of this. Therefore, it almost certainly should not determine her decision.

Freedom: Harry's life story will be enhanced through his knowing that his son is coming home.

Objectivity: If Harry believes that his nurse will not advise his family of his prognosis, and she does, then she violates the standard of objectivity by undermining Harry's objective awareness. In the nature of the case, she cannot ask for Harry's advice. She cannot ask him whether he wants to know that his son is coming home without letting him know that his son is coming home.

Self-assertion: If she informs him, Harry will have better control of how he wants to use his time and effort.

Beneficence: There is no sense in which the standard of beneficence calls for a nurse to do the greatest good for the greatest number. It calls for her to do the greatest good for her patient. Harry's nurse does this by going to Harry and discussing the situation with him.

Fidelity: The nurse can assume that Harry would desire to know that his son is safe and coming home. This knowledge would enhance the remainder of his life and, perhaps, even make the dying process easier for Harry. This is the nurse's professional responsibility.

A nurse's overriding agreement is with her patient. Fidelity requires that she be true to this agreement. The nurse–patient agreement will not allow Harry's nurse to do nothing. She must discuss the situation either with Harry or with his family. She cannot discuss it with his family without Harry's permission. She must discuss it with Harry.

She might begin somewhat like this: "Harry, I want you to let me tell your family about your condition. There are a number of things they will want to discuss with you. Harry, I am going to ask you to trust me. Honest to God, if you let me talk to them, you will be very glad you did." However, Harry must know of his son's homecoming.

Dilemma 11.4, page 215

Whose life is it anyway?
How would you explain to the young benefactor's family that they should feel no sorrow but pride and gratification at the contribution their son made to the happiness and prosperity of the village? The drawback to this practice is that to save potential victims it makes actual victims.

Autonomy: If the family believes that a relatively small benefit for a very large number of people is better than a large benefit for an individual, they will understand. If they understand this, they can understand anything however absurd.

Freedom: You can explain to them that their son lost his freedom, but the villagers as a whole gained a far greater measure of freedom, and when they see the joy on the faces of the villagers, they will be glad at what their son was able to accomplish.

Objectivity: Objectively the entire village is a greater number than their son.

Self-assertion: Because of their son's achievement, everyone will have greater control of their time and effort. The villagers will treat them with gratitude and a greater respect. Their son was a soldier fighting the unending war against mindless, tyrannical brutality.

Beneficence: It is well known throughout the village that they are people of good will with a desire to do what is best for others. Most people never have this opportunity, but through their good fortune, they have had it.

Fidelity: You can explain that you know they had a great affection for their son, but now they can glory in the knowledge that the affection they had for the sum total of the villagers, they were able to express through the sacrifice of their son and you know how gratified they must be.

All of this may sound perfectly ridiculous, but some research experiments followed this logic. The most infamous of which was the Tuskegee syphilis experiment (1932–1972) where treatment was withheld from some subjects, even though it was known that penicillin would have cured them, so that the researchers could observe the course of the illness. This was, in effect, another form of telishment.

Dilemma 11.5, page 220

Was a bride justified in seeking asylum to avoid female circumcision?
If rational self-interest is wrong, then Fauzuja Kassindja was wrong. And she should not have been given asylum.

Assuming that there is nothing in the nature of women from her country that makes them natural play things, the fate Fauzuja Kassindja faced in her native country violated all of the bioethical standards. This would set a precedent permitting anyone to do anything that whimsy urged them to do. Under this standard, what she did could not have been wrong.

On the other hand, if there is something in the nature of female rational animals such that they are excluded from the rights agreement, this has never been shown. And this practice of female circumcision would nullify individual rights or, at least, place the recognition of rights on an arbitrary basis.

Dilemma 11.6, page 221

Are the parents justified in having another baby under these unusual circumstances?

This is a case of several human beings, two at a time, discussing together, deciding together, and coming to an agreement—an ethical agreement—and under the circumstances the best possible agreement.

This is a life and death dilemma. In this dilemma the embryo, obviously, will not be able to make a decision for herself so, as surrogates, we must make the decision for her. We must not frolic about with figures of speech or cultural platitudes as if they were analytic processes. We must not content ourselves with an automatic, formalistic resolution. It would be unworthy of a professional to make a decision out of context and without analysis.

These are not the only temptations we face. To make the dilemma easier to deal with, it is natural to imagine that the embryo is someone we know. If we analyze this case according to the standards of agreement, our analysis might lead to the decision that the embryo should not be conceived. But this would be a mistake. In making a bioethical decision for a patient, it is necessary to get as close as possible to the patient. In making a bioethical decision for an embryo, it is necessary to get much closer to the embryo than to any other patient. We will analyze it according to the bioethical standards and then according to the elements of autonomy.

Many nurses, with the best intentions in the world, will take what they learn dealing with adult patients, or what they observe between nurses and adult patients, and transpose this onto the situation of the embryo. Onlookers will analyze the case from the outside and come to the wrong decision. They analyze, from an external point of view, one or two of the standards. The analysis ought to come from an internal point of view—the embryo's point of view—from the elements of human autonomy. The Ayalas analyzed the case from the inside and came to an objectively justifiable decision.

Nearly always when an ethical agent makes a decision, she makes it against the background of the standards of agreement: freedom, objectivity, and the rest. On some level of awareness, she is aware of the importance of these standards. But in cases involving an embryo, or a neonate, analysis through the standards can be misleading.

First, we will analyze the case through the bioethical standards. For the reasons we discussed, this will be a faulty analysis.

Autonomy: To conceive for the purpose of obtaining bone marrow would be a violation of the embryo's independence and autonomy. She would be treated as the mere instrument of someone else's purpose. She would be subjected to something to which she has not consented.

But the fact that she has not consented, in this circumstance, does not mean that the action should not be taken. It means nothing more than that serious reasoning should be given to the circumstance—reasoning for the embryo that the embryo cannot do for herself.

It is very important to notice here that when the case is analyzed on the basis of the embryo's autonomy, without reference to the elements of autonomy, something is omitted.

The embryo is virtually regarded as unreal. Without sufficient reason, it is assumed that this real person would refuse this interaction. The fact is the embryo cannot consent to all of this. Another fact is she cannot voice a refusal. These facts are the horns of the dilemma. The fact that the embryo will become an independent and autonomous human being ought not be disregarded. The question to be answered is this: If the embryo could communicate her desires, would she refuse life and this interaction with her sister?

This blunder in the analysis from autonomy exemplifies a blunder that is epidemic in what passes for contemporary bioethical analysis. The decision maker's analysis becomes an analysis of the word *embryo* rather than an analysis of a human being's life.

To conceive for the purpose of obtaining bone marrow is not a violation of the embryo's independence or autonomy. It is a reason to assist the embryo in the forming of an agreement that will have the most desirable consequences. In return for an intrusion, the evil of which is little more than symbolic, she will receive a lifetime and all the possibilities of a human lifetime.

Imagine an 8-year-old faced with a dilemma. She is dying from renal failure. Her brother is dying of leukemia. He proposes to her that if she will donate marrow for a transplant, he will in return give her a kidney. It is inconceivable that the 8-year-old would refuse this agreement.

The Ayala embryo is in a position very similar to the 8-year-old. But she gains an entire lifetime. If the embryo could make an informed decision, it is not likely that she would refuse the agreement that gives her life.

Our analysis from autonomy was a blunder. The analysis was an analysis of an abstract concept. It was not the analysis of a person's autonomy. That which was analyzed was not the possibility of joy and happiness in a human existence. That which was analyzed was the meaning of a word totally isolated from rational human concerns. The same will hold true of the rest of the analysis.

Freedom: The embryo will have no voice in the matter. She will have no freedom to decide and act on her individual purposes. But she does have a voice in the matter. It is the rational and caring voice of her parents and of free and insightful biomedical professionals. This is the next best thing to her own freedom.

It is not true that she is entirely lacking freedom. By being conceived, she gains the capacity and the freedom to develop ontogenetically.

She cannot decide and act on her own. This does not establish that a decision and action through which she will gain life is either forbidden or that it has no importance to her. It certainly does not mean that her life has less importance than free-floating ethical formalities.

Objectivity: A decision to conceive will not be based on objectivity for it cannot be based on communication. But this is not true. The decision to conceive *is* based on objectivity. It is based on the Ayalas' honest and courageous observation of all of the objective facts of the situation. It is based on a true realization that what must be analyzed is not the nature of an abstract standard. What must be analyzed is a question of life or death for a real, albeit potential, human person.

Self-assertion: The embryo's self-governance will be taken away. She will not be treated as an end in herself but as a means to the ends of others. Her right to control her time and effort will be disregarded.

But the embryo's self-governance will not be taken away. She will be endowed with all the time and effort of a life to control. The expectation that a party to an agreement will perform her part of the agreement is not an alienation of her self-governance. Whenever an agreement is formed, each party to the agreement becomes, in a way, a means to the ends of the other. There is nothing sinister in this.

Beneficence: In regard to the embryo it is maleficent to invade her body without her consent and with no direct benefit to her.

But it is not maleficent to invade the body of this embryo. For contextual reasons, no explicit consent can be obtained, but there is an overwhelmingly high probability that, if she could give consent, she would.

If a life-saving operation were performed on an embryo, her body would be invaded without her consent, but no substantive bioethical dilemma would be involved.

As the circumstances of anyone's life change, the story of their life changes. In this case, the onset of their daughter's sickness required a change in the story of the Ayala family, a change over which they took active and thoughtful control. Under different circumstances, they might not have conceived a child. This provides no reason to believe that, once their decision had been made, they would be indifferent to the child. Their concern for their living daughter is strong evidence to the contrary.

Fidelity: To do this will be to betray and to violate the rights of this potential person. This would be a valid point only if the implicit agreement that establishes individual rights precludes any further agreement or if the "voluntary consent objectively gained" were always direct and explicit. It is quite obvious that it cannot always be direct and explicit. This is no reason to sink back into the moonless night of formalism. It is a reason to exercise analysis and enlightened judgment.

If we analyze six words (the words symbolizing the bioethical standards), and if we take our analysis out of context with no regard to the circumstances of the people involved and without concern for the nature of human life, we may come to the conclusion that we ought to advise against the conception. This resolution, although based on a diligent analysis, would disregard several vital factors. And it begins with a mistake. The mistake is in attempting to make the situation easier and more familiar than it can actually be under the circumstances. We cannot directly communicate with the embryo. She is not a friend, someone we know.

The embryo has had no life experiences, has formed no values has no established purposes or goals. Regarding the embryo as a person capable of communication completely falsifies the situation.

If the embryo were a mere blob of protoplasm, there would be no dilemma. But there is a dilemma. The embryo is a blob of protoplasm but with the potential for future life. And precisely because of this potential, a resolution of the dilemma in favor of conception is a resolution in favor of the embryo. A resolution against conception is a resolution in favor of an out-of-context and meaningless taboo.

A headline in a national news magazine declared that the Ayalas' action created one child to give life to another. It is possible to describe the situation in these terms. It is much more accurate to describe the Ayalas' action as creating one child to give life to two.

The standards by which we analyzed the dilemma are the standards of agreement. And no verbalized discourse or agreement with the embryo is possible. If the dilemma involved a fully mature person who refused this interaction, that would be the end of it. We would have the only justifiable resolution. But the dilemma does not involve a fully mature person. This is a crucial difference. In order to analyze the case, we must let the embryo "speak" for herself through us.

We must have recourse to a thought experiment. We must speak for the embryo herself, and to do this, we must have recourse to the elements of autonomy, the elements that describe what it means to be an individual human being.

Desire: Everything about a person—or any living being—can be regarded as a manifestation of desire. All life arises from life's desire for itself. After conception, all of the embryo's ontogenetic processes are a form of desire—the desire for her future life and her mature state.

Some people, at some time in their lives, decide that it would have been better had they never been born. But, for this specific person, there is absolutely no evidence that she would prefer not being born. All the processes of human development suggest that she will want to come into existence.

Reason: If the embryo could be brought to the age of reason, to maturity, and if she could think over the question of whether being conceived and born under these peculiar circumstances was or was not better than the alternative—never being at all—the odds are overwhelming that she would favor being conceived. It is virtually unimaginable that she would want to return to a time 18 or 19 years earlier to undo everything—never be conceived, never be born, and never be alive.

Life: At the present moment, the potential infant has no hopes or plans for her life. But there is every reason to believe that in time she will form, as everyone forms, a life plan. In the meantime, the Ayalas face a very important alternative. They must choose between two lives and one death.

In this situation, it is better to analyze realities rather than words. It is better to analyze objective facts rather than irrelevant formalities or catch phrases. If we do, it will not be terribly daring to assume that in the context of this human reality, two lives, as an alternative, is preferable to one death. There is no acute ethical dilemma in the human realities of this situation.

Purpose: The child who needs the bone marrow transplant has purposes right now. In time, the other child will form purposes in relation to the world. These purposes will make her donation of bone marrow utterly insignificant. Decide and advocate against conception and neither will be better off. Neither will be able to form and pursue purposes. Quite obviously each will be significantly worse off. The entire family will be significantly worse off. Each child gives life to the other. The children give life to the family. The fact that an ethical agent can make an ethical analysis and choose one alternative, an alternative that leaves everyone involved worse off, should alarm an agent and make her aware that something is wrong with her ethical decision making.

Ethics is not a matter of numbers. It is a matter of individuals. Choose conception and this individual, the living child, will be better off, and that individual, the embryo, will be better off. The choice to be made is a choice between ethical formalism and an ethic that is appropriate to human life and the real world.

Agency: When two people get together and work together to increase their agency, this is a process of interaction. Interaction is precisely what is happening here. Through this interaction, the embryo is being given a benefit. She will be given the benefit of being born into a loving family in return for a benefit to the embryo herself—her sister's being.

A senseless formalism might reject this decision. But if a nurse is to be a rational advocate, if her perspective, as she argues for her patient, is going to be based upon agreement and the welfare of her patient, then she must argue for this decision. The probabilities are overwhelming that if the embryo herself could speak, this is the decision she would desire. It is inconceivable that, under these circumstances, she would not opt to live. And a nurse may have the exalted opportunity to act as her voice.

There is never a question of aborting the baby if it is not an acceptable donor. Whatever the outcome, the Ayala family will increase by one. Mrs. Ayala, at the age of 42, is not in good health and has been advised against having another baby. Mr. Ayala will have to undo a vasectomy. Despite these obstacles they try to conceive and do. They give birth to a healthy baby girl—a new member of the Ayala family who is an acceptable donor.

Dilemma 11.7, page 223

Does a flawed decision making method reveal a flawed character?
A mistaken decision is not the same as a flaw in one's character. Evelyn's mistaken decision was that an emotion was a judgment. An emotion is not a judgment. Before she declares war on her character, she ought to declare war on her badly flawed decision. It is not her capacity to but her method of making decisions that is at fault.

Dilemma 11.8, page 223

How are emotions an attack on the decision maker's reasoning power?
When people turn away from the contemporary ethical systems, they go into emotivism, which leaves them entirely disoriented. They are unable either to pursue or to serve their rational self-interest. This is another version of the same thing. They never knew how to face the dilemma life presented them. Often, they were advised to something obviously against their best interest; blindly following their emotions became another way of slapping their own face.

Their faces represent their reasoning capacity. It is a way of expressing one's anger at oneself. One has achieved nothing but to discover another source of frustration. Unfortunately, this is a common occurrence. Devastation follows on emotions and frustration follows on devastation.

Dilemma 12.1, page 233

Should a nurse intervene on behalf of her patient against the physician's decision?
Every health care professional is limited in the actions he can take. Every nurse must come to terms with this fact. Nurses today practice within a pluralistic society and in the bureaucracy of the health care system. It would be unreasonable for a nurse to expect that she can remake the system in her image. This is a dilemma where a nurse must make a judgment as to what she is willing to risk. But, ethically, she owes her greatest fidelity to her patient.

Marilu may decide that there is nothing that she can do. Based on this decision she may do nothing. Marilu has no ethical obligation to do the impossible. She does have an obligation to know the difference between the right thing to do—the thing that her agreement calls for her to do—and the wrong thing to do. She also has an obligation to know why it is impossible to do it.

In this situation, for Marilu to continue to dispute with the physician would not make sense. It would be a formalistic action that might make Marilu look very good in her own eyes. It probably would not do much to help Lillian. The best thing for Marilu to do may be to contact Lillian's daughter and explain the situation to her.

Dilemma 12.2, page 239

Should a noncompliant patient be punished by his family?
Autonomy: Tyler's cause-and-effect actions are unintelligible, so the standard of autonomy gives him no support. But the same holds true of his family, so autonomy must be set aside.

Freedom: If the physician's plans involved taking resources for someone more likely to be compliant, then there is a problem. If a noncompliant patient is given full freedom, he would exercise it in a way that would make him a nonpatient. His actions would conflict with the nature of the health care system. But, in this case, the treatment the patient is given takes nothing away from anyone. And to deny him freedom entirely would make no sense.

Objectivity: There is no obvious objective reason why the patient should not receive the treatment the physician plans. If he recovers, what his objective judgments would be cannot be known. But it is reasonable to hope for the best. The patient's mother and sister have no objective reason to deny him treatment, and their wishes should be disregarded.

Self-assertion: If the patient was denied self-assertion, the outcome would be predictable and, for him, unfavorable. If his self-assertion is given all the support possible, the outcome might possibly be favorable.

Beneficence: The benefits to the patient's relatives, whatever they might be, are completely irrelevant. There ought to be a much more significant reason for denying beneficence to a patient in the health care setting.

Fidelity: Obviously, the patient's relatives feel no fidelity to his best interest. The patient may not either. But a decision should not be made through rationalizing over what is not known.

Dilemma 12.3, page 240

Who should get the heart?
The ideal way to establish who is to be the recipient would be to establish that everyone concerned has an obligation to accept one person (Mr. X or Ms. Y) as the rightful recipient. Calling in Hank, a nursing assistant, to flip a coin will not establish an obligation. The judgment of an ethics committee will have some weight but not enough to establish an obligation. One of the candidates could have given a significant contribution to the hospital, but this is not sufficient to establish an obligation.

The hospital team offered both candidates an agreement—an explicit one in the case of Mr. X and an implicit one with Ms. Y. Only one accepted the offer. The hospital team offered an agreement to Mr. X in the form of a warning about his habits. He repeatedly rejected the offer saying that it was "too hard." Had he accepted this offer, the team would have been obligated to keep the terms of the agreement and act to sustain or protect his life.

Ms. Y could be told the circumstances and wait for another heart to become available. However, she is under not obligation to do this. She was offered the same agreement as Mr. X, albeit, implicitly. She accepted and kept her part of the agreement. And now the hospital team has an obligation to keep that offer.

Looking at this in another way, the heart donor has made an implicit agreement. It is unlikely that he would donate his heart expecting it to be given to someone as indifferent to the donor's bequest as Mr. X promises to be. There seems to be a perfect meeting of the minds between the donor and Ms. Y. If Ms. Y does not feel it would be too hard to care for her new heart, she is the one morally entitled to it.

Dilemma 12.4, page 241

What should be done when the family and the patient have different agendas from benevolent motives?
Autonomy: The Mrs. C. that the family visits can be either one of two persons. One person would not be alert and interactive. But she would be free from suffering. The other Mrs. C would be (may be) alert and interactive. If she were, she would undergo significant suffering. The choice is between the pleasure of small talk and the comfort of knowing that Mrs. C. is not suffering.

Freedom: The pleasure of planning for the future is not a real possibility. Mrs. C. has no future. There is no enjoyment that could possibly justify the suffering Mrs. C. would endure.

Objectivity: The family seems incapable of maintaining an objective awareness of what is transpiring. There is no reason to continue Mrs. C. suffering until they stumble onto the reality of the situation.

Self-assertion: The family would violate Mrs. C's right to self-assertion. They would be indifferent to what she is experiencing and hope that she would join them in their indifference.

Beneficence: The family's desires would cause Mrs. C. positive harm and provide her with no benefit. Chatting with her family who is indifferent to what one is going through is not a benefit. She has defined benefits in her desire to be kept pain free.

Fidelity: The only fidelity to the family relationship that Mrs. C can count on is the fidelity that she exercises toward herself in refusing the desires of the family. She has to count on the health care professionals to maintain her fidelity to herself.

Reference

President's Commission for the Study of Ethical Problems and Medicine and Biomedical and Behavioral Research. (1982). *Making health care decisions: The ethical and legal implications of informed consent in the patient-practitioner relationship* (Vol. I). Washington, DC: U.S. Government Printing Office.

Glossary

abstract Refers to the more general and less contextual. *John* is an individual concrete. *Boy* is an abstraction. *Male* is still more abstract. *Person* more abstract still. "A nurse ought to be faithful to her agreement with every patient who comes under her care" is more abstract (more general and less contextual) than "This nurse ought to be faithful to her agreement with this patient."

acceptance Positive response to the offer of an agreement. Engagement with another agent in order to realize a purpose.

action A behavior arising in the decision of an agent to which the agent assigns a personal meaning. A behavior that an agent initiates from within and that remains under the agent's control.

affinity A state of approval of the character and motivations of another agent to the point of being willing to emotionally identify with the other.

agent One who initiates action or one who is capable of taking internally generated action.

agency The capacity of an agent to initiate and sustain action.

agreement A propensity or formal potentiality in existents to behave in specific ways when they are interacting. A shared state of awareness—a meeting of the minds—on the basis of which interaction occurs.

analysis The process whereby one seeks to understand a whole by examining its basic parts or a process of directed awareness aimed at understanding.

animal For purposes of bioethical analysis, any organism capable of moving about from place to place on its own power. This obviously includes humans.

animality That which an animal organism has in common with other animal organisms.

apathy Lack of interest in the things that a person generally considers worthy of attention.

appropriate Whatever gives an agent a greater power of agency is appropriate for that agent; for instance, an understanding of the nature of a dilemma is appropriate for its solution. Freedom from suffering and disability are appropriate to every human being. That which produces intelligibility in the relations between ethical causes and effects (responses). Those conditions under which an agent's virtues can flourish, that which makes an increased or more certain understanding possible, that which supports the continuation of causal chains and enables an agent to realize his purpose is appropriate to the agent's agency.

arbitrary A belief, conclusion, or decision is arbitrary when it is not based upon compelling evidence—when another belief, conclusion, or decision could have been chosen just as well.

autonomy As a bioethical standard, the independent uniqueness of every individual person. This uniqueness is the specific nature—the character structure—of that person. One's autonomy includes one's specific identity and consequent ethical equality with all other rational agents. Primarily, however, it refers to an agent's uniqueness.

balance The property of an interaction whereby there is a mutual exchange of values—reciprocity. Balance and proportion are maintained when there is a parity between benefit given and benefit received. Balance and proportion are lacking when there is a disparity or when a harm is returned for a benefit or vice versa. In one sense, balance and proportion are beneficence. In the same sense, they are justice.

benefactor An agent who acts so as to bring about a benefit to a beneficiary.

beneficence The act of assisting a patient's effort to attain that which is beneficial. The desire to benefit one with whom one empathizes. As a bioethical standard, the power of a patient (or professional acting as the agent of a patient) and the necessity he faces to act to acquire the benefits he desires and the needs his life requires.

beneficiary One who benefits from an action. The recipient of a benefit.

benefit "Something that enhances or promotes well-being" (*American Heritage Dictionary*, 1997).

benevolence A psychological inclination to beneficence.

bioethical standards The character structures of a person that serve as measuring rods of the justifiability of his motives and actions.

bioethics A system of standards arising with the professional agreement to determine, sanction, and justify the interaction of a biomedical professional and patient.

burnout "A syndrome of physical and emotional exhaustion involving the development of a negative self-concept, negative job attitude, and loss of concern and feeling for patients" (Pines & Maslach, 1978).

caregiver strain A deleterious effect of witnessing the suffering of patients and being unable to alleviate this suffering.

caring A devotion to a patient beyond that which is demanded by one's professional practice.

category The aspects of professional action by which the skill or competence of that action can be judged.

causal Pertaining to cause and effect.

certainty A state, following upon analysis, where understanding has a visual quality that adds justified confidence to one's judgment. All certainty depends upon what the context allows.

character structure Every standard taken as a virtue plays a part in structuring the individual nature of a person. Each standard, in this sense, is a character structure. The interlocked virtues that produce and explain the individual's characteristic actions are his or her character structure.

choice The intentional resolution of an alternative.

codependence This is a way of caring in which the nurse tries to find her sense of ethical worth by working to make herself and her patient mutually dependent on the other.

coercion The act of compelling someone, by threats or force, to act in a particular manner. The act of forcibly restraining, compelling, or controlling another person.

cognition The act of grasping the defining or relevant properties of an object or aspects of a situation.

cognitive agreement An agreement of the understanding with the object that is understood—the agreement between a knowing mind and its known object.

coherence A theory of truth that holds that a belief is true if it is logically coherent with the collection of one's other true beliefs.

concept A mental sign, held in the mind, signifying something existing in reality; the idea of that which is known. That which relates a knower to that which is known.

conceptualism The theory that concepts are formed by virtue of the similarity of similar things.

conditions The effect on a person of circumstances that have been brought about by oneself or another and have an effect on a person.

conflict The opposite of harmony.

consequences That which follows as the result of a cause; the moral effects of an initiated cause.

considerations Purposes, context, and causal progression. It includes the facts of the situation, the facts of awareness, and the facts of one's knowledge.

context The interweaving of the relevant facts of a situation—the facts that are necessary to act upon to bring about a desired result, the knowledge one has of how to most effectively deal with these facts, and one's awareness of what is relevant.

> **(of awareness)** An agent's present awareness of the relevant aspects of the situation.

> **(interpersonal context)** A context involving more than one person.

> **(of knowledge)** An agent's preexisting knowledge relevant to the situation.

(of the situation) The interwoven aspects of a situation that are fundamental to understanding the situation and to acting effectively in it.

(solitary context) A context involving only one person—the agent.

continuity The connectedness of events in a process. The continuing existence of a state of affairs.

correspondence A theory of truth that holds that a belief is true when it arises from, is formed according to, and corresponds with the state of affairs that is the object of the belief.

courage The habit of responding to the possible gain or loss of a value with action motivated to an appropriate degree given the worth of the value.

decision A choice made between alternative values and consequent courses of action.

deontology "The theory that . . . actions in conformance with . . . formal rules of conduct are obligatory regardless of their results" (Angeles, 1992).

desire One's psychological orientation toward a purpose. The capacity of an organism whereby it acts to retain its values, including its own life.

determine To bring something—a state of awareness or a state of being—into existence; to direct a course of action.

determinism The doctrine that human choices are the effects of necessitating conditions; the theory that all conscious behavior is a response to outside forces in the same way that the behavior of physical entities is a response to external forces.

dilemma A situation in which one is faced with a conflict of purposes or with purposes whose value is not clear.

doubt The state of mind in relation to a belief when there is both reason to accept the truth of belief and reason not to accept the truth of the belief and no objective way to decide which is valid.

duty An ethical sanction demanding adherence to a rule without regard to consequences.

element "The fundamental, essential, or irreducible constituent of an object" (*American Heritage Dictionary*, 1997). Thus the roundness of a ball is an element of a ball. Its color is not.

emotivism The doctrine that holds feelings or emotions as forms of ethical knowledge. The doctrine that every ethical judgment is nothing more than a disguised description of a person's feelings.

epistemology The study of how truth is identified, how knowledge is acquired, and how knowledge is validated.

ethical Pertaining to ethics.

ethical agreement An agreement between persons concerning vital and fundamental values.

ethical noncognitivism The theory that ethical terms cannot be defined or understood, hence ethical judgments can be neither true nor false.

ethical nonnaturalism Ethically good and bad properties form no part of the world in which we live. Properties in things that we consider ethical properties are not in the thing but merely in our preference or aversion.

ethicist One engaged in the theoretical study of ethics.

ethics A system of standards to motivate, determine, and justify actions directed to the pursuit of vital and fundamental goals. Ethics is not convenience and it is not etiquette, and it is not that which brings on a state of self-satisfaction.

evasion The refusal or failure to give appropriate consideration to facts that ought to be factored into a decision-making process.

evil The evil in relation to an ethical agent is that which negates (blocks) its efficient functioning as the kind of thing it is (failure and the violation of rights, for instance, are evils); disruption of an intelligible, causal sequence in knowledge or action; inappropriate or disproportionate to the context.

existential Concerning human existence.

explicit Actually spoken or agreed to—not merely understood implicitly.

extremes A method of analysis through which a health care professional can clarify a bioethical context by identifying the relationships—the rights and responsibilities—of the people involved in the context.

fidelity Adherence to the terms of an agreement. An individual's faithfulness to his autonomy. For a nurse, it is a commitment to the obligation she has accepted as part of her professional role.

flourishing The realization of human development and its potentialities (e.g., happiness); enjoying happiness based on circumstances desirable and appropriate to one's time of life.

foreseeable Predictable according to that which is given in the context—probable.

formal agreement An agreement made between persons to interact on the basis of complementary motivations.

formalism The theory that ethical action is action that conforms with certain forms of behavior; an ethical formalist is one who concentrates entirely on the abstract category into which an action can be placed, without regard for the context or the effects of the action.

freedom As a bioethical standard, self-directedness. An agent's capacity and consequent right to take independent, long-term actions based on the agent's own evaluation of his circumstances.

fundamental Essential to making or revealing a thing as the kind of thing it is; the fundamental element of a thing is that which best explains its behavior. For instance, roundness is essential to the rolling of a ball; therefore, roundness is a fundamental property of a ball. The roundness (globularity) is also the defining property of a ball.

fundamental element That element in a context that determines what will occur, how it will occur, and the foreseeable outcomes.

gentle (as in "gentle coercion") Simple coercion destroys a patient's ability to act on his understanding of his situation, on his notion of self-ownership, or on his conception of benefit and harm. *Gentle coercion* involves dialogue with a view to persuasion—but persuasion by means of activating, or at least not destroying, a patient's understanding and self-ownership. A form of persuasion that is neither disinterested nor an attempt to take over control of a person's time and effort. Gentle coercion does not attack a person's reasoning power. It is an appeal to that person's reasoning power.

Golden Mean That middle state or action that is appropriate to a context and, therefore, a virtue. The extremes of excess and deficit are vices, inappropriate to the context.

good The good of a thing is that which assists its efficient functioning as the kind of thing it is (i.e., success, fidelity, respect for rights, and health care are all goods); appropriate or proportionate to the context.

habit Behavior, associations, or inclinations acquired by repetition (Angeles, 1992).

hedonism The ethical theory that only those actions that produce pleasure in the agent are appropriate ethical actions. Pleasure being the only value worthy of pursuit.

implicit Understood, but not as a focus of intention. Understood without being openly expressed; that of which one is not consciously aware but which can be brought to conscious awareness.

indeterminate That which is not subject to precise analysis and identification.

indirection That which characterizes bargaining with a patient in a way that avoids predictable conflict.

in-general An action that is taken in a way that is appropriate to a situation of a type in which it is taken rather than a way that is specifically appropriate to the concrete situation, it is taken in-general.

integrity A virtue that characterizes an ethical agent in his fidelity to his own objective values and agreements—fidelity to oneself; the causal connection between experience, belief, description, and action.

intelligible Structured in such a way as to be understandable.

intelligibility That aspect of an object or state of affairs whereby it is recognizable as the kind of thing it is (if the fundamental nature of a state of affairs is easily recognizable, then the state of affairs is intelligible; if any aspect of a state of affairs makes the state of affairs recognizable, then that is its fundamental aspect).

intention The state of affairs that an agent acts to bring about; a mental act of attention to an object.

interaction A chain of actions arising from agreement and interwoven in a cause-and-effect sequence.

interpersonal ethics Ethics as it pertains to interaction between two or more persons. A system of standards arising with an agreement to motivate, determine, and justify the implicit presuppositions of interaction.

interwoven Systematic; composed of interacting, interrelated, or interdependent facts that form a complex whole (e.g., sweaters are made up of interwoven strands of yarn; ethical contexts of the interweaving of circumstances and awareness).

introspection The act of directing one's attention back into one's own subjectivity; the act of reflecting back onto one's own psychological processes.

intuitionism Any theory that attributes ethical insight to a spontaneous event vis-à-vis a process, for example, the theory that ethical agents possess an ethical sense analogous to the five senses.

justice The concept justice can, perhaps, be best understood by analogy to a much more basic concept—the concept of physical causality. Physical objects act and interact on the basis of what their nature permits them to do—and they cannot act contrary to this. Justice, then, is to ethical agents as causality is to physical objects. Physical objects cannot interact acausally or unjustly. Ethical agents, however, have the power to choose, and they can choose either appropriately (so that, intelligible cause-and-effect relationships are maintained—which is justice; or in such a way that the intelligible cause-and-effect relationships between actions and reactions are lost—this is injustice).

justifiable That in a choice or decision that makes it subject to approval upon being explained.

justification A description in terms of how something meets a purpose—the purpose as formulated in a decision or agreement; demonstration that something is correspondent with the terms of an agreement.

justify To describe or explain in terms of or as related to an agreed-upon purpose.

lenses The bioethical standards serve as a sort of lens insofar as analysis conducted on their basis serves to reveal the justifiability of motivations, decision, choices, and so forth.

life The process wherein an organism generates and sustains actions directed toward the attainment of its needs and purposes according to its potential; a process whose natural product is flourishing.

logical According to the demands of understanding; intelligible.

logical positivism The theory that statements have cognitive value if, and only if, they can be, at least in principle, verified by sense experience.

meaning (in ethics) Relation to a purpose. The meaning of X to an agent is the way X assists or hinders an agent's purpose or an agent's flourishing.

metaphysics In the tradition—"The study of being qua being" (Aristotle as quoted in McKeon, 1941); the study of what is real in reality. For instance: That everything is what it is, that nothing is what it is not; a demonstration of why something is what it is. Or that something has a foundation in reality. For instance: Symphonology has a foundation in reality since, throughout reality, agreement produces harmony. The lack of agreement either produces nothing or produces discord.

more or less Out of context; inexact; without a purpose.

mores Rules or standards of behavior as related to a certain society; the ethical conventions of a society.

motivation The reason that an agent takes an action. As the desire not to get wet is the motivation for opening one's umbrella; fear is one's motivation for taking flight; the desire to gain benefits only possible or more easily acquired through cooperation, is one's motivation for entering into an agreement.

natural agreement An agreement among things that they will interact according to the nature of each. For instance, a leaf will be carried by the wind. Natural agreements arise through the nature of each existent.

necessary It is probably not necessary to define *necessary*. But if a certain state of affairs, A, can be an actual state of affairs only if another state of affairs, B, is actual, then B is necessary to A. This is the thrust of *necessary* throughout the book.

normative "Having to do with an established standard of behavior" (Runes, 1983); having to do with ethics.

nurse (or any health care professional) The agent of a patient, doing for the patient (given education and experience) what he would do for himself if he were able.

nurturing Affording professional treatment in order to bring a patient to a better state of life, health, and well-being.

objective Existing apart from a perceiving subject; having actual existence or reality; as in objective awareness; directed outward to the characteristics necessary to establish cognition of an object.

objective awareness Awareness directed outward to the characteristics necessary to establish cognition of an object.

objectivity As a bioethical standard, a desire to know something as it is in itself and apart from distorting conditions or misleading prejudgments; a patient's need to achieve and sustain the exercise of his objective awareness.

obligation A condition that (ethically) necessitates the obliged to perform some action.

offer The state of mind of another ethical agent that seems to promise to serve a purpose if one engages with it.

paradox A paradox is a description of a state of affairs that apparently cannot exist, but which, in fact, can exist or apparently can exist, but which, in fact, cannot exist.

passion A behavior that an agent undergoes through a force external to self and not as the outcome of his or her act of self-determination.

paternalism The practice of assuming an authority that one does not possess. The acting toward one as if you were a parent and they were your child.

patient One who has lost or suffered a decrease in agency. One who is unable to take the actions his survival or flourishing requires. An agent, but in relation to a biomedical professional. One whose actions are affected by the actions of an agent.

perfect agreement An objective agreement is an agreement to interact made between two agents when their interaction is based on an objective awareness of the circumstances influencing their interacting and its foreseeable result. A perfect ethical agreement is an objective agreement where each agent is objectively certain that the other is the right person with whom he should be interacting.

perfection Intrinsic desirability, appropriateness to survival and flourishing.

person A rational animal, independent, able to act on the basis of decisions and agreements, and able to discover meaning in things.

power A capacity to bring about a state of affairs.

practical reason Intelligent in matters of ethics; when the aim of ethics is action.

precondition "A condition that must exist before something else can occur" *(American Heritage Dictionary,* 1997). That which is related to something else in such a way that it is necessary to the existence of that second thing. Parents are the precondition of a child, language is a precondition of literature, objectivity is a precondition of an agreement.

presupposition Very much like precondition but having more to do with the context of one's knowledge. That which must be assumed if that of which it is a presupposition is assumed. For example, knowledge of the fact that Paul is or was a child presupposes knowledge of the fact that Paul had parents. Knowledge of the fact that a culture has produced literature presupposes knowledge of the fact that the culture possesses a language. Knowledge of the fact that one has formed an agreement presupposes knowledge of the fact that one is free to form an agreement.

pride The objective conviction that one is worthwhile. The pleasure that one takes in one's virtues.

principle The motivating ground of an action. A basic fact, truth, or law from which other facts, truths, or laws proceed. A basic cause from which other causes arise.

probability When the evidence for an alternative significantly outweighs the evidence against it, the first alternative is more probable than the second—foreseeability.

professional One who has, by virtue of education, training, and experience to enter a profession and to act effectively in it.

proper Appropriate to a context; meeting a requisite standard.

proportion A measure of benefit or value between one action or the product of the action in comparison with another action, or the product of another action according to reciprocity. In one sense, balance and proportion are beneficence. In the same sense, they are justice.

purpose That state of affairs that is the object of an action motivated by desire; the psychological condition that accompanies an orientation toward bringing about this state of affairs.

rational Tending to appropriate proportions; well reasoned; appropriate to the context.

rational self-interest An agent's rational self-interest is defined in terms of one's understanding of one's individual nature against the background of what is needed for personal development. It also requires a complete acceptance of the nature, motivations, and the self-interest of one's "trading partners."

realism–moderate The theory that concepts are formed through the abstract sameness of things.

reason The faculty of thinking; thinking being a process of awareness directed toward (a) what is relevant, (b) what is appropriate, (c) what is balanced, and (d) what is proportional in the demands of a context and the agent's responses to these demands.

reciprocity An appropriate balance between value given and value received. A balanced interchange of benefits or values.

relevant Necessary to the understanding of a context. Serving to bring about balance and ethical proportion (something is relevant to a context if the context cannot be fully understood without it).

responsibility The ethical link connecting an agent to the consequences of the changes he has caused to come about.

rights The product of an implicit agreement among rational beings made and held by virtue of their rationality not to obtain actions nor the products or conditions of actions from one another except through voluntary consent objectively gained. Rights means, in one sense, the product (freedom from aggression) of an agreement (not to aggress). In another sense, rights is the agreement itself. In either sense, the generic term (freedom from aggression; agreement) is singular. Therefore, the term rights is a singular term. It is a grave ethical mistake to regard the term rights as a political rather than a more fundamental, ethical term, and to regard it as plural—an ever-changing product of legislation.

ritualistic ethic An ethical system that holds that ethical principles are right or wrong without regard for the desires, choices, and purposes of the people involved or the consequences of ethical action.

sameness Although individual things are not the same as individuals, they are the same as members of the same genus. John and Mary are merely similar to each other as individuals, as members of the genus, person, they are the same.

sanction The word *sanction* has various meanings. In ethics, it is used to mean "agreement" or "cooperation" in a broad, metaphorical sense. For instance, criminals do not have the sanction of reason. Nature sanctions actions taken with foresight. Reality does not sanction irresponsible actions.

self-assertion The power and right of an agent to control his time and effort. It implies a person's self-ownership (self-governance). As a bioethical standard, the right of an individual to be free of undesired or undesirable interaction; the right to control one's time and effort; the right to initiate one's own actions.

sequentiality Pertaining to a series of future events, intelligibly and causally linked to a series of past events.

sincerity The quality of one's motivation in forming an agreement when one is fully committed to the agreement.

social relativism The theory that what is ethical and what is unethical is determined by the customs, beliefs, and practices of a society.

solitary ethics A system of standards to motivate, determine, and justify decisions and actions taken in the pursuit of an agent's own vital and fundamental goals.

standard That by which the ethical appropriateness of an action can be measured. Various standards that have been proposed are: Socrates, knowledge of that which is beneficial; Plato, the Form of the Good; Aristotle, the actions that noble and virtuous people would take; Aquinas, happiness; Spinoza, the preservation and enhancement of the agent's life; Kant, duty; Bentham, the greatest good for the greatest number; Ayn Rand, the preconditions of "man's life qua man."

sufficient One thing, A, is sufficient to another thing, B, if the existence of A, in and of itself, makes necessary the existence of B. For instance, the existence of lightning is sufficient to the existence of thunder. Thunder cannot exist without lightning. Lightning cannot exist without producing thunder. Desire is not sufficient to action—one may feel desire without acting. But action is sufficient to justify a belief in the existence of desire. Action is a behavior motivated by desire, action implies desire.

symphonology A system of ethics based on the terms and presuppositions of agreement. In any specific case, this will be the agreement that establishes the nature of the relationship between the parties involved in interaction.

system The interrelationships of the elements that make up a whole.

tacit That which is hidden from direct view; relying on focal and subsidiary awareness; unspoken but ever-present knowledge, guides us to comprehension of something real; based on experience. "We know more than we can say" (Polanyi, 1966).

telishment The practice of reducing crime by subjecting criminals to death by slow torture and revealing to potential criminals what their fate will be by gently torturing an innocent person to death. This last being telishment.

term "A condition or stipulation that defines the nature and limits of an agreement" (*American Heritage Dictionary*, 1997).

triage A triage situation is a situation calling for choices to be made when the benefits that can be brought about in the situation are limited. The choices may be choices among benefits or beneficiaries or both.

truth The relationship of correspondence between an idea and the object of the idea.

uncertainty The mental context of a dilemma. The right or best course of action may be action A or action B. But the superiority of one over the other is not clearly evident to the person who has to make the choice.

uniqueness Difference from others of the same kind.

utilitarianism "The theory that one should act as to promote the greatest happiness (pleasure) of the greatest number of people" (Angeles, 1992).

utility Greatest good for the greatest number.

value The object of an action that is motivated by an autonomous desire; that which is instrumental in the realization of a purpose.

vice The opposite of virtue. A habit produced by an inferior or corrupt character. A habit established on irrational desire.

vicious Tending to vice; unable to live rightly and well.

violate To violate a standard is to ignore or act against the character structure that is signified by the standard. More generally, whenever one ignores or acts against that which is appropriate to an agreement, one violates the agreement.

virtue A human excellence. "Action according to the nature of that which acts" (Spinoza, 1675/1949). For instance, it is a virtue in a horse to run swiftly; it is a virtue in a boat not to sink; it is a virtue in a person to live rightly and well. According to a purposive ethic, *virtue* refers to a person's ability to act to fulfill his or her rational desires.

virtuous Tending to virtue; habituated to living rightly and well.

vital Essentially related to the preservation or enhancement of life, as, for instance, a vital need or a vital desire.

vital agreement An agreement between the life of a living thing and the organic conditions necessary to its life or survival. It is life's agreement with itself.

volition The power to take uncompelled and purposeful actions.

vulnerable Unprotected, capable of being harmed.

whim A decision made on the analysis of subjective factors. A decision motivated by one's feelings or attitudes apart from the context.

wisdom Prudent judgment as to how to use knowledge in the everyday affairs of life (Angeles, 1992).

Note: The various philosophic systems that we have described above are not complete descriptions. In some cases, we would not claim "ballistic accuracy." Our purpose is not to provide the reader with a complete understanding of contemporary philosophy but to include everything that separates symphonology from it. However, the descriptions of the ethical systems are reliable.

References

American heritage dictionary (3rd ed.). (1997). Boston: Houghton Mifflin.

Angeles, P. A. (1992). *Dictionary of philosophy* (2nd. ed.). New York: Harper Collins.

McKeon, R. (Ed.). (1941). *The basic works of Aristotle.* New York: Random House.

Pines, A., & Maslach, C. (1978). Characteristics of staff burn-out in mental health setting. *Hospital Community Psychiatry, 29,* 233–237.

Polanyi, M. (1966). *The tacit dimension.* Garden City, NJ: Double Day.

Runes, D. D. (Ed.). (1983). *Dictionary of philosophy.* New York: Philosophical Library.

Spinoza. (1949). *Ethics.* (J. Gutmann, Ed.). New York: Hafner. (Original work published 1675)

Index